Screening for Cancer

Contributors

George H. Anderson
Alan A. Bassett
R. A. Cartwright
Richard Costlow
Robert B. Fath, Jr.
Martin Fleisher
Robert S. Fontana
Gary D. Friedman
Isaburo Fujimoto
Peter Greenwald
Matti Hakama
Elizabeth Herbert
Takeshi Hirayama
Shigeru Hisamichi
Heizaburo Ichikawa
William H. Kern
Nagi F. Khouri
Toshiji Kobayashi
F. A. Macrae
Anthony B. Miller
David Mock
Duncan Neuhauser
Akira Oshima
Philip Prorok
David Schottenfeld
Morton K. Schwartz
Edward J. Sondik
Frederick P. Stitik
Philip Strax
Melvyn S. Tockman
Suketami Tominaga
C. B. Williams
Sidney J. Winawer
Lewis B. Woolner
Tatsuya Yamada

Screening for Cancer

Edited by

Anthony B. Miller
NCIC Epidemiology Unit
University of Toronto
Toronto, Ontario, Canada

1985

ACADEMIC PRESS, INC.
(Harcourt Brace Jovanovich, Publishers)
Orlando San Diego New York London
Toronto Montreal Sydney Tokyo

ACADEMIC PRESS, INC.
Orlando, Florida 32887

United Kingdom Edition published by
ACADEMIC PRESS INC. (LONDON) LTD.
24–28 Oval Road, London NW1 7DX

Library of Congress Cataloging in Publication Data
Main entry under title:

Screening for cancer.

Includes index.
1. Cancer–Prevention. 2. Medical screening.
I. Miller, A. B. (Anthony B.) [DNLM: 1. Mass Screening–methods. 2. Neoplasms–prevention & control.
QZ 200 S433]
RC268.S38 1985 362.1'96994 84-24162
ISBN 0–12–496720–5 (alk. paper)

PRINTED IN THE UNITED STATES OF AMERICA

85 86 87 88 9 8 7 6 5 4 3 2 1

Contents

Contributors xv

Preface xix

I Fundamentals of Screening

1 Principles of Screening and of the Evaluation of Screening Programs

Anthony B. Miller

I. Introduction 3
II. Definition of Screening 4
III. The Validity of a Screening Test 5
IV. General Principles Governing the Introduction of Screening Programs 9
V. The Ethics of Screening 13
VI. The Population to Be Included in Screening Programs 15
VII. Diagnosis and Treatment of the Discovered Lesions 15
VIII. Evaluation of Screening Programs 16
IX. Conclusion 22
References 22

2 Screening in the Context of Cancer Control

Peter Greenwald, Richard Costlow, Philip Prorok, and Edward J. Sondik

I. Cancer Control and Screening 25
II. Phases of Cancer Control Research 27
III. Review of Screening Programs 29
IV. New Methods for Screening and Detection . . 36
V. Policy Analysis and Screening Evaluation . . 37
VI. General Considerations 45
References 46

3 Economic Aspects of Screening

Duncan Neuhauser

I. Introduction 49
II. The Benefits of Screening 50
III. Benefits Now and Later 51
IV. Externalities and Equity 52
V. Societal Costs versus Charges 53
VI. Average versus Marginal Costs and Benefits 53
VII. Application of Such Models in Practice . . . 55
VIII. Conclusion 56
IX. Bibliographic Sources 56
References 57

4 The Problem of Identification of High-Risk Subjects for Selective Screening

Matti Hakama

I. Introduction 59
II. Success Measures 59
III. Selective Screening and Validity 61
IV. Effect of Selective Screening in Quantitative Terms 61
V. Attempts to Combine Risk Factors 63
VI. Prospects for Selective Screening 65
References 66

5 Application of Screening, Including Multiphasic Screening, to Target Populations

Gary D. Friedman

I. Introduction 70
II. Brief Historical Perspective 70
III. Secondary Advantages of Multiphasic Screening 71
IV. How to Select a Target Population 73
V. How to Select an Appropriate Screening Test 74
VI. How to Invite the Target Population to Be Screened 74
VII. How to Maintain Patient Satisfaction 75
VIII. How to Maintain Provider Satisfaction . . . 75
IX. General Principles for Implementing Multiphasic Screening 76
X. Pitfalls to Be Avoided 77
XI. Multiphasic Health Testing Services as Part of a Health Care Delivery System 78
XII. Specialized Health Examinations 78
XIII. Quality Control of Screening Procedures . . . 79
XIV. Conclusion 82
References 83

II Screening Tests

6 Cervical Cytology

George H. Anderson

I. History of the Pap Smear 87
II. Requirements for a Pap Smear Screening Program 88
References 102

7 Pulmonary Cytology in Lung Cancer Screening

Lewis B. Woolner and Robert S. Fontana

I. Introduction 105
II. Sputum Cytology Test: Technical Aspects . . 106
III. Processing of the Sputum Specimen 107

IV. Morning "Pooled" Spontaneous-Cough Sputum . . . 108
V. Adequacy of the Specimen . . . 108
VI. Preparation of Slides . . . 109
VII. Microscopic Screening . . . 109
VIII. Cytologic Reports . . . 110
IX. Management of Subjects with an Abnormal Sputum Specimen . . . 112
X. Discussion . . . 114
XI. Sensitivity and Specificity . . . 117
XII. To Test or Not to Test? . . . 118
References . . . 119

8 Screening Tests for Bladder Cancer

William H. Kern

I. Introduction . . . 121
II. Cytologic Screening . . . 122
III. Other Screening Procedures . . . 134
IV. Summary . . . 137
References . . . 138

9 Mammography

Philip Strax

I. Introduction . . . 141
II. Rationale . . . 142
III. Historical Review . . . 143
IV. Technical Factors . . . 144
V. Radiation Risk . . . 147
VI. Interpretation . . . 148
VII. Conclusions . . . 159
References . . . 160

10 Chest Radiology

Frederick P. Stitik, Melvyn S. Tockman, and Nagi F. Khouri

I. Introduction . . . 163
II. Radiographic Techniques . . . 164
III. Quality Control . . . 173

IV. The Value of Screening Radiography in Detecting Lung Cancer 174
V. Conclusions 182
References 189

11 Double Contrast Radiography of the Stomach

Heizaburo Ichikawa and Tatsuya Yamada

I. Introduction 193
II. Method 194
III. Presentation of Films Taken with the Double Contrast Method 196
IV. Results 207
V. Discussion 208
VI. Summary 213
References 213

12 Ultrasound: Screening for Early Breast Cancer by Echography

Toshiji Kobayashi

I. Introduction 215
II. History of Breast Echography 216
III. Equipment for Gray-Scale Echography . . . 218
IV. Technique Used for the Water-Bag Examination 220
V. Echographic Characteristics of the Normal Female Breast 220
VI. Diagnostic Criteria 223
VII. Demonstration of Typical Echograms in Various Abnormalities 226
VIII. Malignant Disease (Breast Cancer) 226
IX. Application of Ultrasound to Screening for Breast Cancer 231
X. Conclusion 234
References 235

13 Fecal Occult Blood Testing

Martin Fleisher, Morton K. Schwartz, and Sidney J. Winawer

I. Introduction 237
II. Test Characteristics 238

III. Diet 240
IV. Sensitivity 241
V. Storage and Rehydration 242
VI. Quality Control of Fecal Occult Blood Tests 242
VII. Available Tests 244
References 246

14 Sigmoidoscopy and Other Tests for Colorectal Cancer

F. A. Macrae and C. B. Williams

I. Choice of Techniques: Risk Evaluation . . . 250
II. Technical Aspects 256
III. Sensitivity and Specificity 262
IV. Logistics 264
V. Training 265
References 265

15 Physical Examination of the Breast and Breast Self-Examination

Alan A. Bassett

I. Introduction 271
II. The Technique of Physical Examination of the Breast 272
III. Breast Self-Examination 284
IV. Conclusion 290
References 290

III Screening for Specific Cancer Sites

16 Screening for Cancer of the Cervix

Anthony B. Miller

I. Introduction 295
II. Natural History 296
III. Evaluation of the Outcome 303
IV. Risk Groups for Screening 312
V. Optimal Screening Schedules 313

VI. Research Issue 319
VII. Conclusion 319
References 320

17 Screening for Cancer of the Breast

Anthony B. Miller

I. Introduction 325
II. Problems in the Evaluation of Screening for Breast Cancer 326
III. The Health Insurance Plan (HIP) Study . . . 328
IV. The Breast Cancer Detection Demonstration Projects (BCDDP) 330
V. The International Union Against Cancer (UICC) Workshop 332
VI. Further Studies on Breast Screening 332
VII. Other Modalities for Screening for Breast Cancer 337
VIII. Future Application of Breast Cancer Screening 338
IX. Conclusion 342
References 343

18 Screening for Colorectal Cancer

Sidney J. Winawer, Robert B. Fath, Jr., David Schottenfeld, and Elizabeth Herbert

I. Introduction 347
II. High-Risk Groups 348
III. Screening Tests and Trials 353
IV. Guidelines for Screening and Case Finding . . 360
V. Summary and Future Studies 363
References 364

19 Screening for Gastric Cancer

Takeshi Hirayama, Shigeru Hisamichi, Isaburo Fujimoto, Akira Oshima, and Suketami Tominaga

I. Introduction 367
II. Rate of Screening by Age Groups 368

III. Method of Mass Screening 369
IV. Results of Mass Screening 370
V. Evaluation of Mass Screening 371
VI. Side Benefits of Mass Screening 373
VII. Declining Detection Rate 373
VIII. Improving the Cost Effectiveness of Mass Screening 374
IX. Approaches Used to Minimize the Side Effects of Mass Screening 374
X. Summary and Conclusion 375
References 376

20 Screening for Lung Cancer

Robert S. Fontana

I. Introduction 378
II. Design of the Mayo Lung Project (MLP) . . 381
III. Results of the MLP Screening Program . . . 382
IV. Discussion 390
V. Summary 394
References 394

21 Screening for Bladder Cancer

R. A. Cartwright

I. Overview of Bladder Cancer Epidemiology as Relevant to Screening Programs 398
II. Survival in Bladder Cancer 403
III. Screening for Bladder Cancer 407
IV. Analyses of Bladder Cancer Screening . . . 412
V. Future of Bladder Cancer Screening 415
References 416

22 Screening for Oral Cancer

David Mock

I. Introduction 421
II. Epidemiology and Etiology 422

III. Squamous Cell Carcinoma 426
IV. Verrucous Carcinoma 431
V. Characteristics of Premalignancy and Early Carcinoma 432
VI. Malignant Tumors of the Salivary Gland 434
VII. Malignancies of Other Tissue 435
VIII. Oral Examination 435
IX. Diagnostic Procedures 436
X. Summary and Conclusions 439
References 440

Index 445

Contributors

Numbers in parentheses indicate the pages on which the authors' contributions begin.

George H. Anderson (87), Director of Laboratories, A. Maxwell Evans Clinic, Cancer Control Agency of British Columbia, Vancouver, British Columbia, Canada V5Z 3J3

Alan A. Bassett (271), Assistant Professor of Surgery, University of Toronto, Toronto, Ontario, Canada M5G 1X5, and Department of Surgery, Mount Sinai Hospital, 600 University Avenue, Toronto, Ontario, Canada M5G 1X5

R. A. Cartwright (397), Epidemiologist, Yorkshire Regional Cancer Organisation, Yorkshire Regional Health Authority, Cookridge Hospital, Leeds LS16 6QB, England

Richard Costlow (25), Chief, Cancer Detection Branch, Division of Cancer Prevention and Control, National Cancer Institute, National Institutes of Health, Bethesda, Maryland 20205

Robert B. Fath, Jr. (347), Fellow, Gastroenterology Service, Department of Medicine, Memorial Sloan-Kettering Cancer Center, New York, New York 10021

Martin Fleisher (237), Attending Clinical Chemist, Department of Clinical Chemistry, Memorial Sloan-Kettering Cancer Center, New York, New York 10021

Robert S. Fontana (105, 377), Professor of Medicine, Mayo Medical School, and Consultant, Division of Thoracic Diseases and Internal Medicine, Mayo Clinic and Mayo Foundation, Rochester, Minnesota 55905

Gary D. Friedman (69), Assistant Director for Epidemiology and Biostatistics, Department of Medical Methods Research, Kaiser-Permanente Medical Care Program, Oakland, California 94611

Isaburo Fujimoto (367), Director, Department of Field Research, Center for Adult Diseases, Osaka, Osaka 537, Japan

Peter Greenwald (25), Director, Division of Cancer Prevention and Control, National Cancer Institute, National Institutes of Health, Bethesda, Maryland 20205

Matti Hakama (59), Professor of Epidemiology, Department of Public Health, University of Tampere, SF-33101, Tampere 10, Finland

Elizabeth Herbert (347), Program Coordinator, Memorial Sloan-Kettering Cancer Center, New York, New York 10021

Takeshi Hirayama (367), Chief, Epidemiology Division, National Cancer Research Institute, Tokyo 104, Japan

Shigeru Hisamichi (367), Professor, Department of Public Health, Tohoku University, School of Medicine, Sendai 980, Japan

Heizaburo Ichikawa (193), Director, National Cancer Center Hospital, Tokyo 104, Japan

William H. Kern (121), Director of Pathology, The Hospital of the Good Samaritan, Los Angeles, California 90017, and Clinical Professor of Pathology, Department of Pathology, University of Southern California School of Medicine, Los Angeles, California 90033

Nagi F. Khouri (163), Assistant Professor of Radiology, Department of Radiology and Radiological Science, The Johns Hopkins Medical Institutions, Baltimore, Maryland 21205

Toshiji Kobayashi (215), Professor and Chairman, Department of Central Clinical Laboratory, School of Medicine, University of Occupational and Environmental Health, Kitakyushu City 807, Japan

F. A. Macrae (249), Applied Health Sciences Fellow, National Health and Medical Research Council (Australia), Department of Gastroenterology, The Royal Melbourne Hospital, Victoria 3050, Australia

Anthony B. Miller (3, 295, 325), Director, NCIC Epidemiology Unit, Faculty of Medicine, University of Toronto, Toronto, Ontario, Canada M5S 1A8

David Mock (421), Associate Professor, Department of Oral Medicine and Pathology, Faculty of Dentistry, and Assistant Professor, Department of Pathology, Faculty of Medicine, University of Toronto, Toronto, Ontario, Canada M5G 1G6

Duncan Neuhauser (49), Professor of Epidemiology and Community Health, Professor of Medicine, Adjunct Professor of Organizational Behavior, Keck Foundation Senior Research Scholar, and Associate Director, Health Systems Management Center, Department of Epidemiology and Community Health, School of Medicine, Case Western Reserve University, Cleveland, Ohio 44106

Akira Oshima (367), Department of Field Research, Center for Adult Diseases, Osaka, Osaka 537, Japan

Philip Prorok (25), Chief, Screening Section, Biometry Branch, Division of Cancer Prevention and Control, National Cancer Institute, National Institutes of Health, Bethesda, Maryland 20205

David Schottenfeld (347), Chief, Epidemiology and Preventive Medicine Service, Department of Medicine, Memorial Sloan-Kettering Cancer Center, New York, New York 10021

Morton K. Schwartz (237), Chairman, Attending Clinical Chemist, Department of Clinical Chemistry, Memorial Sloan-Kettering Cancer Center, New York, New York 10021

Edward J. Sondik (25), Chief, Operations Research Branch, Division of Cancer Prevention and Control, National Cancer Institute, National Institutes of Health, Bethesda, Maryland 20205

Frederick P. Stitik (163), Professor of Radiology, Eastern Virginia Medical School, Norfolk, Virginia 23505, and Clinical Associate Professor of Radiology, The Johns Hopkins Medical Institutions, Baltimore, Maryland 21205

Philip Strax (141), Clinical Professor, Department of Oncology, University of Miami School of Medicine, Miami, Florida 33101, and Associate Clinical Professor, Community and Preventive Medicine, New York Medical College, Valhalla, New York 10595, and Lecturer, Department of Environmental Medicine, New York University School of Medicine, New York, New York 10016, and Medical Director, Guttmann Breast Diagnostic Institute, New York, New York 10001

Melvyn S. Tockman (163), Associate Professor, Department of Environmental Health Sciences, The Johns Hopkins University, School of Hygiene and Public Health, Baltimore, Maryland 21211

Suketami Tominaga (367), Chief, Division of Epidemiology, Aichi Cancer Center Research Institute, Nagoya 464, Japan

C. B. Williams (249), Consultant Physician, St. Mark's Hospital for Diseases of the Rectum and Colon, London EC1V 2PS, England

Sidney J. Winawer (237, 347), Chief, Gastroenterology Service, Department of Medicine, Memorial Sloan-Kettering Cancer Center, and Memorial Hospital for Cancer and Allied Diseases, New York, New York 10021

Lewis B. Woolner (105), Emeritus Professor of Pathology, Mayo Medical School, and Emeritus Consultant, Section of Surgical Pathology, Mayo Clinic and Mayo Foundation, Rochester, Minnesota 55905

Tatsuya Yamada (193), Chief, Department of Diagnostic Radiology, National Cancer Center Hospital, Tokyo 104, Japan

Preface

Ideally the control of cancer should be achievable either by preventing the disease from occurring or, if it does occur, by curing those who develop it with appropriate treatment. Complete success of one of these two approaches would make the other unnecessary. Currently it seems unlikely that either will be completely successful, and that they will continue to complement each other. However, for a number of cancer sites, an alternative approach may prove to be more appropriate, at least in the short term. This approach is to attempt the control of cancer by screening. This book has as its goal the presentation of the current state of the art on screening for cancer. It is not all-inclusive, but it covers an unusually wide range of issues. In some respects it builds on the presentation of the workshop on Screening in Cancer held under the auspices of the International Union Against Cancer (UICC) in Toronto, Canada, in 1978 (Miller, 1978). It also complements the activities of a project on Screening for Cancer which has been set up as part of the Programme on Detection and Diagnosis of the UICC, and which will report its activities in a series of summary papers and UICC Technical Reports over the next four years (Prorok *et al.*, 1984).

This volume (in contradistinction to the forthcoming UICC Technical Reports) largely focuses on screening for cancer in "Western" nations. It should be of value to those involved in the planning, management, and conduct of screening programs, to those in voluntary agencies who need to know about the background for possible public education activities, and to those in government who may be considering continuing the support of existing screening programs or beginning new ones. We trust it will prove to be a useful teaching aid for epidemiologists and others concerned with professional, and possibly particularly graduate, training.

The book is divided into three parts. Part I is concerned with the general principles of screening and of its evaluation. It is important to recognize here that it is impossible to evaluate screening without first setting up a screening program. Part II is concerned with established and potential screening tests.

This section should be interpreted in the light of the definition of screening of the U.S. Commission on Chronic Illness (1957), "the presumptive identification of unrecognized disease or defect by the application of tests, examinations or other procedures that can be applied rapidly." A screening test is not intended to be diagnostic. Rather a positive finding will need to be confirmed by special diagnostic procedures. Part III is concerned with screening for specific cancer sites. In this section it is clear that our knowledge of screening for the cancers considered is at different stages of development. Further, in a few sites, it seems likely that the promise of screening using existing tests has not been fulfilled. This should increase our determination to continue to evaluate existing and all future screening programs.

As editor, I recognize my great indebtedness to my colleagues in this endeavor, who have adhered to my requests for the timely submission of manuscripts and who have tolerated and complied with my requests for changes. We trust our readers will find the resulting product worthwhile and useful, and that you will inform us of our errors and of advances in knowledge in this field so that we can produce an even more valuable edition in the future.

Anthony B. Miller

Miller, A. B., ed. (1978). Screening in cancer: A report of a UICC international workshop, Toronto, Canada, April 24–27, 1978, UICC Technical Report Series, Vol. 40. International Union Against Cancer, Geneva.

Prorok, P. C., Chamberlain, J., Day, N. E., Hakama, M., and Miller, A. B. (1984). UICC workshop on evaluation of screening programmes for cancer. *Int. J. Cancer* **34**, 1-4.

U.S. Commission on Chronic Illness (1957). "Chronic Illness in the United States," Vol. 1. Harvard University Press, Cambridge, Massachusetts.

Screening for Cancer

I

Fundamentals of Screening

1

Principles of Screening and of the Evaluation of Screening Programs

ANTHONY B. MILLER

I. Introduction 3
II. Definition of Screening 4
III. The Validity of a Screening Test 5
IV. General Principles Governing the Introduction of Screening Programs 9
A. Importance of the Disease 10
B. Natural History 11
C. Treatment for the Disease 12
D. Acceptability and Safety of the Screening Test 13
V. The Ethics of Screening 13
VI. The Population to Be Included in Screening Programs 15
VII. Diagnosis and Treatment of the Discovered Lesions 15
VIII. Evaluation of Screening Programs 16
A. Bias in Evaluating Survival 16
B. Classification of Approaches to Evaluate Screening 18
C. Randomized Trials 18
D. Quasi-Experimental Studies 19
E. Case-Control Studies 19
F. Risks and Benefits of Screening 20
G. Summary of Evaluation Issues 21
IX. Conclusion 22
References 22

I. INTRODUCTION

Because of the deep-rooted belief that early diagnosis of disease is beneficial, many tend to regard screening as bound to be effective. For cancer of the cervix, for example, it was optimistically assumed for a while that appropriate screening

ISBN 0-12-496720-5

would eventually prevent all mortality from the disease. This is now believed unlikely (Miller, 1978). The purpose of this chapter is to attempt to define some of the fundamental issues which we now appreciate are relevant to the consideration of screening and its evaluation; to discuss some of the theoretical bases for solutions of these issues; and to describe some approaches to evaluating the effectiveness of screening before it can be accepted as an established cancer control measure in any site.

II. DEFINITION OF SCREENING

It is first necessary to establish what we mean by *screening*. As indicated in the preface to this volume, screening was defined by the U.S. Commission on Chronic Illness (1957) as "the presumptive identification of unrecognized disease or defect by the application of tests, examinations or other procedures that can be applied rapidly." A screening test is not intended to be diagnostic. Rather, a positive finding will need to be confirmed by special diagnostic procedures.

Throughout this volume, screening is considered in the context of mass application to populations. Indeed, some would regard mass screening as being restricted to use as a public health measure and offered either in special clinics or at least by public health authorities. Nevertheless, it has to be recognized that many of the screening programs considered in this volume have not been offered in this way, but rather in the context of routine, general health care, sometimes purely as an adjunct to health care directed primarily to other circumstances. For example, screening for cancer of the cervix in the province of British Columbia, Canada, is done almost entirely by family physicians, although it is also offered under special circumstances, such as in clinics for the treatment of sexually transmitted diseases or in medical care facilities concerned with women in prison. Nevertheless, a distinction can be drawn even in this program between screening and *case finding;* the latter was defined by Sackett and Holland (1975) as "the utilization of a special procedure to identify existing but, up until then, unsuspected disease which may be unrelated to their chief complaints, when someone attends a physician in the context of seeking medical care." In case finding, the encounter is initiated by the patient and the purpose is a comprehensive assessment of health. Many women, however, go to their physicians primarily to obtain a Pap smear. Others go for a general health examination, during which the opportunity is taken to obtain a Pap smear or to conduct an examination of the breasts. I believe that these approaches can be included in our definition of screening, and that it should not be necessary to set up a special procedure through a public health department, requiring people to attend specific clinics, in order to include this approach within the context of screening.

It is important to recognize that some organizations have advocated screening largely in such a context. Thus, the American Cancer Society (1980) advocates screening as a physician-based approach. Although at times it may be difficult to draw a distinction between case finding and screening, I believe we should recognize that for efficient conduct of screening programs, it is necessary to utilize existing health care systems and at times, such as in identifying women at high risk of cancer of the cervix who are sexually active, use the opportunities provided by physician visits for other purposes to ensure that the individual has been appropriately screened.

These questions have been considered by others. The working group for the review of the U.S. Breast Cancer Detection Demonstration Projects (Beahrs *et al.*, 1979) stated that "similar scientific and ethical considerations are applicable when 'a mass screening program' or periodic general health monitoring by physicians is under consideration. In fact, the monitoring may currently account for most of the 'screening' underway in the United States." However, Eddy (1980) feels screening should be limited to those conditions or tests in which the judgment of a physician is not needed to determine if a test should be conducted. This requires enough knowledge of the benefits and risks to ensure that the physician recognizes the appropriate circumstances under which he should perform a screening test. It seems appropriate to resolve this question on the basis of the need for judgment by the physician. If the physician exercises judgment in deciding whether or not a test (which may or may not be known to be of value) is used, then it is not screening. However, once something becomes part of a routine medical examination, it is considered screening.

It is therefore in this context that the fundamental issues relevant to screening and its evaluation will be considered in the remainder of this chapter, and in the chapters that follow.

III. THE VALIDITY OF A SCREENING TEST

Two measures suffice to describe the validity of screening tests: sensitivity and specificity. *Sensitivity* is defined as the ability of a test to detect all persons with the disease in the screened population. This is expressed as the proportion of those with the disease in whom a screening test gives a positive result. *Specificity* is defined as the ability of a test to identify correctly those persons free of disease in the screened population. This is expressed as the proportion of those free of the disease in whom the screening test gives a negative result. These two measures may be further expressed in terms of test results as follows: sensitivity is calculated as the true positives divided by the sum of the true positives and false negatives and expressed as a percentage; specificity is calculated as the true negatives divided by the sum of the true negatives and false positives and expressed as a percentage (Table I).

In practice, the difficulty with these measures arises in distinguishing true

TABLE I

The Relationship between Sensitivity, Specificity, and Predictive Value

	Disease status	
Test result	Present	Absent
Positive	True positive (TP)	False positive (FP)
Negative	False negative (FN)	True negative (TN)

$$\text{Sensitivity} = \frac{TP}{TP + FN} \times 100\%$$

$$\text{Specificity} = \frac{TN}{TN + FP} \times 100\%$$

$$\text{Predictive value positive} = \frac{TP}{TP + FP} \times 100\%$$

$$\text{Predictive value negative} = \frac{TN}{TN + FN} \times 100\%$$

positives from false positives and true negatives from false negatives. It is well recognized that the position of the boundaries that are set between disease and health can considerably influence the numerical values placed on sensitivity and specificity. A relatively imperfect test of a quantitative, continuously distributed measurement can be artificially given a very high sensitivity by setting the boundaries to incorporate a high proportion of those who are eventually found to have the disease in the positive category, but at a substantial cost in terms of false positives and therefore low specificity. Conversely, the same test can be made to appear highly specific, but will then become insensitive if the boundary between positive and negative is shifted in the opposite direction, with a high cost in terms of false negatives.

Many have sought special indices to express this reciprocal relationship between sensitivity and specificity. One approach is to plot the relationship between the true positives (sensitivity) and the false positives (1 minus the specificity) when the decision boundaries to define these functions are varied. These curves are called *receiver operating characteristic (ROC)* curves. A comprehensive treatise discussing the use of ROC curves in the evaluation of diagnostic systems is that of Swets and Pickett (1982).

However, difficulties in defining sensitivity and specificity may be enhanced by uncertainty as to what truly constitutes an abnormality in the context of the findings from a screening program. In order to come to such a decision, it is essential to know the natural history of the conditions identified as a result of screening. However, such knowledge may not be available at the initiation of a screening program, and may be obtained only as a result of careful study of the program's findings.

Nevertheless, the definition of disease is crucial in order to determine sensitivity and specificity. Most people have a clear idea of what constitutes disease in terms of what surfaces in standard medical practice. Cancers in general present with recognizable characteristics in symptomatic individuals. By definition, screening is conducted on asymptomatic individuals, so that most cancers that are identified through screening are likely to be in an early stage and may not have the generally recognized clinical characteristics. Further, screening usually tends to identify a number of other conditions which fall under the heading of preclinical or even precancerous lesions, often covering a wide spectrum of abnormalities. The definition of the true precursor condition(s) identified by screening, for which the term *detectable preclinical phase (DPCP)* has been proposed by Cole and Morrison (1980), presents a number of difficulties. For example, for cancer of the cervix, most would include *in situ* carcinoma in the DPCP. Most would also include the moderate and severe dysplastic lesions. In a laboratory which did not regard mild dysplasia as indicating disease, the specificity of cervical cytology would be regarded as much lower than it would in a laboratory which included mild dysplasia within the DPCP.

A common error in evaluating potential screening tests is to determine the sensitivity in relation to people who have clinical disease. A test which, under these circumstances, may appear to be highly sensitive may later be found to be much less sensitive when its ability to detect the DPCP is evaluated. In the screening context, therefore, sensitivity may vary according to whether it is estimated for early invasive carcinomas, *in situ* cancers, or precancerous lesions; and specificity may vary according to whether it is estimated in a clinical series which may include related pathological conditions or in an essentially healthy population. Both should therefore be determined under actual screening conditions. To do so is far easier for specificity than for sensitivity (May, 1974). This is because the diagnostic processes that follow a positive screening test generally identify those who truly have the disease fairly rapidly, and thus distinguish the false positives from the true positives. Since, under most circumstances, the proportion of those screened who are expected to have the disease is low, a good approximation of specificity is reached by calculating the proportion of all those who tested negative expressed as the sum of the test negatives plus the false positives. Including the false negatives in both the numerator and the denominator in these calculations introduces little error.

Sensitivity, however, is a difficult measure to determine initially in a screening program. The reason is that the false negatives are not immediately apparent. Retesting all those who test negative either with the same or, preferably, a more sensitive test to identify the false negatives is rarely possible. Even retesting a sample of the negatives may prove difficult and, if the disease is of low prevalence, may result in wide confidence limits on the estimated proportion of false negatives. Only by following up the total population who screened negative may it be possible eventually to identify those who had the disease at the time the test was administered but were not so identified. Indeed, in many circumstances, it may not be possible to identify the false negatives with precision. If test results are retained, for example, if cervical smears can be reexamined or mammography films reassessed, then it may be possible, when an individual who tested negative later presents with disease, to look back and determine whether an abnormality was present on the initial examination which could have been identified. Even this process, however, is subject to some error, since with hindsight it is much easier to see something when we know from subsequent experience where to look. However, for physical examinations as a screening modality for breast cancer and for what we have called the *biological component* of false negatives in cervical cytology—i.e., that disease which was indeed present but which, for some reason, did not exfoliate, or that disease which was not incorporated in the smear because it was taken inefficiently (Boyes *et al.,* 1982)—a direct identification of false negatives is not possible. It is then necessary to determine the proportion of those who, it is anticipated, were false negatives by relating the detection rates on successive screens to the expected incidence (Boyes *et al.,* 1982; Walter and Day, 1983).

Two recommendations were made in a workshop held under the auspices of the International Union Against Cancer (UICC) with regard to the validity of screening tests (Miller, 1978). First, "The sensitivity and specificity of the screening test to be used should have been evaluated and their expected values stated"; second, "There should be an acceptable program of quality control to ensure that the stated levels of sensitivity and specificity are attained and maintained." The second recommendation raises the issue of the problems that can arise in a screening program if adequate quality is not maintained. Quality control involves issues which concern the validity of the screening test and its safety, e.g., the need to ensure that radiation exposure does not drift upward in a mammography screening program. It includes the training of those who will actually administer and read screening tests, their supervision, and the introduction of procedures to check on the extent to which those who are positive or negative are misclassified. In general, these issues fall outside the scope of this chapter, but they are considered for cervical cytology by Anderson in Chapter 6. It must be emphasized, however, that quality may also suffer because of overwork and boredom. One of the reasons why it was felt desirable to recommend changing the frequency of examination for most women in cervical cancer screening programs in Canada was to avoid the repetitive rescreening of normal women, with the flooding of laboratories with unnecessary, unrewarding work (Task Force, 1976). That such issues are not simple is underlined by considerations of observer variation on mammography (Boyd, *et al.*, 1982). Particularly relevant to breast cancer screening programs is the extent to which abnormalities are identified and appropriate recommendations are made on their further management. Dual reading helps to increase specificity without loss of sensitivity. This permits the division of recommendations into two groups, "suspicion of malignancy" or "satisfactory (normal) examination (repeat in one year)," and results in far greater consistency.

Most commentators in the past, when considering the relative weight to be placed on sensitivity and specificity for cancer screening programs, tended to encourage high sensitivity even at the cost of relatively low specificity, since it was felt important to attempt to avoid missing individuals who truly had malignant disease. However, this is probably an error. Although the objective of screening for cancer is to identify disease in the DPCP while it is still curable, if a test is made so sensitive that it begins to pick up lesions which would never have progressed in those individuals' lifetime, it may involve a substantial additional cost. There is no point in identifying through screening a cancer which would never have presented in that individual's lifetime and little point in identifying a cancer which, if it did present, would be curable. Also, if high sensitivity is bought at the expense of low specificity, then a considerable number of nonmalignant lesions may be identified which may appear to require treatment, which may involve some risk, though the lesions might have been allowed to persist in the individuals without detriment to their health.

The *process measure,* as distinct from a measure of validity which most clearly expresses this difficulty, is the predictive value of a positive test (Table I). This measure is defined as the proportion of those who test positive who truly have the disease. This measure is most influenced by the specificity of the test and the prevalence of disease in the population (Miller, 1982). If tests are administered under circumstances in which a low predictive value positive results, then not only the costs of correctly identifying those who are falsely positive, but also the potential hazard, may be high, since an individual classified as false positive derives no benefit but incurs a potentially substantial risk from the procedures associated with subsequent diagnosis. A test with a low predictive value positive thus rapidly falls into disrepute.

IV. GENERAL PRINCIPLES GOVERNING THE INTRODUCTION OF SCREENING PROGRAMS

The principles which should govern the introduction of screening programs were reviewed during the UICC workshop on screening for cancer (Miller, 1978). These will be considered in certain broad subject areas.

A. Importance of the Disease

As noted during the UICC workshop, "The disease should be common and should be the cause of substantial mortality and/or morbidity." In most people's minds, these prerequisites definitely exist for cancer. However, it is important to recognize that the overall life expectancy of a screened population may be little changed even if the program is successful. In most technically advanced countries, if all cancer were eradicated, the effect of other competing causes of death is such that the life expectancy would be increased by only about 2.5 years. Nevertheless, the life expectancy of an individual otherwise destined to die of the specific cancer will be increased considerably, and screening for cancer of the breast and cervix has been believed to be worthwhile because of the predilection of these diseases for younger women (Table II). Further, the economic importance of reducing death at younger ages leads to consideration of the potential years of life lost at different ages as an index of premature mortality (Table III). Such an analysis confirms that cancer of the colon and rectum tends to affect an older population that is more at risk from death from other causes, so that premature mortality is less than for breast and lung cancer at every age. It also shows the greater contribution of deaths from cancer of the cervix to premature mortality than cancers of the colon, rectum, and lung up to age 40 (for lung cancer) and 45 (for colon and rectum cancer).

Nevertheless, there may be certain circumstances in which the major benefit from screening may follow not from the reduction of mortality but from the reduction of morbidity consequent upon the diagnosis of a cancer in a more treatable phase in its natural history. This could mean that less treatment would be required and the possibility that treatment may be debilitating or mutilating would be greatly reduced. Such advantages may be difficult to quantify, al-

TABLE II

Cumulative Incidence (Percentage) of Cancer of the Colon and Rectum, Lung, Breast, and Cervix in Women, Canada (Excluding Ontario), 1978

Age	Cancer of the colon and rectum	Cancer of the lung	Cancer of the breast	Cancer of the cervix[a]
Less than 50	0.31	0.17	1.59	0.52
50–69	2.22	1.10	4.48	0.58
70–84	4.80	0.80	4.55	0.45
Total	7.33	2.07	10.62	1.55

[a] Cases coded to cancer of the uterus (unspecified) allocated to cancer of the cervix in the ratio of the number of cases coded to cancer of the cervix : cancer of the corpus.

TABLE III

Potential Years of Life Lost before Age 70 from Cancer of the Colon and Rectum, Lung, Breast, and Cervix in Women, Canada, 1981

Age	Cancer of the colon and rectum	Cancer of the lung	Cancer of the breast	Cancer of the cervix[a]
20–24	0.0	0.0	47.5	142.5
25–29	212.5	212.5	765.0	595.0
30–34	225.0	375.0	1725.0	522.0
35–39	520.0	650.0	3055.0	973.0
40–44	825.0	1650.0	3987.5	932.0
45–49	1530.0	2295.0	5332.5	833.0
50–54	2152.5	3815.0	6072.5	829.5
55–59	2837.5	3625.0	5725.0	601.0
60–64	1950.0	2745.0	3645.5	570.0
65–69	902.5	927.5	1177.5	151.5
Total	11155.0	16295.0	31532.5	6149.5

[a] Deaths certified to cancer of the uterus (unspecified) allocated to cancer of the cervix in the ratio of the number of deaths certified to cancer of the cervix : cancer of the corpus.

though there may be considerable psychological advantages to individuals. There may also be considerable advantages to communities in the lowering of requirements for extensive rehabilitation services, and these may be measurable in economic terms.

B. Natural History

In the UICC workshop, it was emphasized that the natural history of the condition should be known. Ideally, such a requirement, particularly for cancer, implies that it is known at what stage in the natural history of the disease progression and death can no longer be prevented. If such information were available, and if the stage of the disease in individuals was determinable, it would be possible to decide precisely when a screening test should be applied in order to achieve maximum benefit and minimal overutilization of resources. Unfortunately, it seems unlikely that knowledge will be accumulated to determine the natural history of disease in individuals in such a precise fashion. It is recognized that the progression of clinically detected disease, from the time of diagnosis to cure or to death, varies substantially in different individuals. It seems almost certain that the distribution of growth rates of preclinically detectable disease which might be identified by screening is equally wide. Thus, although a research objective for screening must be to determine the extent of the distribution of what was described in the UICC workshop as the "time to escape from curability," in considering the introduction of screening programs and the scheduling of tests within programs, it is necessary to encompass a wide range of possibilities. It should also not be assumed that disease processes are inevitably progressive. For cancer of the cervix, for example, a large proportion of *in situ* carcinomas may undergo regression (Boyes *et al.*, 1982). Such a conclusion has implications for the optimum periodicity of screening examinations (Yu *et al.*, 1982). Designing a program for those lesions that will progress and escape curability more rapidly is the appropriate approach.

C. Treatment for the Disease

In the UICC workshop, two recommendations relevant to treatment were made: first, "There should be evidence of the effectiveness of treatment of lesions discovered as a result of screening in reducing mortality and the level of improvement expected should be stated"; second, "There should be reasonable expectation that recommendations for the appropriate management of the lesions discovered from a screening program will be complied with both by the individual with the lesion and by the physician responsible for his health care."

Underlying these recommendations was the concern that programs be set up only when there were adequate facilities for treating lesions discovered as a result of screening and functioning referral systems to secure such treatment. This, unfortunately, has at times not been true for cancer screening programs, particularly in some developing countries. There is obviously no point in establishing a screening program and identifying lesions which should be treated if the facilities are not available or if the infrastructure for referral, confirmation of diagnosis, and treatment is not in place. In general, this is not a problem in technically advanced countries, although, unfortunately, allied problems have occurred. Thus, on occasion, it has not been certain whether lesions identified as a result of screening should be regarded as truly malignant. Indeed, it has to be recognized that when lesions are first identified in a screening program, information may not be available on their appropriate treatment and special studies may be required. Otherwise, errors in terms of observation rather than treatment, on the one hand, or too extensive treatment, on the other, are possible.

A different sort of difficulty could arise when, as a result of screening, lesions are diagnosed earlier in their natural history but death is still inevitable. If this is so, i.e., if all available screening methods will not succeed in diagnosing more lesions before they have metastasized widely and are outside the range of current therapy, then screening in order to detect such lesions is not worthwhile. Earlier studies of screening for lung cancer suggested that this condition was not amenable to screening for this reason (Weiss, 1978; see also Chapter 20).

D. Acceptability and Safety of the Screening Test

One of the desirable attributes of screening tests is their acceptability both to the population to which they are offered and to those who administer them. It is perhaps surprising that cervical cytology should have achieved such widespread acceptability, since it involves a potentially unpleasant and embarrassing examination. Presumably, the reason for its acceptance is that cancer of the cervix is regarded as an unacceptable disease to many women, and many health-conscious women are prepared to go to the trouble of seeking out and taking the test. Paradoxically, however, those who are least at risk for the disease seem to be most likely to accept the test.

Breast cancer screening, on the other hand, has encountered problems of acceptability in North America, but not to the same extent in Europe (see Chapter 17). Initially, because of the concern of women over breast cancer, the demonstration projects in the United States were often overwhelmed with those who wished to take advantage of the screening. More recently, in Canada, however, where adverse publicity stated that mammography might involve substantial risk, particularly in younger women, and that in some women it might induce the condition which it was designed to prevent, much resistance was encountered.

Screening for colon cancer also has its difficulties, particularly in view of the inevitable distaste of individuals for a procedure which involves the manipulation of feces. In a number of pilot programs, therefore, the return rates for fecal occult blood slides have been disappointingly low.

A screening procedure, therefore, has to be acceptable to the population in its widest sense. The test should be simple and as easy to administer as possible, the procedure involved should be acceptable, and there should be no unpleasant or potentially hazardous implications for its use. In spite of the necessity for a blood test, the initial enthusiasm over tumor markers such as carcinoembryonic antigen (CEA) arose over the realization that a relatively simple blood test for cancer may have widespread appeal. Its failure to live up to its potential, however, was due to a combination of low specificity and low sensitivity (Miller, 1974; Schottenfeld *et al.*, 1978). Nevertheless, complex procedures are unlikely to be acceptable as screening tests.

V. THE ETHICS OF SCREENING

In general medical practice, the special nature of the relationship between a patient and his physician has dictated the need to build up a core of ethical principles which govern this relationship. Further, in the last few decades, it has been appreciated that particular issues may arise when a patient becomes the subject of a research investigation which is superimposed on his search for and receipt of appropriate medical care. It was initially not appreciated, however, that screening created a completely new spectrum of issues that may require more restrictive boundaries of behavior than currently apply in medical practice. For example, when a patient goes to see a physician for relief of a symptom or treatment of an established condition, the physician is required to exercise his skills only to the extent that knowledge is currently available. In screening, however, those who are approached to participate are not patients, and most of them do not become patients. The screener believes that as a result of screening, the health of the community will be better. He does not necessarily imply that the condition of every individual will be better. However, screening is often promoted as implying a benefit to each screenee. In fact, in some circumstances, individuals included in a screening program may be placed at a disadvantage. At the very least, therefore, those planning to introduce a screening program should be in a position to guarantee an overall benefit to the community and a minimal risk that certain individuals may be disadvantaged by the program. It was the inability to guarantee overall benefit and lack of disadvantage to those screened which led to the proscription of mammography in women under the age of 50 in the U.S. breast cancer detection demonstration projects in the absence of certain indications (Beahrs *et al.*, 1979).

A second ethical issue which is directed to the obligation to provide appropriate care in a community rather than individuals concern the equitable distribution of limited resources across the whole community to obtain maximum benefit. Under certain circumstances, the offer of screening could actually diminish the total level of health in a community. This may be a particular problem for developing countries when resources are diverted from one area to another. Thus, resources devoted to cancer screening, which might be regarded as prestigious, high-technology projects, could divert attention from the appropriate provision of routine health care for more important health problems. Even in technically advanced countries, this issue could arise. Indeed, one of the considerations in the nonadoption of routine breast cancer screening for women under the age of 50 in North America is the high cost of the procedures involved if extended over the total community (Bailar, 1978).

Screening programs, therefore, carry an ethical responsibility at least as great as that for medical practice, since invitations to participate are given to ostensibly healthy people. Indeed, the burden of proof regarding the efficacy of the procedures and the necessity to avoid harm are greater than those that may be required for diagnostic or therapeutic procedures carried out when a patient presents with symptoms to a physician. Although several screening programs have been introduced in technically advanced countries, there is a particular need for caution and care when such programs are considered for developing countries in order to ensure that they do not overbalance the health care system in the area in which they are introduced.

VI. THE POPULATION TO BE INCLUDED IN SCREENING PROGRAMS

For a screening program to be successful, the population to be included should be one in which the disease is known to have a high prevalence. This will not only encourage a high predictive value for a positive test, but will also tend to promote a higher quality of performance and assessment of test results and will result in lower costs per case detected. Thus, in all screening programs, it is desirable to attempt to include only those who are at risk of the disease, and to ensure particularly that those who are at high risk are included. This approach was recognized by the Canadian Task force (1976) on cervical cancer screening programs. This group carefully defined those who it believed were at such low risk for the disease that they need not be included, thus defining the remaining at-risk population. However, it has to be recognized that it may be difficult to identify the high-risk group for screening with sufficient precision to justify concentrating on high-risk groups only (see Chapter 4).

One possible approach to concentrating the population at risk would be to administer a "prescreening" test. For example, thermography has been considered but largely discarded as a means of concentrating women at risk for mammographic breast cancer screening programs (Beahrs *et al.*, 1979), although an initial mammogram to identify parenchymal patterns for those more precisely at risk of breast cancer may have greater potential (Wolfe, 1976). Such approaches have to be carefully evaluated. Thus, it is possible that cancers occurring in persons identified as being at risk by a prescreening test might behave differently from other cancers, and this could affect the success of the program. If, for example, the prescreening test tended to concentrate persons with slower-growing cancers, then the major yield from the screening program might be lost.

VII. DIAGNOSIS AND TREATMENT OF THE DISCOVERED LESIONS

Since a screening test is not diagnostic, the success of the program will ultimately depend upon the extent to which those identified as abnormal accept the procedures offered for further evaluation.

A number of areas may create difficulty. For example, in the initial phases of many breast cancer screening programs, it has been necessary to demonstrate to the community of medical practitioners that the abnormalities identified were indeed of importance and should be treated seriously (Miller and Bulbrook, 1982). This is one of the problems that arise over the fact that lesions may be identified initially in screening programs whose biological features, natural history, and other characteristics may be in doubt. Further, it should not be automatically assumed that those identified as having an abnormal lesion will comply with recommendations for its treatment. Thus, the subjects in the screening program may require some education as to the approaches that should be followed. It is, therefore, not sufficient to set up public education programs to encourage people to attend for screening and ignore the problems of subsequent management that will arise for those with identified abnormalities.

In the UICC workshop (Miller, 1978), a number of recommendations were made with regard to these issues:

1. The target population should be clearly defined and selected in such a way that, given the likely sensitivity and specificity of the test, an acceptable predictive value will be achieved.
2. As far as possible, the target population should be limited to those at particular risk of the disease in order to give a reasonable prevalence of detection when such individuals at risk can be identified.
3. There should be a reasonable expectation of reaching the target population and of achieving reasonable compliance in response to invitations to attend. The expected level of compliance should be stated.
4. There should be a reasonable expectation that recommendations for further diagnostic evaluation will be complied with by individuals who have a positive test.
5. There should be an agreed-upon policy on the classification of borderline abnormalities and also on their management, as well as on recommendations for their follow-up.
6. There should be a reasonable expectation that recommendations for appropriate management of lesions discovered by a screening program will be complied with both by the individual with the lesion and by the physicians responsible for his health care.

VIII. EVALUATION OF SCREENING PROGRAMS

A. Bias in Evaluating Survival

A number of issues have to be considered when evaluating programs. Almost invariably, individuals with disease identified as a result of screening will have a longer survival time than those diagnosed in the normal way following the appearance of symptoms. Two concepts explain this fact. The first is *lead time,* defined as the interval between the time of detection by screening and the time at which the disease would have been diagnosed in the absence of screening. In other words, it is the time by which screening advances diagnosis of the disease. For example, if, as a result of screening, the point of diagnosis is pushed back one year, then inevitably persons diagnosed by screening will survive 1 year longer even if there is no long-term benefit. Lead time can also be an important factor if survival is compared among subgroups of patients, e.g., those detected by different screening modalities. Lead time is likely to be different in various subgroups, thus making survival comparisons difficult.

The other concept which explains the differential survival of those identified in screening programs compared to those diagnosed in normal clinical practice has been called *length-biased sampling.* This concerns the fact that screening tests inevitably identify selectively the slowly developing abnormalities in the population and miss the rapidly progressive abnormalities that are more likely to present with symptoms before the initiation of the program or between screening examinations. This bias is most likely to be expressed at the initiation of a screening program. Eventually, after appropriate follow-up, providing all individuals are kept under observation and disease which is diagnosed and treated between screenings is identified, the effect of length bias on incidence or mortality will be reduced. It is an important bias for programs of short duration and has been identified in a clinical series (Boyd, 1978). It can, however, be important in longer-term programs, especially when considering the incidence and mortality over the total period of the program, depending on the relationship between the natural history of the disease and the interval between screenings. Bailer (1978) has indicated how the length bias effect in the U.S. breast cancer detection demonstration projects may have loaded the series with individuals who were unlikely to have had much benefit from screening.

A further bias of concern is *selection bias.* This refers to the fact that people who enter screening programs have a different probability of developing (and dying from) disease than the general population. This has been well demonstrated (in opposite directions) in screening programs for cancer of the cervix and cancer of the breast (see Chapters 16 and 17). Another type of selection bias has some similarities to length bias and relates to the fact that individuals who develop rapidly progressive disease and who are thus probably more likely to die than the majority of individuals with disease are unlikely to be found in a population which presents for screening. Indeed, although some individuals take advantage of a screening program if they have symptoms, these symptoms are likely to be rather slowly progressive, and those with more severe symptoms will go elsewhere for diagnosis and treatment.

One further aspect of selection of individuals for screening programs causes difficulty in their evaluation, even if mortality is used as an outcome measure, unless mortality is determined in the total population screened, including those who both accept and reject the procedure. This concerns the fact that those who already have the disease of interest will not be regarded as eligible for the screening test. Yet it is from this group that the majority of deaths from the disease are initially derived. Thus, in the first few years of a screening program, there will be few deaths from the disease, although this can hardly be regarded as a benefit of screening. This can be regarded as an extreme example of length-biased sampling.

Morrison (1982a) has described a method whereby the effects of lead time and length-biased sampling on the mortality of screen-detected persons can be analyzed. The numbers of diseased persons benefiting from screening and lead time can be estimated by comparison of the number of deaths and number of diagnosed cases in the entire screened population and an otherwise comparable unscreened population. Such a comparable situation, is however, rarely obtained outside of a controlled trial.

B. Classification of Approaches to Evaluate Screening

Bearing these biases in mind, it is possible to classify the various approaches that have been used to evaluate the results of screening. A simple count of screen-detected cases is least reliable, and computing the distribution of stages of disease and comparing this with that expected from an unscreened population is hardly better. Assessing the survival of screen-detected cases in comparison with an unscreened population also has little validity. However, determining the absolute number (or the rate, not the proportion) of cases of advanced disease in the screened population in comparison with an unscreened population is of more value, since advanced cases are indicative of potential mortality from the disease (Miller and van Slooten, 1983; Chamberlain, 1984).

Thus, the only truly valid outcome measure for assessment of the results of a screening program is mortality from the disease in the total population screened in comparison with the mortality that would be expected in the same population without screening.

C. Randomized Trials

The design of choice for assessing the effectiveness of screening is a controlled trial in which the population is randomly divided into a study group offered the screening program and a control group that receives the currently accepted program of routine diagnosis and medical care. Randomization of individuals is preferred if the objective is to assess the effectiveness of a screening test, but randomization of groups may be necessary if the objective is to assess the effectiveness of a screening program. Group randomization may be essential if public education is integral to the administration of the screening test (as in the promulgation and use of breast self-examination) (Prorok and Miller, 1984).

D. Quasi-Experimental Studies

A second-best method of measuring effectiveness is to compare mortality in a defined population before and after the introduction of a screening program, providing that the information on mortality is reliable and is believed to be predictable for the future and that the screening program can be rapidly introduced to apply to the whole population at risk. In such quasi-experimental studies, interarea comparisons should be mandatory, i.e., comparing intensively screened and nonscreened areas, and should also include evaluation of time trends. Such studies are not a cheap and easy way out, but demand the same methodological accuracy as randomized controlled trials. In view of the substantially larger populations that may have to be studied in quasi-experimental studies compared to randomized trials, they may be more expensive than the preferred design.

Nevertheless, ethical issues may preclude the utilization of randomized trials, particularly for programs which were introduced before the necessity of such studies was appreciated. This is particularly true for screening for cancer of the cervix (see Chapter 17) and may now be true for screening for cancer of the stomach in Japan (see Chapter 19). Hence, a number of attempts have been made to evaluate the effectiveness of screening programs in the absence of controlled trials. The approaches that have been generally appropriate for cancer of the cervix may not apply to other sites, and many have attempted to develop other approaches. However, they have usually based their estimates of effectiveness on what Prorok *et al.* (1981) have called *pseudo variables*. These are variables which in a controlled trial would be determined only after randomization, and are therefore at least potentially affected by treatment. They include improved stage distributions of screen-detected cases over what would be anticipated from experience in a nonscreened population. As indicated above, such improved distributions are necessary to demonstrate effectiveness, but are not sufficient because they are influenced by lead time and length-biased sampling.

E. Case-Control Studies

Another approach to evaluation, which can be applied only when a screening program has been in operation for some time, is a case-control study. This method has been applied in the evaluation of screening for cancer of the cervix (Clarke and Anderson, 1979) and in several studies evaluating breast self-examination (see Chapter 17); the problems that arise over the selection of cases and controls in such designs have been considered in detail by Morrison (1982b).

Essentially, the objective of the approach should be to mimic as far as possible the situation in a controlled trial in which mortality is the endpoint (Weiss, 1983). The cases should therefore be selected by criteria which represent as closely as possible those that result in death. Thus, advanced disease cases should be selected, prevalent in the population which has been screened, and not newly diagnosed cases, which could include those diagnosed as a result of screening and subject to lead-time bias. The controls should be selected at random from the population in which screening was offered, and cases of early disease, which happen to be sampled, should be retained in the control series. The *exposure* variable is the extent to which the screening test was used in cases and controls, and a protective effect of screening will be demonstrated by a significant reduction in screening test utilization in cases compared to controls, measured by the odds ratio determined in the usual way, as in etiologic case-control studies. Providing the cases and controls were derived from the total population in which screening was offered, an additional strength of this approach is its ability to measure the *attributable benefit,* i.e., the extent to which the use of screening results in a reduction in the prevalence of advanced disease in the population. Unfortunately, so far, no study has been reported which includes all of these desirable features. In particular, the case-control studies that have sought to evaluate the use of breast self-examination have, by including early cases of disease, not eliminated lead-time bias.

One difficulty with the case-control approach for evaluation of screening, which explains why it has been used so seldom up to now, is the frequent strong correlation between risk factors for the disease and the likelihood that individuals will be screened. The correlation is positive for breast cancer and inverse for screening for cancer of the cervix. Nevertheless a case-control interview study will permit the acquisition of data on risk factors that will facilitate control for them in the analysis. Clarke and Anderson (1979) addressed this issue by partially matching for socioeconomic status, using neighborhood controls, and by stratification within their analysis by identified risk factors. Their selection of five controls per case facilitated this process. However, for some diseases, in which risk factors predict risk or attendance for screening rather poorly, and in which compliance with invitations to attend for screening have been shown to be correlated with risk for the disease (e.g., breast cancer), this may still be a residual concern.

F. Risks and Benefits of Screening

One important evaluation issue is determination of risk versus benefit. The group that achieves benefit in the screening program comprises those in whom screening succeeds in identifying disease at the point in its natural history when cure is still possible, whereas if the disease had not been identified as a result of screening, presentation with symptoms subsequently would have resulted in death. Those individuals with true positive tests who would have been cured if their disease had been allowed to present normally may have some benefit from reduced morbidity, but those with disease who might never have presented during their lifetime and those who will inevitably die whatever the results of screening will be disadvantaged by the program. All persons with false positives will also be disadvantaged, the extent of hazard depending upon the test and the diagnostic procedures that become necessary as a result of the test. Persons with false negatives will also be disadvantaged if they fail to take early action after the occurrence of symptoms because of the false reassurance they received from the screening. Careful balancing of risks versus benefits is therefore required in the evaluation of any screening program.

G. Summary of Evaluation Issues

Following a workshop on screening for cancer held by the UICC in 1983, a statement summarizing the issues relevant to evaluation of screening for cancer was developed (Prorok and Miller, 1984, pp. 3–4). This reads as follows:

1. State of the Art
   a. The preferred approach to evaluation of screening for cancer is a randomized controlled trial. Randomization should be individual if the aim is to evaluate the efficacy of the screening test. If the aim is to evaluate the effectiveness of the screening program, group randomization is acceptable.
   b. In the absence of randomization, screening programs can be evaluated by non-experimental methods either on an individual or group basis, such as by a saturation approach in defined geographic areas with no screening offered in comparable control areas. Before and after comparisons as well as assessment of time trends of mortality should be employed.
   c. Mortality from cancer is the preferred and always applicable endpoint for evaluation of screening. Incidence of cancer is only applicable as an end-point for evaluating screening if a precursor is detected by the application of the screening test and reduction in the incidence of clinically invasive cancer which would otherwise result in death can be anticipated.
   d. Other approaches sometimes used in the past to evaluate screening, including assessment of survival, distribution by stage, or counts of cases are influenced by biases including lead-time, length bias and selection bias, and are not applicable in the evaluation of screening.
2. Research Issues
   a. Case-control studies are being introduced in the evaluation of screening programs. This is a new methodology that needs to be further assessed. Case-control studies can be evaluated in the context of a randomized clinical trial evaluating screening.
   b. New statistical methodology needs to be employed in evaluating the extent to which assessment of deaths in cases diagnosed in a screening program mimics mortality reduction. This should be addressed both in situations where case numbers screened and control groups equalize, and where they do not.
   c. Evaluation of surrogates for mortality in the assessment of the effectiveness of screen-

ing, especially the absolute number or rate of advanced cases in a population offered screening compared to a comparable control population.

d. Approaches to statistical modelling based on the observed natural history of the detectable preclinical phase identified by cancer screening tests. Such models may be utilizable in evaluating issues such as periodicity of screening, age at onset and cessation of screening, which would probably not be subjected to evaluation in randomized clinical trials.

3. Applicability

a. Screening for cancer is demanding of health care resources. Unless reduction in mortality from the disease can be demonstrated by appropriately designed research studies, screening for cancer cannot be recommended as a public health policy for any cancer site.

b. Even where research studies have demonstrated mortality reduction, it will be necessary to assess the level of this benefit with any morbidity and resource costs arising from the screening program, in policy decisions about its widespread provision.

IX. CONCLUSION

In conclusion, there are a number of fundamental issues which have to be resolved when considering evaluation of screening. The general principles which govern the introduction of programs include the following: (1) the disease should be an important health problem; (2) the natural history of the lesions identified by screening should be known; (3) there should be a recognized treatment for such lesions; and (4) the test used should be acceptable and safe.

The other issues range from ethics to economics. Critical components include the definition of the disease to be identified by screening and the population to be included in the program. It cannot be assumed that a screening program for cancer will necessarily benefit the population to which it is applied. The underlying assumption that the detection of disease before symptoms develop improves the chances of preventing death and disability has to be tested each time a program to screen a different cancer is proposed. Further, the benefits devised from the program must be clearly shown to exceed the costs, in terms of both ill health induced by the test and accompanying procedures and the cost of the program. The other chapters in this volume will indicate the extent to which these principles have been realized in screening for cancer.

REFERENCES

American Cancer Society (1980). Guidelines for the cancer-related check-up. Recommendations and rationale. *Ca—Cancer J. Clin.* **30,** 194–240.

Bailar, J. C., III (1978). Mammographic screening, a reappraisal of benefits and risks. *Clin. Obstet. Gynecol.* **21,** 1–14.

Beahrs, O. H., Shapiro, S., and Smart, C. (1979). Report of the working group to review the

National Cancer Institute—American Cancer Society breast cancer detection demonstration projects. *JNCI, J. Natl. Cancer Inst.* **62,** 640–709.
Boyd, N. F. (1978). A preliminary appraisal of the effects of length biased sampling and observer variability on screening. *In* "Screening in Cancer" (A. B. Miller, ed.), UICC Tech. Rep. Ser., Vol. 40, pp. 40–50. Int. Union Against Cancer, Geneva.
Boyd, N. F., Wolfson, C., Moskowitz, M., Carlile, T., Petitclerc, M., Ferri, H. A., Fishell, E., Grégoire, A., Kiernan, M., Longley, J. D., Simor, I. S., and Miller, A. B. (1982). Observer variation in the interpretation of xeromammograms. *JNCI, J. Natl. Cancer Inst.* **68,** 357–363.
Boyes, D. A., Morrison, B., Knox, E. G., Draper, G. J., and Miller, A. B. (1982). A cohort study of cervical cancer screening in British Columbia. *Clin. Invest. Med.* **5,** 1–29.
Chamberlain, J. (1984). Planning of screening programmes for evaluation of non-randomized approaches to evaluation. *In* "Screening for Cancer" (P. Prorok and A. B. Miller, eds.), UICC Tech. Rep. Ser., Vol 78, pp. 5–17. Int. Union Against Cancer, Geneva.
Clarke, E. A., and Anderson, T. W. (1979). Does screening by "Pap" smears help prevent cervical cancer? A case-control study. *Lancet* **2,** 1–4.
Cole, P., and Morrison, A. S. (1980). Basic issues in population screening for cancer. *JNCI, J. Natl. Cancer Inst.* **64,** 1263–1272.
Eddy, D. M. (1980). "Screening for Cancer: Theory, Analysis and Design." Prentice-Hall, Englewood Cliffs, New Jersey.
May, D. (1974). Error rates in cervical cytological screening tests. *Br. J. Cancer* **29,** 106–113.
Miller, A. B. (1974). The joint National Cancer Institute of Canada/American Cancer Society study of a test for carcinoembryonic antigen (CEA). *Cancer* **34,** 932–935.
Miller, A. B., ed. (1978). "Screening in Cancer," UICC Tech. Rep. Ser., Vol. 40. Int. Union Against Cancer, Geneva.
Miller, A. B. (1982). Fundamental issues in screening. *In* "Cancer Epidemiology and Prevention" (D. Schottenfeld and J. F. Fraumeni, Jr., eds.), pp. 1064–1074. Saunders, Philadelphia, Pennsylvania.
Miller, A. B., and Bulbrook, R. D. (1982). Screening, detection and diagnosis of breast cancer. *Lancet* **1,** 1109–1111.
Miller, A. B., and van Slooten, E. A. (1983). Screening and diagnosis in breast cancer; workshop report. *Eur. J. Cancer Clin. Oncol.* **19,** 1711–1716.
Morrison, A. S. (1982a). The effects of early treatment, lead time and length bias on the mortality experienced by cases detected by screening. *Int. J. Epidemiol.* **11,** 261–267.
Morrison, A. S. (1982b). Case definition in case-control studies of the efficacy of screening. *Am. J. Epidemiol.* **115,** 6–8.
Prorok, P. C., and Miller, A. B., eds. (1984). "Screening for Cancer," UICC Tech. Rep. Ser., Vol. 78. Int. Union Against Cancer, Geneva.
Prorok, P. C., Hankey, B. F., and Bundy, B. M. (1981). Concepts and problems in the evaluation of screening programs. *J. Chronic Dis.* **34,** 159–171.
Sackett, D. L., and Holland, W. W. (1975). Controversy in the detection of disease. *Lancet* **2,** 357–359.
Schottenfeld, D., Winawer, S. J., and Miller, D. G. (1978). Screening and early diagnosis of large bowel cancer. *In* "Screening in Cancer" (A. B. Miller, ed.), UICC Tech. Rep. Ser., Vol. 40, pp. 307–327. Int. Union Against Cancer, Geneva.
Swets, J. A., and Pickett, R. M. (1982). "Evaluation of Diagnostic Systems: Methods from Signal Detection Theory." Academic Press, New York.
Task Force Appointed by the Conference of Deputy Ministers of Health (1976). Cervical cancer screening programs. *Can. Med. Assoc. J.* **114,** 1003–1033.
U. S. Commission on Chronic Illness (1957). "Chronic Illness in the United States," Vol. 1. Harvard Univ. Press, Cambridge, Massachusetts.

Walter S. D., and Day, N. E. (1983). Estimation of the duration of a preclinical disease state using screening data. *Am. J. Epidemiol.* **118,** 865–886.
Weiss, N. S. (1983). Control definition in case-control studies of the efficacy of screening and diagnostic testing. *Am. J. Epidemiol.* **118,** 457–460.
Weiss, W. (1978). Problems in screening for lung cancer. *In* ''Screening in Cancer'' (A. B. Miller, ed.), UICC Tech. Rep. Ser., Vol. 40, pp. 216–232. Int. Union Against Cancer, Geneva.
Wolfe, J. M. (1976). Risk for breast cancer development determined by mammography parenchymal pattern. *Cancer* **37,** 2486–2492.
Yu, S. Z., Miller, A. B., and Sherman, G. J. (1982). Optimizing the age, number of tests and test interval for cervical screening in Canada. *J. Epidemiol. Commun. Health* **36,** 1–10.

2

Screening in the Context of Cancer Control

PETER GREENWALD, RICHARD COSTLOW, PHILIP PROROK, AND EDWARD J. SONDIK

I. Cancer Control and Screening 25
II. Phases of Cancer Control Research 27
III. Review of Screening Programs 29
A. Breast Cancer 30
B. Lung Cancer 31
C. Colorectal Cancer 33
D. Uterine Cancer 34
E. Genitourinary Cancer 35
F. Other Cancer Sites 35
IV. New Methods for Screening and Detection 36
V. Policy Analysis and Screening Evaluation 37
A. The Design and Evaluation of Screening Programs 38
B. Disease Factors 41
C. Selecting the Population 41
D. Implementation of Program Components 43
VI. General Considerations 45
References 46

I. CANCER CONTROL AND SCREENING

Cancer control and prevention are now feasible for several cancers, and many cancer control and prevention research opportunities hold great promise. For example, prevention is feasible for lung cancer caused by smoking; and cervical cancer deaths are largely preventable because of the Pap test and curative therapy

ISBN 0-12-496720-5

for early disease. Also, we know more about mammography. On the other hand, many gaps still exist in our knowledge of cancer control and of screening for cancer control. Therefore, in the National Cancer Institute's (NCI) Division of Cancer Prevention and Control (DCPC), with the help of the scientific community, we have been reviewing cancer control research opportunities and restating the research objectives of DCPC's programs. We have based our activities on the premise that the scientific method applies to cancer control as much as it does to other research areas. Close observation, measurement, quantitative analysis, and analytic thought are as important here as in basic laboratory or clinical research.

Assigning priorities to the numerous opportunities for cancer control research requires a clear definition of *cancer control.* We have developed a one-sentence definition which we feel captures the meaning of this term: "Cancer control is the reduction of cancer incidence, morbidity, and mortality through an orderly sequence from research on interventions and their impact in defined populations to the broad, systematic application of the research results." A few points in this definition warrant some explanation. The goal is expressed as rates: the reduction of cancer incidence, morbidity, and mortality; the aim is to reduce these rates in the whole population. "Through an orderly sequence" means the use of the scientific method in a progression from basic or clinical investigations to wide application. *Interventions* is a key word: cancer control, by this definition, must involve an intervention. For example, an epidemiologic study that examines an etiologic factor, but does not involve interceding for public or patient benefit, would not be cancer control according to this definition. On the other hand, the definition would include the application of a screening technique, a preventive strategy, a medical treatment, or a rehabilitation technique in an effort to see if it can be effectively adopted in the community. The phrase "their impact in defined populations" is included because research on cause-and-effect relationships does not necessarily tell us how to achieve an effective, wide-scale impact. Research is needed on how best to achieve changes in large populations—in other words, defined population research.

In this context, then, the basis of any cancer screening program must be sound quantification of the extent to which incidence, morbidity, and mortality are reduced. Information on the reduction of mortality by screening is probably the most glaring lack in screening programs. Until such information is available for any cancer site, wide-scale efforts must be preceded by a sequence of research phases aimed at gathering the necessary information on the efficacy, potential impact, and cost effectiveness of potential screening programs. In this chapter, we discuss a sequence of five phases, review the merits of existing screening methods and programs, summarize the chief elements requisite to implementing a cancer screening program, and argue that evaluation of screening is fundamental to policy decision making.

II. PHASES OF CANCER CONTROL RESEARCH

To approach cancer control research systematically, we are now classifying all cancer control research efforts into an orderly sequence of five phases of an overall research process. The classification applies to all cancer control research, both for prevention and for management. *Prevention* refers to people for whom there is no diagnosis of cancer; it includes primary prevention and screening. *Management* refers to treatment, continuing care, and rehabilitation of patients with a diagnosis of cancer.

The five phases are (I) hypothesis development, (II) methods development, (III) controlled intervention trials, (IV) defined population studies, and (V) demonstration and implementation studies. Hypothesis development is simply an assessment of where the research leads are; many come from basic science and clinical research. These leads tell us where to focus in cancer control. Methods development and testing is the first step in cancer control research; for example, if a diagnostic procedure is to be adapted for population screening, modifications of equipment and procedures for screening might be tested first. Controlled intervention trials tell us if something is potentially effective; however, the conclusions cannot be generalized to other populations. For example, thousands of controlled studies show a cause-and-effect relationship between smoking and cancer, and some indicate factors which contribute to smoking behavior but do not provide information on how to lower smoking rates. If we had been classifying research into the phases described above, we probably would have stopped duplicative studies long ago and instead would have encouraged defined population studies. Defined population studies test and compare the effects of interventions in a sample population that is adequately representative of a larger population to warrant generalizing about the probable effectiveness of the interventions on a broader scale. To conduct defined population studies, there must be methods for identifying the population denominators and the occurrence of cancer within the population.

The orderly sequence of the first four phases will provide a better basis for making decisions about demonstration and implementation studies, a necessity illustrated by the recent breast cancer screening program. The Health Insurance Plan (HIP) of Greater New York, which conducted an excellent study of the effectiveness of breast cancer screening, showed that periodic screening could reduce breast cancer mortality. We then jumped, perhaps prematurely, to a national policy of promoting breast cancer screening. As with other scientific studies, demonstration and implementation studies are research, and careful evaluation of their effects is essential.

In the field of screening, we have been reviewing programs and think that there is a need for more research and for systematic application of selected modalities. For example, population screening programs generally do not endure when they are not integrated into the usual practice of medicine. Most people see a doctor every year or two, especially older people, who are at the highest risk for cancer. One of the most effective approaches, therefore, may be to build selective screening techniques into the usual practice of medicine.

TABLE I

Cancer Control Phases in Screening/Early Detection Research

	Phases				
Reference	I	II	III	IV	V
Breast cancer					
Andersson (1981)			X		
Baker (1982)					X
Doll (1981)				X	
Lundgren *et al.* (1982)		X			
Miller (1982)			X		
Shapiro *et al.* (1982a)			X		
Shapiro *et al.* (1982b)			X		
Tabar and Gad (1981)			X		
Lung cancer					
Band *et al.* (1982)					X
Kotin and Paul (1982)					X
Levin *et al.* (1982)			X		
Martini (1982)			X		
Sanderson and Fontana (1982)			X		
Colorectal cancer					
Gilbertsen *et al.* (1980)			X		
Winawer *et al.* (1980)			X		
Uterine/cervix cancer					
Boyes (1981)					X
Navarre (1982)		X			
Nogouchi *et al.* (1982)		X			
Genitourinary cancer					
Betkerur *et al.* (1980)		X			
Nemoto *et al.* (1982)		X			
Prostate cancer					
Catalona and Menon (1981)		X			
Thyroid cancer					
Schneider *et al.* (1980)			X		
Shiamoka *et al.* (1982)			X		
New methods					
Computed tomography		X			
Diaphanography		X			
Nuclear magnetic resonance		X			
Thermography		X			
Ultrasound		X			

Another effective approach for selective screening might be to seek out high-risk and industrial populations. An examination of Papanicolaou (Pap) testing in New York State indicated that to reach the women at high risk of cervical cancer—that is, the poor, the blacks, the Puerto Ricans—it may be most practical to identify where these people go for medical care. Women at highest risk for cervical cancer are found in hospital emergency rooms. These patients often do not have a regular doctor, and many emergency rooms are used for regular medical care and not for emergencies. Thus, it appears that doing Pap testing in emergency rooms might be particularly valuable.

Quality control of screening and testing methods also seems to be worth investigating. For example, across the country, the false-negative Pap test rate is about 30%. Many women who have been diagnosed with invasive cervical cancer or who have died from it had a negative Pap test 2 or 3 years before the diagnosis. It is not known if the tests were really negative, or if the collection of cells was inadequate, or if the Pap smears were improperly done, or if the slides were misinterpreted.

In the next section, studies of screening methods for various cancers are reviewed and are classified by the phase of research they represent in the cancer control phases.

Table I illustrates a distribution of ongoing studies in cancer screening. The distribution correlates fairly well with current practices in screening. Further, it can be seen that some screening practices have been applied prematurely considering their meager scientific basis, as in lung cancer. This table also illustrates the dearth of Phase IV studies and areas which are in need of more intensive applied research to bring them to the point where Phase V can be applied, i.e., where the process is ready to be implemented as a public health measure.

III. REVIEW OF SCREENING PROGRAMS

All too often, screening for cancer is confused with early, definitive diagnosis and is presumed to result in reductions in cancer incidence, morbidity, or mortality. The U.S. Commission on Chronic Illness defines screening as "the presumptive identification of unrecognized disease or defect by the application of tests, examinations or other procedures that can be applied rapidly" (see Chapter 1). Although this definition clearly implies that screening requires only "presumptive identification" of disease, further conditions must be fulfilled in the context of cancer control: there must be proof that screening reduces the incidence, morbidity, or mortality of the disease and that there is a means for broad, systematic application of screening to the public at large. Since cancer is manifested in a variety of ways and in numerous anatomical sites, screening efforts must be "customized" to reflect the unique characteristics and problems for each cancer site; hence, research studies on screening for cancer have been reported individually by cancer site. Regardless of the site, however, the same fundamental technical issues for screening apply; these have been adequately discussed by Miller in Chapter 1.

A. Breast Cancer

Cancer of the female breast continues to be the leading cause of cancer death among women [Surveillance, Epidemiology, End Results (SEER), Horm *et al.*, 1984], but is amenable to screening and early detection, which have been demonstrated to reduce mortality. Screening with physical examination and mammography is beneficial for women 50 years of age and older, and there is suggestive evidence (Baker, 1982; Shapiro *et al.*, 1982a) that younger women may also benefit; however, randomized, controlled trials are likely to be the only way in which that benefit can be quantified. Even with successful screening in randomized trials, breast cancer survival rates differ for various races (Shapiro *et al.*, 1982b), an observation requiring further study to explain.

No ongoing, randomized, controlled trials on breast cancer screening are being conducted in the United States; however, several trials are underway in other parts of the world. The information derived from these trials will provide further bases on which to make decisions about breast cancer screening in the context of cancer control. A controlled, randomized trial has been initiated in Canada (Miller, 1982) to examine the benefit of mammography and physical examination in women aged 40 to 49 and to determine the independent effect of mammography in women aged 50 to 59. Conservative estimates indicate that it is reasonable to expect that the benefit from screening for breast cancer by mammography and physical examination will significantly exceed any possible hazard from the radiation (Miller, 1982).

In the United Kingdom, a large-scale, nonrandomized trial has been started by an Early Detection of Breast Cancer Group (Doll, 1981) to evaluate the effectiveness of different methods of detection. One group of 25,000 women aged 45 to 64 are invited for annual clinical examinations of the breast, or mammography, or both. Two other groups of 25,000 and 40,000 in the same age range are invited to education sessions on breast self-examination. Four control populations totaling 120,000 are offered no special services beyond conventional diagnostic facilities.

In Malmo, Sweden, a randomized radiographic screening trial for 15,748 women 45 to 69 years of age was conducted between January 1977 and September 1978 (Andersson, 1981). One oblique and one craniocaudal mammographic view for each breast was obtained. Conclusions from the study indicate that the detection rate of breast cancer with a tumor diameter less than 1 centimeter was 7.5 per 1000; 16% of these cancers were noninvasive and 43% were invasive. With a reported radiographic sensitivity of 91.5%, a specificity of 99.2%, and a predictive value of 47%, radiographic mammography seemed to be an effective screening method for detecting early breast cancer; however, the preliminary findings in this study must await an assessment of a long-term follow-up.

Another randomized, controlled trial in Sweden in two separate counties was begun in 1977 by the National Board of Health and Welfare (Tabar and Gad, 1981). The trial is being conducted among 94,000 women over 39 years of age with an age-matched control population of 67,000 women. The only screening method used in the study population is a single mediolateral oblique view by mammography. One round of screening has been completed. Preliminary analyses reflect a 94.5% sensitivity and a 95.9% specificity. Information on the periodicity of examination and the benefit to women aged 40 to 49 is expected when the trial is completed.

A third study in Sweden was begun in 1974 among 6845 women 40 years of age and older (Lundgren and Helleberg, 1982). This study was not randomized and was undertaken to reach a conclusion about the optimum interval of time (periodicity) for effective screening by single-view mammography. The population was screened in 1974, 1977, and 1980. During the 6-year period, 111 breast cancers were detected at screening, 15% as interval cancers and 7% among nonresponders. The predictive value for biopsy recommendations was 78%; 63% of the women had clinical Stage I tumors and 59% had tumors equal to or less than 1 centimeter. The authors' conclusion was that this method was suitable for screening; acceptance of this method, however, is not universal among radiologists.

Finally, a word must be said about self-examination of the breast and its potential as a screening method. It is not the means for the *earliest* detection of breast cancer. The efficacy of this approach has yet to be proven by means of a randomized, controlled, prospective trial, and given the promise of newer techniques for detecting smaller lesions and the number of years such a trial would require, we may not have a trial with the endpoint of reduction in mortality.

B. Lung Cancer

Lung cancer continues to be an immense public health problem as the leading cause of cancer death in men, second only to breast cancer in women (Horm *et al.*, 1984). Cancer control efforts to reduce mortality from lung cancer have consisted of primary prevention such as smoking prevention and cessation, avoidance of exposure to asbestos, and avoidance of exposure in occupational settings such as uranium mines. Today, the only available means of identifying presymptomatic lung cancers are chest radiography and sputum cytology, and unfortunately, these methods are more applicable to diagnosis than to early detection. When lung cancer is detected by either chest X ray or sputum cytology, there is no assurance that the disease is in an early stage. Several studies are in progress to determine the efficacy of these screening methods in reducing the mortality from lung cancer. To date, however, the results of such screening studies have not shown clear benefits, and mortality has not been significantly reduced by screening or therapeutic interventions at an earlier stage of disease.

In the early 1970s, NCI sponsored three large clinical trials of lung cancer screening in high-risk populations of men 45 years or older who were chronic, excessive cigarette smokers. An interim report of one randomized study (Sanderson and Fontana, 1982) indicates that three times as many Stage I lung cancers were detected in the screened group (chest radiography and sputum tests at 4-month intervals) than in a nonscreened control group. Although observed survival seems to have improved as a result of screening, no significant difference in mortality has yet been found between the screened and nonscreened groups. Further follow-up on this study may determine the usefulness of this screening procedure.

In a second study, a population of 10,000 high-risk men (chronic smokers aged 45 or older) were randomized into two groups after entry into the program. One group was offered annual chest X ray examinations for 5 years, and the other group was offered annual chest X ray and cytological examination of aerosol-induced sputum collected every 4 months. The results of this study thus far (Levin *et al.*, 1982) provide no evidence that mass screening by chest X ray and sputum cytology followed by prompt, appropriate therapy reduces mortality from lung cancer.

The third study of lung cancer screening in high-risk men had two groups of subjects; one group was given a chest X ray annually, and the other group had annual chest X rays and cytological examinations of sputum samples every 4 months. An interim report (Martini, 1982) states that the effect of screening on lung cancer mortality can be estimated only indirectly by the apparent increase in survival time.

Studies of lung cancer screening programs in industrial settings among workers at high risk (Kotin and Paul, 1982; Band *et al.*, 1982) have also shown that reduction of mortality has not been significant.

Research on screening for lung cancer indicates clearly that at present the most desirable approach for reducing mortality from this disease is primary prevention (Carter, 1981). Of all environmental bronchogenic carcinogens, cigarette smoking is known to contribute most to the annual increase in mortality from lung cancer. Cancer control efforts, therefore, are best placed in areas that lead to the largest reduction in exposure to known bronchogenic carcinogens such as cigarette smoke.

C. Colorectal Cancer

In the United States, cancer of the colon and rectum is the second highest cause of cancer deaths in men and the third highest in women (Horm *et al.*, 1984). The relative 5-year survival rate from this disease has increased about 7% during the last decade for whites and about 4% for blacks. Colorectal cancer is responsive to therapeutic interventions; these increase the survival rate, especially when the disease is detected at an early stage. Screening for early detection of colorectal cancer would therefore appear to have potential for reducing mortality. Most of the literature on early detection of colorectal cancer concerns relatively sophisticated diagnostic procedures rather than techniques applicable to mass screening. In recent years, however, attention has been given to the use of tests for fecal occult blood, which may indicate the presence of colorectal cancer prior to overt symptoms.

The test for fecal occult blood depends upon the pseudoperoxidase activity of hemoglobin, which interacts with hydrogen peroxide to oxidize guaiac on a test slide, turning it blue (Winawer *et al.*, 1982). Several slide tests are now available, including a single Hemoccult and a Hemoccult II slide (Smith, Kline, and French, Inc.) with six areas or "windows" for smears. The Hemoccult II slide is somewhat more sensitive because it uses a more highly purified guaiac which ordinarily contains a whole family of guaiac compounds. Although many fecal occult blood slide tests are available commercially, they are all based on the same principle (Winawer and Sherlock, 1982). The test appears to be more sensitive for cancers than for adenomas, but will detect more adenomas if they are bleeding. A summary of clinical data on the fecal occult blood test shows that its predictive value for neoplasia ranges from 18 to 50%, the false positivity with hydrated slides is up to 20%, and the false negativity for cancer with hydrated slides is 9%. Sufficient quantities of blood anywhere in the gastrointestinal tract can, therefore, elicit a positive test. Moreover, since peroxidase activity is the basis for the test, certain dietary foods containing high peroxidase activity, for example, uncooked vegetables and fresh fruits, can also cause a positive test; ascorbic acid can also interfere with the oxidation of guaiac and produce false-negative results. All in all, the test must be performed under careful conditions, and interpretation must be made with many conditions in mind. At present, only two controlled clinical trials are in progress to test the efficacy of screening with the fecal occult blood test (Winawer *et al.*, 1980; Gilbertsen *et al.*, 1980). Neither study is complete, and available data are inconclusive about the reduction of mortality as a result of screening with the fecal occult blood test.

Several basic issues must be resolved before a comprehensive cancer control program of screening for colorectal cancer can be implemented (Sherlock *et al.*, 1980). First, the expected benefit from this type of screening will have to be quantified. Perhaps the completion of ongoing trials will provide this answer.

Second, a suitable means is required to identify high-risk individuals in a given population who can be targeted for screening. Third, the techniques of screening must be refined for acceptable limits of sensitivity and specificity. Fourth, a careful cost-benefit analysis must be done which includes the safety of diagnostic tests that must be used to diagnose definitively cases identified by screening. Therefore, it appears premature to advocate the mass use of screening by fecal occult blood testing.

D. Uterine Cancer

The incidence of cervical cancer in the United States has been steadily decreasing but, combined with endometrial cancer, still accounts for about 5% of cancer deaths among women (Horm *et al.*, 1984). In 1985 there will be about 7000 deaths from cervical cancer and 3000 from endometrial cancer (American Cancer Society, 1985). The decreasing death rate from uterine cancer is attributed largely to the use of the Pap test and regular health checkups. The continuous progress that has been made in reducing the incidence and mortality of cervical cancer gives hope that many more deaths can be averted with appropriate public health and education programs.

Probably more epidemiologic work has been done on uterine cancer than on any other gynecological cancer, and space does not permit a comprehensive review of that literature. For our purpose, it is sufficient to cite the most recent report by the Canadian Task Force on Cervical Cancer Screening Programs (Task Force, 1982). One of the task force's most striking observations is the relatively poor reliability of cytologic diagnosis in laboratories other than standard reference laboratories, a significant point when considering cancer control programs that include screening for cervical cancer. Efforts to attain more standardized laboratory techniques and more uniform technology should have a high priority in screening programs for cervical cancer. The report further emphasizes the need to pay more attention to the high-risk groups of women and to expand the high-risk group in annual screening to include younger women 18 to 35 years of age who have had intercourse. The recommendations of this task force are based on what is recognized as the best available information.

Among the newer technologies for early detection of cervical cancer, colposcopy has been suggested as a useful adjunct in evaluating individuals with abnormal Pap smears (Navarre, 1982). The advantages of colposcopy are that patients are spared extra visits and the trained physician can arrive at a quicker diagnosis than with the Pap smear report. Training in the use of the colposcope is necessary for appropriate application of this technique. In British Columbia, a screening program has contributed to a reduction in incidence and mortality from carcinoma of the cervix (Boyes, 1981). This program has been running for more than 30 years and recently included colposcopy for small, directed biopsies. The introduction of colposcopy to the program significantly changed the diagnostic criteria in the program, and subsequent analyses will have to take this fact into consideration.

As the efforts to reduce mortality from cervical cancer continue, new technology, improved efficiency, and reduced cost of obtaining specimens must be carefully monitored. Japanese investigators have described a self-collection device (the Kato technique) for obtaining cervical specimens that may be useful in remote and rural areas (Noguchi *et al.*, 1982). Unlike former collection methods that required irrigation, the Kato technique uses mechanical scraping and immediate fixation of the specimen in a mailable plastic container. The only difference in results between the Kato self-collection specimens and those obtained by physicians in the study was the degree of severity of the lesions detected, not between positives and negatives.

E. Genitourinary Cancer

In the United States, cancer of the urinary bladder accounts for 5% of cancer deaths in men and about 3% in women. Population groups that are at higher risk for bladder cancer than the general population include workers in the chemical, rubber, and dye industries and cigarette smokers. To date, efforts to obtain early detection of bladder cancer have either been impractical for mass screening or have had equivocal results when reduction of mortality was analyzed as an endpoint. For cancer control purposes, primary prevention by avoiding exposure to known or suspected bladder carcinogens seems to be the most fruitful approach. At this time, there are no practical methods for mass screening to detect cancer of the urinary system.

In a study (Betkerur *et al.*, 1980) of techniques—urine cytology, urinary cholesterol, urinary carcinoembryonic antigen (CEA), and urinary immunoglobulin levels—urinary cytology appeared to have the most potential for detecting bladder cancer; however, false positives were unacceptably numerous considering the risks of therapeutic interventions. A study in Japan of 16,062 inpatients and outpatients selected randomly provided urine specimens for cytologic examinations after toluidine blue staining (Nemoto *et al.*, 1982). The detection rate was 1 case of bladder cancer in 5000 patients. No evidence was presented, however, to predict a reduction in mortality or an increase in survival time.

F. Other Cancer Sites

Cancer of the prostate accounts for about 10% of cancer deaths in men but has not been amenable to mass screening procedures. Screening for prostatic cancer is complicated by the existence of a clinically occult and often biologically latent form, as well as a clinically overt form which is often lethal. Thus, the true prevalence of this disease is difficult to determine. About 1 patient in 30 with prostatic cancer ever shows clinically manifest disease, and about 1 in 100 dies of his disease. For this reason, decisions about appropriate therapy, if any, would be difficult even if highly sensitive screening methods were applied. Numerous biochemical tests have been suggested, but none has been outstanding as a potential method for screening and early detection of prostate cancer (Catalona and Menon, 1981). Enzyme tests that have been investigated for prostatic cancer screening include acid and alkaline phosphatase, creatine phosphokinase, lactic dehydrogenase, and ribonuclease. Proteins such as oncofetal proteins, alpha-fetoprotein, and many others have also been tested, but for one reason or another have not been suitable as a prostatic cancer screening procedure.

Cancers at other anatomical sites such as the thyroid gland, testicle, skin, and oral cavity have been reported to be detectable by screening and early detection methods. Most of these reports have been confined to high-risk groups, but we lack data on reduced mortality as a result of these types of screening. For thyroid cancer, populations at high risk because of prior head and neck X ray irradiation have been screened (Schneider *et al.*, 1980). Whether or not the detection of cases in such programs reduces mortality has not been assessed. In another similar study begun in 1977, a follow-up evaluation concluded that screening by physical examination, with palpation of the thyroid, was effective in identifying earlier disease, but no conclusions were possible about reduction of mortality from screening (Shimaoka *et al.*, 1982).

IV. NEW METHODS FOR SCREENING AND DETECTION

The applicability of several newer methods of visual imaging is being explored for mass screening, especially nuclear magnetic resonance (NMR), ultrasound, thermography, diaphanography, and computed tomography (CT) scanning. These techniques have typically been used as an adjunct for definitive diagnosis to locate potentially malignant tumors and to direct biopsies. Their application to mass screening has not yet been tested sufficiently; thus, their potential for reducing mortality, as well as their risk or cost versus their benefit, are uncertain. Most screening studies of these techniques have been conducted in an attempt to find noninvasive techniques to replace ionizing radiation imaging. Except for CT scanning, none of these techniques use ionizing radiation and, thus far, there are no known major risks with their use.

Interest is increasing in the newest of these techniques, NMR, introduced in 1971. The basis of the detection is the observance of the difference between spin-lattice relaxation times (T) for normal and malignant tissue by producing an electronic image that can be viewed. A preliminary report on the use of this technique (Ross *et al.*, 1982) indicated that T values can distinguish normal breasts and those with extensive fatty replacement from breasts with other types of lesions. The major difficulties with this technique are the length of the examination (the average total time per patient is 1 hour), the specific localization of lesions, and the discrimination between T values for dysplasia and neoplasia. Although preliminary results from this technique are exciting, much remains to be done before it can be used for mass screening.

Ultrasonic and thermographic imaging appear to have the greatest potential for application to mass screening. Comparisons of ultrasound with mammography have reported a sensitivity of 69% for ultrasound mammograms and 74% for radiographic mammograms (Cole-Beuglet *et al.*, 1981). These values, however, were not statistically different. Thermography has been shown to be a sensitive marker for local thermal and vascular abnormalities in the breast, but is not a specific test for the presence of carcinoma or for diagnosis of other breast diseases (Nyirjesy, 1982). Thus far, none of the new techniques have approached the resolution of detail obtained by X ray mammography, but further research and clinical testing should continue.

Diaphanography utilizes a cool, bright, light surface to transilluminate the breast; it is applied after adaptation in a completely darkened room. This technique has been reported to detect breast tumors as small as 5–6 millimeters (Mallard, 1981). Obviously, controlled trials and further clinical application must be done to assess the efficacy of this technique for mass screening. Its simplicity and noninvasiveness are distinct advantages, and new developments with color imaging and TV cameras may enhance its potential for breast cancer screening.

Although CT scanning has been used to detect breast carcinomas, it has not yet taken the place of conventional mammography (Chang *et al.*, 1982). It is likely that the time for examination, the cost, and the availability of the equipment will preclude its application to mass screening for cancer.

V. POLICY ANALYSIS AND SCREENING EVALUATION

In this section, we turn to the evaluation of screening programs and examine, in a general fashion, the decision on whether or not to implement particular screening programs. As discussed in the earlier sections, the role of screening is to provide information to individuals about the likelihood that they may have or may develop cancer. The role of evaluation of screening is to determine the significance of the gain and the information afforded by earlier detection, together with the *a priori* projection of the various outcomes associated with the screening test. Four categories of factors must be addressed before a decision is made about whether or not to implement a screening program: the health consequences of the disease; knowledge of the natural history of the disease; availability of a valid, acceptable, safe screening test; and availability of effective treatment (Miller, 1978, 1982). Subsequently, the question of implementation should focus on the choice of population(s) to be screened and on the quality of available evidence about the cost and effectiveness of screening that particular population.

A. The Design and Evaluation of Screening Programs

The design and evaluation of a routinized screening program depend on how the information gained by screening is to be acted upon; ultimately, the program must be assessed for its effect on cancer morbidity and mortality in the target population.

In discussing general issues concerning screening programs, we will refer to Fig. 1, which is a schematic view, or model, of a screening program for symptom-free individuals. The population participating in the screening program is given a test which yields positive or negative results. If positive, the result may represent a true positive for persons who actually have cancer; however, if the test is flawed, the positive result may be, in fact, a false positive, that is, a positive result for a person who is actually disease free. Similarly, the test results may be negative and represent either a false negative for persons who have the disease or a true negative for persons who are disease free.

Each of the four outcomes has particular significance. The outcome of a positive result would lead, in this model, to further diagnostic testing which, in most but not all cases, will rule out the disease for patients who are disease free. However, some individuals may erroneously enter the treatment phase and undergo unnecessary and perhaps dangerous medical treatment. On the other hand, individuals with true-positive results, as confirmed by subsequent diagnosis, undergo appropriate treatment, the success of which depends on the cancer site and its stage. The outcome of a false-negative result allows the cancer to develop without intervention, possibly to be detected at a later screening test, but in all likelihood the prognosis is poor. The confirmed true-negative outcome is reassuring to the individual. The implications for all of the outcomes are summarized on the diagram.

The evaluation of the screening program must compare that program with the option of no screening at all. In such a case, we must consider, first, the likelihood that a person has cancer, and second, the stage of the cancer at the time the patient seeks diagnosis and treatment. In general, the cancer will be detected at a later stage than it would if the patient were discovered through a screening program which, in most cases, would result in a somewhat poorer prognosis than if the cancer were detected at an earlier stage.

In general, screening involves costs in both fiscal and health terms (such as radiation or perforation of the colon); furthermore, depending on the outcome,

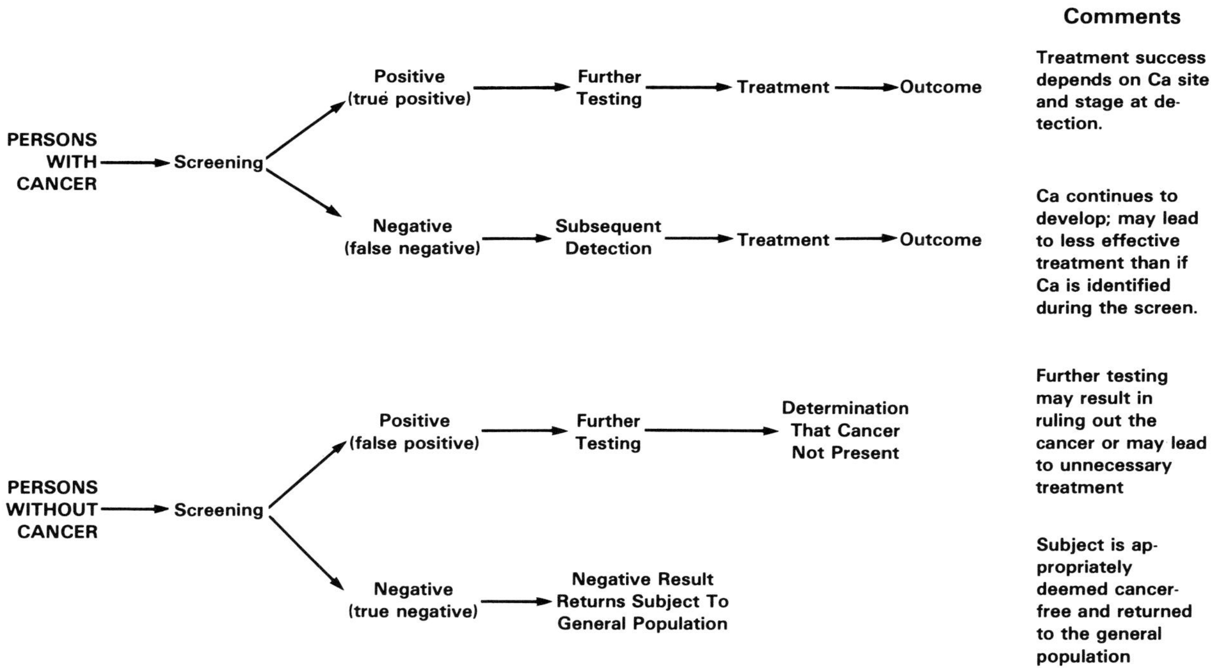

Fig. 1. Schematic view of a cancer screening program and its outcomes.

screening may result in additional, and sometimes unnecessary, health costs or deleterious outcomes. Therefore, the marginal gains in health outcomes compared to the results of not screening must be considered significant enough to justify the control efforts. Evaluation of a screening program takes place at two points in time: first, during the design and conceptualization of the program before it is actually implemented (*a priori* analysis), and second, during or conceivably after the program's operation (*a posteriori* evaluation). Both evaluations are important; they affect key decisions related to the screening program.

The *a priori* analysis determines whether or not the program should be implemented, indicates design modifications, and outlines a subsequent evaluation strategy. In the design context, it is useful to consider that one can select from among a number of screening alternatives, and that the problem in relation to cancer control is to select a screening option that best meets the constraints of a limited budget.[1] An analysis of a program must consider the characteristics (error rates) of the screening test; the population to which the test will be applied; the conditions for applying the test to the population (timing, location); the personnel who will administer the test; special characteristics of the test, including side effects; and treatment strategy and efficacy as indexed by, or predicated on, the results of the test. All of these factors enter into the determination of the marginal effectiveness of screening compared with, for example, no screening at all. In designing the screening program, it is critical to state its design (and evaluation) objectives clearly, because these objectives provide a focus and measurable endpoint for the effects of the program.

The *a posteriori* evaluation affects program operation and management, as well as the design and implementation of further screening programs related to the same problems. In addition, these evaluations show the expected gains from refinements of the tests involved, refinements which include the reduction of both false positives and false negatives.

In designing and evaluating a screening program, the use of mathematical models can be extremely valuable. It is in the mathematical model that the knowledge of the cancer site, the screening program, and the characteristics of the test are all brought together to aid in program implementation and decision making. Eddy and Schwartz (1982) differentiate between deep and surface models of cancer screening, meaning observable cancer events and the pathophysiology of the underlying disease, respectively. They discuss the role of mathematical models and the analysis of screening programs, and point out that there are several different strategies for analysis. They illustrate their argument with two different mathematical models that yield very similar results when applied to the analysis of screening policy for breast cancer. Recent analyses

[1]For the NCI research program on screening, decisions concern the choice between several alternative research strategies involving particular methods and technologies of screening and their evaluation in defined populations.

have resulted in recommendations that various long-established screening rates with respect to both breast and cervical cancer be changed. This is largely the result of the judicious use of mathematical models in the evaluation of screening programs.

B. Disease Factors

Traditional prerequisites for screening have been that the disease be common in occurrence and that it cause substantial mortality or morbidity, but no standards exist for interpreting the terms *common* and *substantial* in this context. For example, should the rates for the cancer in question be compared to those for other cancers or other diseases? An additional prerequisite should be data from intervention trials or defined population studies showing that the proposed screening activity is effective in reducing mortality from the cancer in question. Also, the quality of all available evidence should be analyzed to answer questions such as the following: Were the previous studies randomized trials, saturation studies, geographic comparisons, or observations virtually devoid of experimental content? Which outcome variables were used? Were appropriate methods of analysis used? Was more than one study done, so that confirmatory evidence exists? Were the populations and health delivery systems sufficiently similar to those being considered, so that acceptance, compliance, follow-up, and benefits can be assumed to be comparable? For a discussion of some of these evaluation issues see Cole and Morrison (1980), Prorok *et al.* (1981), and Prorok (1983).

C. Selecting the Population

The conventional wisdom for selecting the population to be screened is that it should be one in which the disease or the phase of the disease detectable by screening has a high prevalence. Screening such a population results in a higher predictive value for the test, fewer false positives, and a lower cost per case found. The implication is that one should concentrate on high-risk groups, provided all other prerequisites of screening are met. Is such an approach practical and successful? How does one identify high-risk populations for screening? The use of epidemiologic risk factors to select groups is an obvious approach. Several examples have been reported for breast cancer screening. In the context of the HIP study, five risk factors were considered: menarche before age 15, first pregnancy after age 29, fewer than three pregnancies, prior breast conditions, and one or more sisters with breast cancer (Shapiro *et al.*, 1974). The results of the study were that, even for women with three or more risk factors, only 33% of breast cancer cases were accounted for. Farewell (1977) used the risk factors of age at menarche, family history, age at first birth, and eticholandone excretion. That study found 82% of the cancers to be concentrated in 55% of the population, or 47% of the cancers in 17% of the population, and concluded that such a high-risk definition was unlikely to be of practical value. Similar conclusions were reached by Soini and Hakama (1978), who examined 20 potential risk variables, and by de Waard *et al.* (1978), who identified 63% of cancers as being concentrated in 37% of the population but felt obligated to examine the remainder of the population, which had 37% of the cancers.

The risk factors for cervical cancer screening may be more straightforward: women who have never had sexual intercourse or who are without a cervix are not at risk, whereas sexually active women are at risk. A detailed discussion of this subject based on a Canadian study appears in the Walton Report (Task Force, 1976), with some refinement given in the report of the reconvened (Task Force, 1982). Despite this analysis, however, one must ask in each instance if the criteria for risk do indeed identify a large enough concentration of the cases in a small enough population to accomplish the cost reductions being sought.

That selective screening may not be applicable in all settings is illustrated by an analysis of data from Finland (Hakama *et al.*, 1979). Fourteen risk indicators associated with fertility, signs and symptoms, other diseases, and other factors were examined both singly and in combination. The best discrimination was achieved by classifying approximately 40% of the cases into about 10% of the population. Other calculations showed that for selective screening to be effective, the relative risk of disease in the high-risk versus the low-risk category must be greater than that implied by the known epidemiology of cervical cancer. A suggested alternative approach is to define the risk according to the type of medical service (Greenwald *et al.*, 1974).

Thus, it would appear that further research on risk group definition in screening is needed for cervical cancer as well as for breast cancer and other major cancers. Similar problems exist for less frequently occurring cancers, which have been less extensively investigated. In a relevant analysis for bladder cancer, Morrison (1979) considers problems which can occur in defining high-risk groups for rare cancers which may be occupationally related, and addresses the trade-offs which must be considered between the potential benefit to a small high-risk group versus the reduction in screening benefit which is then suffered by the larger population from which the high-risk group is selected.

Apart from risk, other factors must be considered in selecting a population to be screened. The anticipated level of acceptance is of prime importance and should be assessed, perhaps in a pilot study. Acceptance of screening and compliance with recommendations for dissemination of scientific information; specifically, the level of education and cultural attitudes and practices could render screening programs ineffective. The amount of previous screening in a potential target population should also be considered as an influence on the type of program to introduce or whether to start a program at all. Several authors contend (for example, Greenwald *et al.*, 1974) that for cervical cancer there should be less emphasis on the continued rescreening of affluent women with a history of negative smears and more emphasis on reaching those women who have not been screened at all. In the United States, this might include women in low-income regions, members of certain minority groups, and older women, perhaps 50 and above, who were not reached previously.

D. Implementation of Program Components

Once the population has been selected, the actual program implementation involves numerous components; we discuss five of these in the following section: recruitment, facilities and personnel, quality control, data management, and funding. Reaching and maintaining the operational stage of a program is a large-scale undertaking, and each step should be well planned for the setting involved. Pilot studies for some or all of the components are advisable.

The first component, and an early step in any program, is recruitment of individuals to be screened. For cancer control purposes, one would hope to screen virtually the entire target population, but this can be difficult to achieve. Recruitment is often more difficult and expensive than was first expected, and the need for repeated efforts should be anticipated. In determining the best approach, careful consideration should be given to the age, cultural, economic, educational, and medical care characteristics of the population. Available approaches range from mass communication campaigns on television and radio, sponsored by government or private organizations, to personal contacts through medical care or by private or religious groups.

The second major component is provision and coordination of the necessary physical resources and personnel. Before putting these resources in place or extending existing ones, however, a needs assessment for resources should be made, based on estimates of the response to the invitation to be screened, of compliance by individuals having a positive test with recommendations to seek further diagnostic evaluation, and of compliance by individuals and physicians with recommendations for appropriate therapy. Given these estimates, planners can determine the best mode of offering the screening tests. Possibilities include adding the test to existing medical care facilities such as physician offices and hospitals, establishing special screening centers, using mobile units to reach rural or remote areas, and establishing centers in industrial complexes. Of primary concern is that the test be accessible to the target group. Special arrangements must be considered if daily routines are to be interrupted for screening. These might include locating centers near the most populous areas, providing transportation, arranging for time off from work for employees to attend screening, providing day care for children, and scheduling weekend hours for screening.

The third component, establishing procedures to interpret the test results and to monitor the quality of test administration and interpretation, should precede or coincide with the initiation of screening. A recent Canadian report on cervical cancer screening (Task Force, 1982) reviewed the quality control issue and outlined the reasons for false-negative results: error in documenting or reporting the smear, inadequate or improper sampling of a lesion due to poor technique or difficult location of the lesion; the presence of interfering substances; technical problems in fixing and staining smears; and errors in the actual reading and interpretation of slides. A related problem is the use of proper terminology in classifying and reporting the results of a test, particularly when the screening test is capable of detecting borderline lesions, such as those in the cervix and breast. A policy for classifying and treating all lesions, particularly the borderline variety, should be established at the start of the program.

Data management is the fourth component that warrants attention before and during screening. Whether or not any part of the program is to be used for research purposes, substantial amounts of data will be generated. It is likely to be necessary to develop, test, and use an automated data processing system. The size and sophistication of the system will depend on the setting and anticipated uses, but provision should be made for the possibility of expansion. Provision should also be made to store the data in secure areas with adequate safeguards for confidentiality. This applies not only to paper records on individuals, but also to cytologic and histologic samples on slides and tissue blocks and to blood and urine samples, some of which may have to be stored at low temperatures for long periods of time.

The final component is financial; someone must pay for the screening program. Private groups, industry, insurance companies, and government are all potential sources of funds. Political considerations will be involved, whether as an issue of jurisdiction between government bodies, or one of regulatory requirements between government and industry. Furthermore, a large-scale cancer control screening program is likely to require a substantial commitment of funds for many years. Because government will probably be involved and because government personnel and policies change, some mechanism should be developed to provide continued funding despite changing governmental priorities. Decision making about the continued operation and funding of a screening program can be facilitated by the adoption of a mechanism to monitor the program continuously. The data management system is central to this undertaking. Such monitoring would minimally include updated estimates of the sensitivity, specificity, and predictive value of the tests, quality control procedures, and compliance with testing, diagnostic follow-up, and treatment. In addition, other elements of the program can be examined if appropriate data have been collected according to a protocol. For example, the cost and availability of material and human resources can be monitored in relation to changing population and disease characteristics. Furthermore, the cumulative benefits of the program can be compared to previous results or costs. Such monitoring and data evaluation can be instrumental in justifying to funding sources the continuation, expansion, or termination of the program. The mechanism for such monitoring would have to be individualized to each setting and is an area for research, but it would likely be associated with the data management facility. For example, a tumor registry covering the entire population is desirable, such as those in Finland and Connecticut. A network of provincial registries has been proposed in Canada (Task Force, 1982), which could be adapted for monitoring. If sufficiently automated, such systems could potentially be used for several cancers or diseases simultaneously.

VI. GENERAL CONSIDERATIONS

In the context of cancer control, numerous issues and questions are relevant to the conduct of any mass screening program. In a broad sense, many of the issues focus as much on whether there is a strong commitment to effective screening techniques, logistics, cost effectiveness, and coverage for these costs as on technological ones. This is true for large screening programs in smaller community clinical settings or in the individual physician's office. Many of the questions can be answered in a finite, scientific way; others are more philosophical and must be addressed with the objective of establishing acceptable policies at the outset that are clear to all those conducting or participating in the screening. In all circumstances, there must be a uniform approach that has sufficient latitude to accommodate local variations without compromising the overall policies and protocols. Close monitoring, quality control, and follow-up are required in such programs, especially if they are large-scale and multicentered nationwide.

Not all issues and questions can be completely resolved for each cancer site. When information is lacking or incomplete, or when a consensus cannot be attained, it is likely that some quantitative *judgment* can be made about the adequacy of information as a basis for making tentative decisions about screening. Qualitative and quantitative judgments for each issue can build an "information profile" relative to screening for each cancer site. Such a profile might not only identify information gaps but might also suggest areas of research of high priority that should be pursued. From the information profile developed for each cancer site, an "action threshold" could be assessed to determine if screening is ready for implementation in the public health arena. For example, if morbidity and mortality are known to be reduced by screening for cancer at a given anatomical site, answers to the following questions are critical: (1) Is the screening method sufficiently sensitive, specific, simple, safe, and convenient? (2) Are the costs reasonable? (3) Are personnel easily trained for consistently high quality and repeatable proficiency? Even if the answers to all these questions are not complete, an action threshold may be reached by considering tradeoffs, for example, specificity may be traded for convenience.

REFERENCES

American Cancer Society (1985). Cancer facts and figures.

Andersson, I. (1981). Radiographic screening for breast carcinoma: I. Program and primary findings in 45–69 year old women. *Acta Radiol., Diagn.* **22,** 185–193.

Baker, L. (1982). The breast cancer detection demonstration projects: Five-year summary report. *Ca—Cancer J. Clin.* **32,** 194–225.

Band, P., Feldstein, M., Watson, L., King, G., and Saccomanno, G. (1982). Lung cancer screening programs in Canadian uranium mines. *Recent Results Cancer Res.* **82,** 153–158.

Betkerur, V., Hlaing, V., Baumgartner, G., Rao, R., Rhee, H., and Guinan, P. (1980). Screening tests for detection of bladder cancer. *Urology* **16,** 16–19.

Boyes, D. A. (1981). The value of a Pap smear program and suggestions for its implementation. *Cancer* **48,** 613–621.

Carter, D. (1981). Screening for lung cancer. *Yale J. Biol. Med.* **54,** 381–385.

Catalona, W. J., and Menon, M. (1981). New screening and diagnostic tests for prostate cancer and immunologic assessment. *Urology* **17**(3); Suppl., 61–65.

Chang, J., Nesbit, D. E., Fisher, D. R., Fritz, S. L., Dwyer, S. J., III, Templeton, A. W., Lin, F., and Jewell, W. R. (1982). Computed tomographic mammography using a conventional body scanner. *Am. J. Radiol.* **138,** 553–558.

Cole, P., and Morrison, A. S. (1980). Basic issues in population screening for cancer. *JNCI, J. Natl. Cancer Inst.* **64,** 1263–1272.

Cole-Beuglet, C., Goldberg, B., Kurtz, A. B., Rubin, C. S., Patchefsky, A. S., and Shaber, G. S. (1981). Ultrasound mammography: A comparison with radiographic mammography. *Radiology* **139,** 693–698.

de Waard, F., Rombach, J. J., and Collette, H. J. A. (1978). The DOM-project for the early diagnosis of breast cancer in the city of Utrecht, the Netherlands. *In* "Screening in Cancer" (A. B. Miller, ed.), UICC Tech. Rep. Ser. Vol. 40, pp. 183–200. Int. Union Against Cancer, Geneva.

Doll, R., Chairman (1981). Working group on early detection of breast cancer, trial of early detection of breast cancer: Description of method. *Br. J. Cancer* **44,** 618–627.

Eddy, D. M., and Schwartz, M. (1982). Mathematical models in screening. *In* "Cancer Epidemiology and Prevention" (D. Schottenfeld and J. Fraumeni, Jr., eds.), pp. 1075–1090. Saunders, Philadelphia, Pennsylvania.

Farewell, V. T. (1977). The combined effect of breast cancer risk factors. *Cancer* **40,** 931–936.

Gilbertsen, V. A., McHugh, R., Schuman, L., and Williams, S. E. (1980). The earlier detection of colorectal cancers: A preliminary report of the results of the occult blood study. *Cancer* **45,** 2899–2901.

Greenwald, P., Feck, G. C., Nasca, P. C., and Polan, A. K. (1974). Epidemiologic basis of regional cancer detection program. *Cancer* **33,** 1732–1736.

Hakama, M., Pukkala, E., and Saastamoinen, P. (1979). Selective screening: Theory and practice based on high-risk groups of cervical cancer. *J. Epidemiol. Commun. Health* **33,** 257–261.

Horm, J., Asire, A. J., Young, J. L., Jr., and Pollack, E., eds. (1984). SEER Program: Cancer incidence and mortality in the United States, 1973–81. NIH Publication No. 85-1837, rev. ed. National Cancer Institute, Bethesda, Maryland.

Kotin, P., and Paul, W. (1982). Results of a lung cancer detection program in an asbestos industry. *Recent Results Cancer Res.* **82,** 131–137.

Levin, M. L., Tockman, M. S., Frost, J. K., and Ball, W. C., Jr. (1982). Lung cancer mortality in males screened by chest X-ray and cytologic sputum examination: A preliminary report. *Recent Results Cancer Res.* **82,** 138–146.

Lundgren, B., and Helleberg, A. (1982). Single oblique-view mammography for periodic screening for breast cancer in women. *JNCI, J. Natl. Cancer Inst.* **68,** 351–355.

Mallard, J. (1981). Silvanus Thompson Memorial Lecture. *Br. J. Radiol.* **54,** 831–849.

Martini, N. (1982). Results of the Memorial Sloan-Kettering lung project. *Recent Results Cancer Res.* **82,** 174–178.

Miller, A. B., ed. (1978). "Screening in Cancer," UICC Tech. Rep. Ser., Vol. 40. Int. Union Against Cancer, Geneva.

Miller, A. B. (1982). Fundamental issues in screening. *In* "Cancer Epidemiology and Prevention" (D. Schottenfeld and J. Fraumeni, Jr., eds.), pp. 1064–1074. Saunders, Philadelphia, Pennsylvania.

Morrison, A. S. (1979). Public health value of using epidemiologic information to identify high-risk groups for bladder cancer screening. *Semin. Oncol.* **6,** 184–188.

Navarre, G. L. (1982). Screening with colposcopy in a prepaid health center. *J. Reprod. Med.* **27,** 98–100.

Nemoto, R., Kato, T., Harada, M., Shibata, K., and Kano, M. (1982). Mass screening for urinary tract cancer with urine cytology. *J. Cancer Res. Clin. Oncol.* **104,** 155–159.

Noguchi, M., Nakanishi, M., and Kato, K. (1982). Appraisal of a newly developed self-collection device for obtaining cervical specimens. *Acta Cytol.* **26,** 633–635.

Nyirjesy, I. (1982). Breast thermography. *Clin. Obstet. Gynecol.* **25,** 401–408.

Prorok, P. C. (1984). Evaluation of screening programs for the early detection of cancer. *In* "Statistical Methods for Cancer Studies" (R. G. Cornell, ed.), pp. 267–328. Dekker, New York.

Prorok, P. C., Hankey, B. F., and Bundy, B. W. (1981). Concepts and problems in the evaluation of screening programs. *J. Chronic Dis.* **34,** 159–171.

Ross, R. J., Thompson, J. S., Kim, K., and Bailey, R. A. (1982). Nuclear magnetic resonance imaging and evaluation of human breast tissue: Preliminary clinical trials. *Radiology* **143,** 195–205.

Sanderson, D., and Fontana, R. (1982). Results of the Mayo Lung Project: An interim report. *Recent Results Cancer Res.* **82,** 179–186.

Schneider, A. B., Pinsky, S., Bekerman, C., and Ryo, U. (1980). Characteristics of 108 thyroid cancers detected by screening in a population with a history of head and neck irradiation. *Cancer* **46,** 1218–1227.

Shapiro, S., Goldberg, J., Venet, L., and Strax, P. (1974). Risk factors in breast cancer—a prospective study. *In* "Host Environment Interactions in the Etiology of Cancer in Man," (R. Doll and I. Vodopija, eds.). IARC Sci. Publ. No. 7, pp. 169–182. Int. Agency Res. Cancer, Lyon.

Shapiro, S., Venet, W., Strax, P., Venet, L., and Roeser, R. (1982a). Ten-to-fourteen-year effect of screening on breast cancer mortality. *JNCI, J. Natl. Cancer Inst.* **69,** 349–355.

Shapiro, S., Venet, W., Strax, P., Venet, L., and Roeser, R. (1982b). (R. Doll and I. Vodopija, eds.). Prospects for eliminating racial differences in breast cancer survival rates. *Am. J. Public Health* **72,** 1142–1145.

Sherlock, P., Lipkin, M., and Winawer, S. J. (1980). The prevention of colon cancer. *Am. J. Med.* **68,** 917–931.

Shimaoka, K., Bakri, K., Sciascia, M., Razack, M., Rao, U., Mettlin, C., Shedd, D., Gajera, R., and Walsh, D. (1982). Thyroid screening program follow-up evaluation. *N.Y. State J. Med.* **82** (8), 1184–1187.

Soini, I., and Hakama, M. (1978). Failure of selective screening for breast cancer by combining risk factors. *Int. J. Cancer* **22,** 275–281.

Tabar, L., and Gad, A. (1981). Screening for breast cancer: The Swedish trial. *Radiology* **38,** 219–222.

Task Force (1976). Cervical cancer screening programs. *Can. Med. Assoc. J.* **114,** 1003–1033.

Task Force (1982). Reconvened task force on cervical cancer screening programs; cervical cancer screening programs. *Can. Med. Assoc. J.* **127,** 581.

Winawer, S. J., and Sherlock, P. (1982). Surveillance for colorectal cancer in average-risk patients, familial high-risk groups, and patients with adenomas. *Cancer* **50,** 2609–2614.

Winawer, S. J., Andrews, M., Flehinger, B., Sherlock, P., Schottenfeld, D., and Miller, D. G. (1980). Progress report on a controlled trial of fecal occult blood testing for the detection of colorectal neoplasia. *Cancer* **45,** 2959–2964.

Winawer, S. J., Fleisher, M., Baldwin, M., and Sherlock, P. (1982). Current status of fecal occult blood testing in screening for colorectal cancer. *Ca—Cancer J. Clin.* **32,** 100–112.

3

Economic Aspects of Screening

DUNCAN NEUHAUSER

I.	Introduction	49
II.	The Benefits of Screening	50
III.	Benefits Now and Later	51
IV.	Externalities and Equity	52
V.	Societal Costs versus Charges	53
VI.	Average versus Marginal Costs and Benefits	53
VII.	Application of Such Models in Practice	55
VIII.	Conclusion	56
IX.	Bibliographic Sources	56
	References	57

I. INTRODUCTION

Is cancer screening worth it?

This simple question has a simple answer: maybe.

A precise answer requires us to use the theories and techniques from medicine, economics, statistics, research design, clinical decision analysis, clinical epidemiology, utility analysis, an understanding of the organization of medical care, cost benefit and cost effectiveness analysis, discounting, the ethical study of society-based values, mathematical modeling, and computer programming.

These topics, at best, and if considered at all, are squeezed into an already crowded medical school curriculum. The number of people who are comfortable with all of these disciplines are perhaps a few dozen worldwide, and that's being very generous.

My assignment is, in these few short pages, to summarize these ideas accurately, clearly, and crisply.

Being "worth it" implies that there is an effort required (called *cost*) and something to be gained (called *benefit*).

ISBN 0-12-496720-5

II. THE BENEFITS OF SCREENING

The first question is: Does screening for cancer result in improved health? Knowing the scientific method is essential, but is also a hinderance to answering this question. According to this method, we never know for certain. We test a null hypothesis and accumulate evidence, but never ultimately prove it.

Evaluation of benefit requires a restatement of the always unproven hypothesis in probablistic terms. Consider this statement: "There is an 80% probability that screening for colon cancer results in prolongation of life and a 20% probability that it does not provide any prolongation of life." Absolute certainty that screening prolongs life would be given a 100% probability here. This is never the case. A zero probability would define the certainty of no benefit. Such probability statements are useful because they can be multiplied by the expected benefit and thereby lower this benefit by the magnitude of our doubt about efficacy.

For example, if the cost per year of life saved by Pap smear screening every 3 years is $600, assuming it works, but if we are only 80% sure that it is effective, then the adjusted cost per year of life saved is $750, which is still a medical care bargain (see Eddy, 1980, p. 260).

Such probability estimates of assurance of benefit are required when a decision must be made to spend more on screening one disease versus another.

Such probability estimates can be derived from the following information:

1. The unsubstantiated opinion
2. The uncontrolled observational study
3. A comparative study
4. A randomized clinical trial

Colon cancer screening has not been subjected to a randomized trial. At least two such trials are underway, but it will be several years before their results are published. While we await these results, what should we do? Add our cumulative experience and transform it into a probabilistic consensus. Everyone who reads the literature on the efficacy of Pap smear screening will derive a different probabilistic estimate.

One attempt to do this is the Report of the Canadian Task Force on the Periodic Health Examination (Task Force, 1979). Screening efforts with clear documentation of efficacy based on well-conducted, randomized clinical trials were given an A rating. Without this kind of evidence, B and C ratings were given. Only A-rated screening programs were endorsed.

"What is the magnitude of benefit?" can be viewed as a separate question.

Medical care benefits can be divided into those that produce changes in the quantity and quality of life.

Most of the evaluative literature is content to demonstrate a statistically significant difference in survival without defining the magnitude of the benefit. If 1000 women with an average age of 45 are screened for breast cancer, how many years of life are "saved"?

A year of life can vary in its quality, and these differences in quality need to be considered, hence the term *quality-adjusted year of life saved (QAYLS).*

Many medical choices are made which, on average, increase the quantity of life but reduce its quality. Life with a radical mastectomy may be longer, but of lower quality compared to life with a lumpectomy. Conversely, other medical choices risk a shorter life in order to improve its quality. Some types of plastic surgery and elective hernia surgery in the elderly are examples.

McNeil *et al.* (1978) show that some patients with lung cancer prefer different treatment depending on how they weigh quantity and quality of life.

Utility analysis is a way of rating patient preferences, usually on a scale of 0 to 1. These scales are best applied to the quality dimension. The worst outcome under consideration is given a 0 value and the best outcome a 1. Other outcomes are given an intermediate value. Such indices can then be used to weigh a year of life saved.

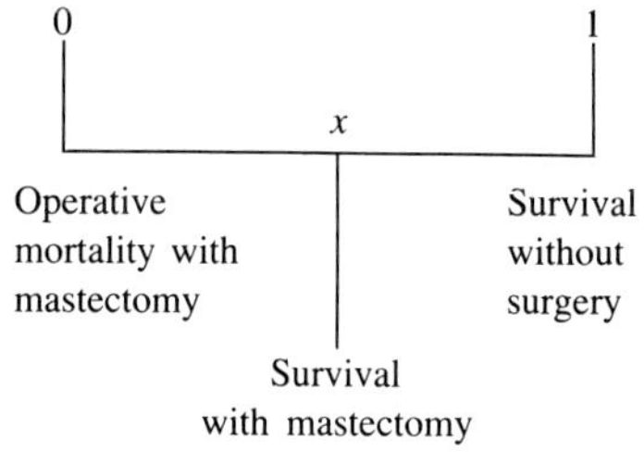

III. BENEFITS NOW AND LATER

The benefits of screening occur later in life. We prefer our benefits and rewards today rather than tomorrow. Taking this preference for the present into account requires *discounting* future benefits into a *present value.*

When it comes to money, the competitive marketplace forces bankers to use a similar discount rate for the money they borrow and lend. Patient preferences can be more idiosyncratic unless society or the government imposes a uniform discount rate. Our society imposes schooling requirements (often something that children would avoid if they could) in order to achieve a minimum level of competence in the future. Imposing a societal discount rate is almost required for a government-supported screening program. When the British National Health Service changed its policy from supporting Pap smear screening once every 3 years to once every 5 years, it implicitly assumed uniform preferences for all clients. However, individuals do choose differently.

IV. EXTERNALITIES AND EQUITY

The classic example of a decision that affects others is the screening and treatment of infectious disease. Your failure to seek vaccination increases my risk of getting the disease. Under such *externalities,* simply weighing your costs and benefits will not necessarily produce a decision acceptable to society. This is a minor problem in cancer screening. However, the equity issue may be more important. To invest in screening for breast cancer rather than lung cancer is almost certainly preferable. Such a decision benefits one group of patients at the possible expense of another. When these groups are disproportionately weighted with men or women, young or old, poor or rich, one ethnic or racial group rather than another, equity issues may become major. For example, it is more cost effective to screen for hypertension among black Americans than other Americans. Ethical, political, and cultural concerns then come to the fore, as do concerns about the relationship of the independent individual and the collective society. Cost-benefit studies are not ethically, culturally, or politically neutral. It is always important to be aware of the often hidden assumptions behind them. One sign of a good cost-benefit study is that these issues are made explicit.

For example, most North American studies assume that a year of life saved is of uniform value, whether that year be for a man or a woman, a year early or late in life, the year of a banker or of a petty thief. When a number of North American researchers went to a Third World country, they were told that the years of an engineer's life are more valuable than the years of life of a peasant farmer, and if their analysis did not take this into account, it would be unacceptable.

Costs are not simply the money spent for screening, follow-up testing, and treatment. They also include the time, trouble, and inconvenience for the patient. The studies should also take into account other changes in the costs of care. Avoiding death by cancer may lead to a more or less expensive death by heart disease.

The *direct* dollar cost of obtaining a Pap smear may be small for some patients compared to the time and inconvenience of this procedure. This is probably the major reason that many women "vote with their feet" and do not return for a lifetime of periodic tests.

Whose costs? the existence of health insurance or a national health service means that the full costs of care are not borne by the patients. Third-party payment exists for just this reason. This vastly complicates the problem. It almost guarantees that the payer's decision will be different from the patient's.

The usual approach to these analyses involves a consideration of societal costs, which are again different. It presumes to measure the resources consumed and to evaluate them in terms of the next best use of these resources thereby foregone. These are called *opportunity costs.* The logic behind this approach is related to the core concepts of microeconomics and is a large topic in itself.

V. SOCIETAL COSTS VERSUS CHARGES

In the United States, the money that a hospital charges may have very little bearing on the actual costs of providing the care. In national health services, as in those of England or Sweden, there is little interest in calculating the costs for particular patients or types of patients within the hospital.

Risks are the dangers associated with treatment. Operations may have mortality; mammography and other X ray procedures yield the hazards of X ray exposure.

The risks of small-dose radiation exposure can be estimated only by extrapolation from large-dose risks. The conservative approach, which uses a linear extrapolation and thereby implies some risk at all levels, appears to be widely accepted. One implication is that the population screened by mammography must have a sufficiently high yield of cancers to offset these risks. Nuclear magnetic resonance (NMR) examination may be equally accurate and avoid radiation exposure. However, they are more expensive than mammography, and the probability is not zero that other risks, now unknown, may be found to be associated with NMR.

In the analysis, risks can either be deducted from the benefit side or added to the cost side, but they must be included.

There are two ways of putting the costs and benefits together. Cost effectiveness equates the costs (usually measured in dollars) with the nondollar units of benefit (years of life saved, QALYS, discounted present values QALYS).

However, a cost per year of life saved ratio does not tell us whether this amount is excessive or acceptable. When costs begin to exceed $20,000 per year of life saved, as in the $2 billion renal dialysis program in the United States, government officials begin to grumble publicly. When the costs per year of life saved are below $10,000, the intervention is usually applauded.

In order to avoid this cutoff problem, the benefits can also be transformed into dollars. Then, with all of the relevent information transformed into dollars, the decision to proceed simply depends on whether the benefits exceed the costs. However, this requires us to turn years of life saved into dollar values. Economists like to equate a human life with its productive contribution, as reflected in a person's income expressed in present-value dollars. Because the elderly, on average, don't earn much, they are little valued by this method. Because of these problems, most medical analyses are presented as cost effectiveness studies.

VI. AVERAGE VERSUS MARGINAL COSTS AND BENEFITS

If a Pap smear is cost effective, why not urge its use every 3 years, every year, twice a year, three times a year? As the time period between screens diminishes, the costs rise almost linearly; further, the yield in detectable cancers diminishes sharply after the first screen, which detects prevalent cases, and later screens, which detect some false negatives and new incident cases. Combining rising costs and declining yields means that the *marginal* cost per case found or the cost per year of life saved rises exponentially. Thus, a Pap smear every 3 years may be very cost effective, but the added or marginal cost per case found when advocating a yearly Pap smear compared with every 3 years may be very large indeed.

Cancer screening decisions require consideration of a large number of variables in combination.

Consider colon cancer. Relevant variables include the prior probability that the patient has colon cancer. This, in turn, is a function of age, family history, other conditions, symptoms, and the prior screening history—the combination of screening tests used, one or multiple occult blood tests, with and without dietary control, straight or flexible sigmoidoscopy, barium enema with or without air contrast, and colonoscopy. Each of these tests has errors (false positives, false negatives), costs, and risks.

What is the effect of early detection on avoiding death? This is a probabilistic function of cancer size. How sure are we that the presumed benefits are not simply lead time bias? What are the costs and risks of treatment? What is the doubling time of colon cancer growth? Does this vary with patient characteristics? What is the expected magnitude of the benefit in quality-adjusted years of life saved discounted to present value? How sure are we that the benefits are real? How are this particular patient's preferences weighed (desire to avoid sigmoidoscopy, fear of cancer, discount rate)? The costs of screening for the patient include travel time and treatment costs, delay and waiting time, and the unpleasantness of the procedure.

There is simply no way that the unaided human mind can weigh all of these variables simultaneously. This requires the use of computer-based decision models which can vary any of these dimensions to match a particular patient. By running such models over and over, systematically changing one variable at a time and observing the effect, if any, on the outcome, one can see which of these variables make a difference. This procedure is called *sensitivity analysis.* The best of these computer-based models for screening are *time-varying Markov models,* which start with a hypothetical 10,000 or so patients and "move" them yearly from one state to another; from unscreened to screened, with cancer, without cancer, rescreened, alive, and ultimately dead. The transitions between one state and another are defined probabilistically based on the kinds of variables listed above. The model is run year by year until all 10,000 patients have died, and a score is kept of the costs and years of life saved. Then the model is rerun using different assumptions, including no screening, and the results are compared.

Such models are only as good as the data applied to them. New data are constantly appearing, and the models must be constantly updated. The models can be run on the hypothetical average patient or modified to fit the individual patient.

VII. APPLICATION OF SUCH MODELS IN PRACTICE

The current approach has been to summarize the key elements of the model into simple decision rules. This was done by the American Cancer Society (ACS) in its revised guidelines of 1980. They concluded that Pap smear screening every 3 years was appropriate. This conclusion was based on a marginal analysis which showed that the added benefits and costs associated with moving from screening every 3 years to every year were about $80,000 per year of life saved.

The ACS was appropriately careful to say that this general decision should not be universal and dogmatic, but should be modified based on the physician's judgment.

Reporting such generalized rules is only a start. The next step is to promote the intelligent discussion of such models among a widening circle of physicians concerned with cancer screening. This procedure has started, but it too is inadequate. The model developed by Eddy (1980) and used by the ACS can be run on a standard 128K home computer. In principle, it could be as easily accessible as your children's PacMan program on a small floppy disk, and as widely distributed.

Such programs could be made easy to use (the jargon term here is *user friendly*), allowing the medical student or physician to run the model, varying the assumptions and observing the results. Only rarely would a physician wish to run such a computer model with a patient present, this being a time-consuming process. The advantage of having the program available is in improved understanding.

Ultimately, such programs could be placed in science museums, high school classes, pharmacies, and doctors' waiting rooms. The PacMan generation is very comfortable with such programs, and they could be an excellent educational device for people with a tenth-grade education or more.

There are now and will continue to be different models for cancer screening. Their relative merits will be an ongoing source of debate and research. These models are only as good as the data they use. However, they can be guides to needed clinical research by pointing out the variables that are critical to the analysis. (This is another use of sensitivity analysis.) Not only do such models point to the need for better data, they also indicate the importance of unique and differing patient preferences.

One can listen to medical education classes day after day without hearing any reference to patient desires that could change a decision. Even if, for most people and for society as a whole, Pap smear screening every 3 years is a reasonable standard, there must be some informed women who would choose an examination yearly or every 5 years. They could have read and understood all of this literature. They could weigh the costs and benefits differently and choose differently. As a surprising consequence, this kind of mathematical clinical decision making may help make medicine more humanistic in its concern for patient preferences.

VIII. CONCLUSION

As a reader, you now realize that I have described a process to approach the evaluation of cancer screening without making a single specific clinical recommendation. My concern is for process now; content will follow. As I have tried to explain, written summaries of screening decision rules are inadequate and well on their way to being obsolete. The ACS report (American Cancer Society, 1980) and the Canadian Task Force Report (1979) are the best of these inadequate summaries, and I refuse to compound this problem here by providing any summary decision rule in writing. The correct presentation of these decision rules will be through interactive computer-based decision models using the methods outlined above and widely accessible through microcomputers. These are within a year or two of being available, and I anxiously await their appearance.

IX. BIBLIOGRAPHIC SOURCES

Assuming a familiarity with basic texts in biostatistics, clinical epidemiology, research methods, and microeconomics, good general introductions include Wilson and Grouch (1982), Warner and Luce (1982), Bunker *et al.* (1977), and Weinstein *et al.* (1980). The long and continuing Office of Technology Assessment series on cost effectiveness and evaluation (1978, 1980) is essential for tracking current work.

The Walton Report (Task Force, 1976), Canadian Task Force (1979), American Cancer Society (1980), and National Institute of Health Consensus reports (e.g., 1979) are the best of the current written decision rules.

For a discussion of quantity versus quality of Life, see McNeil *et al.* (1978). Two elaborate models for cancer screening are presented by Gohagan and Rodes (1982), and Eddy (1980); see also Schweitzer and Luce (1979) and Thompson and Jacobi (c. 1979). The Eddy model was the basis for the ACS 1980 decisions. Reading Eddy requires a knowledge of all of the disciplines listed at the start of this chapter. Another application of the time-varying Markov model in medicine is given by Ransohoff *et al.* (1983). Researchers working in this area tend to belong to the Society for Clinical Decision Making. The society's quarterly journal is *Medical Decision Making*.

The only available medical decision model for a micro (home) computer is that of Littenberg and Smyth-Staruch (1982). Available for $10, this program is appropriate for Apple computers. It gives two examples of the potential of such interactive microcomputer-based medical decision models (pharyngitis and hernia surgery). I am told that an accessible microcomputer-based model for breast cancer screening is nearing completion.

REFERENCES

American Cancer Society (1980). Guidelines for the cancer-related checkup: Recommendations and rationale. *Ca—Cancer J. Clin.* **30**(4), 194–240.

Bunker, J., Barnes, B., and Mosteller, F. (1977). "Costs, Risks and Benefits of Surgery." Oxford Univ. Press, London and New York.

Eddy, D. M. (1980). "Screening for Cancer: Theory Analysis and Design." Prentice-Hall, Englewood Cliffs, New Jersey.

Gohagan, J. K., and Rodes, N. D. (1982). "Early Detection of Breast Cancer: Risk, Detection Protocols, and Therapeutic Implications." Praeger, New York.

Littenberg, B., and Smyth-Staruch, K. (1982). "Sensitivity Analysis Model." Biomatrix, Cleveland, Ohio.

McNeil, B. J., Weichselbaum, R., and Pauker, S. (1978). Fallacy of the five-year survival in lung cancer. *N. Engl. J. Med.* **299**(35), 1397–1401.

National Institute of Health (1979). "Screening and Early Detection of Colorectal Cancer," Consensus Dev. Conf. Proc. NIH, Washington, D.C.

National Institute of Health (1980). "Cervical Cancer Screening: The Pap Smear," Consensus Dev. Conf. Summ., Vol. 3, No. 4. NIH, Washington, D.C.

Office of Technology Assessment, U.S. Congress (1978). "Assessing the Efficacy and Safety of Medical Technologies." U.S. Govt. Printing Office, Washington, D.C.

Office of Technology Assessment, U.S. Congress (1980). "The Implications of Cost-Effectiveness Analysis of Medical Technology." August 1980. U.S. Govt. Printing Office, Washington, D.C.

Ransohoff, D., Gracie, W., Wolfenson, L., and Neuhauser, D. (1983). Prophylactic cholecystectomy or expectant management for silent gallstones. *Ann. Intern. Med.* **99,** 199–204.

Schweitzer, S. O., and Luce, B. R. (1979). "A Cost-Effective Approach to Cervical Cancer Detection," Natl. Cent. Health Serv. Res. U.S. Dept. of Health, Education and Welfare, Washington, D.C.

Task Force (1976). Cervical cancer screening programs. *Can. Med. Assoc. J.* **114,** 1003–1033.

Task Force (1979). Report of the Canadian Task Force on the periodic health examination. *Can. Med. Assoc. J.* **121,** 1193–1254.

Thompson, D. E., and Jacobi, L. W. (circa 1979). "Analysis of Screening Strategies for Colorectal Cancer: An Extension of the Model," Part IV. Michigan Cancer Found., Detroit.

Walton, R. J. (1976). Cervical cancer screening programs. *Can. Med. Assoc. J.* **114,** 1003–1033.

Warner, K. E., and Luce, B. R. (1982). "Cost-Benefit and Cost-Effectiveness Analysis in Health Care. Principles, Practice and Potential." Health Administration Press, Ann Arbor, Michigan (23 C/E, C/B studies up to 1980 related to cancer screening are listed, p. 236).

Weinstein, M., Fineberg, H., Elstein, A., Frazier, H., Neuhauser, D., Neutra, R., and McNeil, B. (1980). "Clinical Decision Analysis." Saunders, Philadelphia, Pennsylvania.

Wilson, R., and Crouch, E. (1982). "Risk/Benefit Analysis." Ballinger, Cambridge, Massachusetts.

4

The Problem of Identification of High-Risk Subjects for Selective Screening

MATTI HAKAMA

I.	Introduction	59
II.	Success Measures	59
III.	Selective Screening and Validity	61
IV.	Effect of Selective Screening in Quantitative Terms	61
V.	Attempts to Combine Risk Factors	63
VI.	Prospects for Selective Screening	65
	References	66

I. INTRODUCTION

Selective screening in a community means applying the screening test to only a subpopulation in that community. The criteria for selection are based on high risk of the disease among those subjected to screening. The purpose of screening high-risk groups only is to reduce the resources required for the program or, sometimes, to reduce the number of those at risk to the adverse effects of the screening test. A selective screening program should detect a substantial proportion of the total number of cancer cases in the entire target population, i.e., only a few cancer cases are assumed to originate in the low-risk groups not subjected to such selective screening.

II. SUCCESS MEASURES

The basic measures of validity for a screening test are sensitivity and specificity. Sensitivity is estimated as the proportion of persons with positive tests among

ISBN 0-12-496720-5

persons with the disease subjected to screening. Specificity is the proportion of persons with negative tests among persons free from the disease. Therefore, sensitivity is the indicator of the yield, and specificity is the indicator of the cost of the screening.

Selective screening cannot be performed without defining the target population from which the high-risk group will be selected. For a successful screening program, performance of the test alone is clearly not sufficient. There are other problems, e.g., in attending the program and in the referral system for the test positives required to confirm the test result.

It is, therefore, useful to define the sensitivity and specificity not only of the test, but of the program as well. Program sensitivity is estimated as the proportion of persons diagnosed as having the disease as a result of screening among all of the persons with the disease in the target population. Program specificity is the proportion of persons not diagnosed as having the disease in the disease-free part of the target population. Not diagnosing the cancer is due either to a negative test or a failure to apply the test, i.e., the person was not screened at all, or the person with a positive test did not have diagnostic confirmation of the test result. A valid test is a prerequisite for a successful program, but the program may fail even if the test is valid. There may be substantial differences in test sensitivity and program sensitivity, on the one hand, and in test specificity and program specificity, on the other.

TABLE I

Sensitivity and Specificity of the Test and the Program

			Diagnostic confirmation	
Attendance	Screening test	Appearing for confirmation	Cancer	Healthy
Yes	Positive	Yes	a	b
Yes	Positive	No	c	d
Yes	Negative	Yes	e	f
Yes	Negative	No	g	h
No	—	Yes	i	j
No	—	—	k	l

$$\text{Test sensitivity} = \frac{a + c}{a + c + e + g} = \frac{a + c}{M_1}$$

$$\text{Program sensitivity} = \frac{a + e + i}{a + c + e + g + i + k} = \frac{a + e + i}{N_1}$$

$$\text{Test specificity} = \frac{f + h}{b + d + f + h} = \frac{f + h}{M_0}$$

$$\text{Program specificity} = \frac{d + h + l}{b + d + f + h + j + l} = \frac{d + h + l}{N_0}$$

Table I illustrates the differences in test and program measures. Screenees who have a positive screening test are referred for confirmation of the result, and all screenees are classified either as having the cancer, denoted by (a), or healthy (b). Sometimes the confirmation process fails, due to problems in the referral system or in the compliance of the screenee. Such failures, denoted by (c) and (d), have no effect on test validity but do have an effect on program validity.

A screening program may identify as positive some cases with a negative test, (e) and (f). The program may take into account other aspects of the individual, such as anamnestic history, clinical examination, and other information in addition to the result of the screening test. Such information has no effect on test validity, but it may increase program sensitivity and reduce program specificity. Even nonattendance for screening at the stage of having the test may have alternative consequences on program validity. Some of those not attending may seek diagnosis elsewhere in the health care system. However, this decision may be due to the activities of the screening program. For instance, some screenees invited to attend the mass screening program may prefer private services and decide to attend them instead of the program for testing.

III. SELECTIVE SCREENING AND VALIDITY

Selective screening has an effect on program validity only. Table II shows an artificial example. One-third of a population of 3000 belongs to a high-risk group with a relative risk of 10. The screening test has a 90% sensitivity and specificity, and the risk of disease in the low-risk group is 1%. The figures in the table result from these assumptions. The sensitivity and specificity of the test are the same: 90% in the high-risk group, in the low-risk group, and in the total population. Program validity will change if selective screening of the high-risk group only is assumed. Program sensitivity will decrease to 75%, and program specificity will increase to 97%. Because sensitivity is the indicator of yield and specificity that of cost, in terms of money or adverse effects, selective screening results in decreased costs, but with a lower yield. In principle, the same would be true if only the low-risk group were screened; program specificity would still be more than 90%, but program sensitivity (and therefore yield) would fall to 15%.

IV. EFFECT OF SELECTIVE SCREENING IN QUANTITATIVE TERMS

The purpose of selective screening is to reduce the cost of the program. Because this inevitably involves a loss in program sensitivity, there is a need to establish a balance between the cost and the yield. No overall optimum exists,

TABLE II

Sensitivity and Specificity of the Test and the Program: Example for Selective Screening

Risk group	Screening test	Diagnostic confirmation: Cancer	Diagnostic confirmation: Healthy	Total
High risk	Positive	90	90	180
	Negative	10	810	820
	Total	100	900	1000
Low risk	Positive	18	198	216
	Negative	2	1782	1784
	Total	20	1980	2000
All	Positive	108	288	396
	Negative	12	2592	2604
	Total	120	2880	3000

High-risk group attending the program	
Test sensitivity	= 90%
Test specificity	= 90%
Program sensitivity	= 75%
Program specificity	= 97%
Low-risk group attending the program	
Test sensitivity	= 90%
Test specificity	= 90%
Program sensitivity	= 15%
Program specificity	= 93%
Total	
Sensitivity	= 90%
Specificity	= 90%

even in principle, but it is useful to find the general relationship between program sensitivity and specificity.

In Table III (based on Hakama *et al.*, 1979), the cost is given in terms of the size of the high-risk group to be screened as a percentage of the total population. The proportion of cases of disease in the high-risk group in the total number of cases in the population is the upper limit of program sensitivity. It depends strongly on the risk of disease in the high-risk group compared to the risk in the low-risk group (relative risk). For example, in order to detect 90% of the cases in a high-risk group comprising 10% of the total population, the risk in the high-risk should be almost 100 times that in the low-risk population.

Very few such strong risk factors are presently known for cancers. The most successful attempts to apply selective screening have been based on a combination of several risk factors at the same time.

TABLE III

Proportion of Total Cases Diagnosed from the High-Risk Group by Size of the Group and Relative Risk (High Risk versus Low Risk)

Size of high-risk group (percentage of total population)	Relative risk					
	2	5	10	20	50	100
1	0.02	0.05	0.09	0.17	0.34	0.50
5	0.10	0.21	0.26	0.51	0.72	0.84
10	0.18	0.36	0.53	0.69	0.88	0.92
20	0.33	0.56	0.71	0.83	0.93	0.96
50	0.67	0.83	0.91	0.95	0.98	0.99
70	0.82	0.92	0.96	0.98	0.99	1.00
90	0.95	0.98	0.99	0.99	1.00	1.00

Some screening programs have failed due to low attendance rates and self-selection of attenders by risk of disease (Foltz and Kelsey, 1980). The figures in Table 3 can also be used to indicate the proportion of cancer cases escaping the screening program, given the proportion of nonattenders (equals the size of the high-risk group) and the degree of self-selection (equals the relative risk). For example, 33% (100 − 67) of the cases will be found if 50% of the population attends and those attending have a risk of cancer that is one-half of those not attending. Thus, the assumed 100% test sensitivity was reduced to 33% program sensitivity. The outcome measure for evaluating the effect of a screening program is the mortality of the disease in the target population. If every second death from cancer could be prevented due to advancement of diagnosis by the screening program, then the effectiveness of the program would be 17 (33/2)%, which might be difficult to detect in the presence of random and potentially confounding effects. Therefore, even if selective screening does not seem to have immediate applicability, the failure of some screening programs is likely to be due to self-selective screening.

V. ATTEMPTS TO COMBINE RISK FACTORS

Apart from the obvious risk factors, such as age and sex, or very rare indicators of risk, there are no known risk factors preponderant enough to have immediate applicability in selective screening. Therefore, several attempts have been made to increase program sensitivity by combining several risk factors and using the combination in defining the high-risk group.

Such a combination should identify persons exposed to several risk indicators at the same time. The combined effect is usually a multiplicative one for which there is also a good theoretical background (Day and Brown, 1980; Peto, 1977). If the risk factors are independent, then the size of the population exposed to several risk indicators decreases rapidly as the number of risk factors increases. Table IV gives an example of this inverse relationship, which implies that the proportion of the total cases found in each high-risk group defined by a simultaneous occurrence of several risk indicators is less than that found by means of a single risk factor.

The best combination of risk indicators can be defined in several ways. Multiple discriminant analysis probably has the widest applicability (Farewell, 1977; Hakama *et al.*, 1979; Soini and Hakama, 1978; Toti *et al.*, 1980). This method defines the best linear combination of the risk indicators which does not assume a simultaneous occurrence of every risk factor or an equal weight for each risk indicator included. Dichotomizing of the risk factor is not required when defining the high- and low-risk groups, but continuous risk variables are assumed and the final cutoff point is defined for the combination score only. The combination score is used to classify the population into a high-risk group subjected to screening and a residual low-risk group. The combination works somewhat better than the most proponderant single risk indicators (Hakama *et al.*, 1979). Furthermore, there is the possibility of continuous selection of the size of the high-risk group; the bigger the group, the greater the proportion of cases included in the high-risk group. The cutoff point for the classification can be selected by the economic resources available (size of the group), by the predetermined yield (proportion of cases in the high-risk group), by maximizing the sum of the program sensitivity and program specificity over the values of discriminant function, or by other criteria.

Most of the studies showed that if the high-risk group was small enough to result in a substantial reduction in cost, then the cases belonging to the low-risk

TABLE IV

Combining Independent Risk Factors: Effect on the Size of the High-Risk Group, on Risk, and on Yield

	Risk factor					
	A	B	C	A and B	B and C	A, B, and C
Size of high-risk groups (%)	50	20	10	10	2	1
Relative risk	2	5	10	10	50	100
Proportion of total cases (%)	67	56	53	53	51	50

group were too numerous (Farewell, 1977; Hakama *et al.*, 1979; Shapiro *et al.*, 1973; Soini and Hakama, 1978), i.e., the program sensitivity was unacceptably low. This seems to be true not only for cancer but for other diseases as well (Kannisto, 1972; Murphy *et al.*, 1982; World Health Organization Expert Committee, 1982).

The risk indicators included in the linear discriminant function differ substantially among different screening programs. Some of the risk indicators are known to the program at the time the high-risk group is identified. These indicators include age, sex, marital status, and occupation if the construction of the high-risk group is based on a population registry or another general population frame. Some risk factors are known only for each individual in the population, but not to the body responsible for the screening program, such as smoking, drinking, and other personal habits, some reproductive characteristics, and some symptoms. Some risk factors require laboratory data, such as previous Pap tests, chest films, and mammograms. Such risk indicators assume first an unselective screening to acquire the basic information for further application of the selective screen. It seems that the most successful selective screenings were based on data related to symptoms (Toti *et al.*, 1980). In such circumstances, it is not clear whether the program was one of selective screening or diagnosis.

VI. PROSPECTS FOR SELECTIVE SCREENING

Cancer is a group of diseases with multiple etiology. In terms of selective screening, this implies that no single etiological factor is likely to be applicable as a basis of selective screening, and that low-risk groups will produce substantial numbers of cancer cases.

There are important exceptions. The identification of high-risk groups does not assume that the etiology of the disease is known; it is sufficient that the high-risk characteristics be mere correlates of the risk yielding high program sensitivity. Age and sex have been used in practically all screening programs as indicators of high-risk groups. Symptoms and diagnostic results based on previous screening may also be used in defining a high-risk group (Hakama and Pukkala, 1977). This applies to the time interval between screenings rather than to an *a priori* definition of a high-risk group. A proposal to screen a subpopulation at shorter intervals assumes that the process of malignant growth is more rapid in the high-risk category. This is likely to be true, e.g., for persons with positive mammography or positive cytology followed by normal histology. Such persons are at high risk, and rescreening at shorter than normal intervals may be warranted. Computer simulation studies also indicate a greater yield with a more frequent schedule of examinations of a high-risk group (Yu *et al.*, 1982).

Smoking of cigarettes deserves special comment. Tobacco smoke is the most important environmental carcinogen affecting the risk of cancer at several sites, and only a few cases of lung cancer appear among persons who have not smoked. However, there is no good evidence that early diagnosis based on screening for lung cancer will reduce mortality from the disease. Smoking of cigarettes should be considered as a subject for regulation and health education, and not as a basis for selective screening for lung cancer at present (see Chapter 20).

We conclude that so far, selective screening based on high-risk populations defined by etiological risk factors has failed. This is true for the approaches based on a single risk factor, as well as those based on a combination of several of them. Several attempts have used risk factors characterizing different aspects of the etiology of a specific cancer. In such cases, program sensitivity was low, i.e., a substantial proportion of the cancer cases diagnosed in the total target population originated in the low-risk group not subjected to screening. The present methods of selective screening for cancer based on risk factors are not likely to be sufficiently effective to be applied in public health programs. If the efficiency and effectiveness of an established program are to be increased, improvements are likely to come from improving the organization, attendance rate, and quality of the test rather than from limiting the activities to high-risk groups only.

REFERENCES

Day, N. E., and Brown, C. C. (1980). Multistage models and primary prevention of cancer. *JNCI, J. Natl. Cancer Inst.* **64,** 977–989.

Farewell, V. T. (1977). The combined effect of breast cancer risk factors. *Cancer* **40,** 931–936.

Foltz, A. M., and Kelsey, J. (1980). The annual pap test: A dubious policy success. *World Health Forum* **1,** 101–116.

Hakama, M., and Pukkala, E. (1977). Selective screening for cervical cancer: Experience of the Finnish mass screening system. *Br. J. Prev. Soc. Med.* **31,** 238–244.

Hakama, M., Pukkala, E., and Saastamoinen, P. (1979). Selective screening: Theory and practice based on high risk groups of cervical cancer. *J. Epidemiol. Commun. Health* **33,** 257–261.

Kannisto, M. (1972). Detection of pulmonary tuberculosis by mass RP surveys: A study of their efficacy. *Scand. J. Respir. Dis.* **81,** Suppl., 1–116.

Murphy, J. F., Newcombe, R. G., and Sibert, J. R. (1982). The epidemiology of sudden infant death syndrome. *J. Epidemiol. Commun. Health* **36,** 17–21.

Peto, R. (1977). Epidemiology, multistage models and short-term mutagenicity tests. *In* "Origins of Human Cancer" (H. H. Hiatt, J. D. Watson, and J. A. Winsten, eds.), Vol. 4, pp. 1403–1428. Cold Spring Harbor Lab., Cold Spring Harbor, New York.

Shapiro, S., Goldberg, J., Venet, L., and Strax, P. (1973). Risk factors in breast cancer—a prospective study. *In* Host Environment Interactions in the Etiology of Cancer in Man" (R. Doll and I. Vodopija, eds.), IARC Sci. Publ. No. 7, pp. 169–182. Int. Agency Res. Cancer, Lyon.

Soini, I., and Hakama, M. (1978). Failure of selective screening for breast cancer by combining risk factors. *Int. J. Cancer* **22,** 275–281.

Toti, A., Piffanelli, A., Pavanelli, T., Buriani, C., Nenci, I., Arslan-Pagnini, C., Zanardi, P., Pecorari, C., Rossi, R., and Barrai, I. (1980). Possible indication of breast cancer risk through discriminant functions. *Cancer* **46,** 1280–1285.

World Health Organization Expert Committee (1982). ''Prevention of Coronary Heart Disease,'' Tech. Rep. Ser. 678. World Health Organ., Geneva.

Yu, S. Z., Miller, A. B., and Sherman, G. J. (1982). Optimising the age, number of tests and test interval for cervical screening in Canada. *J. Epidemiol. Commun. Health* **36,** 1–10.

5

Application of Screening, Including Multiphasic Screening, to Target Populations

GARY D. FRIEDMAN

I.	Introduction	70
II.	Brief Historical Perspective	70
III.	Secondary Advantages of Multiphasic Screening	71
IV.	How to Select a Target Population	73
	A. Prevalence of Disease	73
	B. Cooperativeness	73
	C. Availability of Other Screening and of Follow-Up	74
V.	How to Select an Appropriate Screening Test	74
VI.	How to Invite the Target Population to Be Screened	74
VII.	How to Maintain Patient Satisfaction	75
VIII.	How to Maintain Provider Satisfaction	75
IX.	General Principles for Implementing Multiphasic Screening	76
X.	Pitfalls to Be Avoided	77
XI.	Multiphasic Health Testing Services as Part of a Health Care Delivery System	78
XII.	Specialized Health Examinations	78
XIII.	Quality Control of Screening Procedures	79
	A. Patient Identification and Linkage of Test Results	79
	B. Test Quality Control	80
	C. Instrument Calibration and Standardization	80
	D. Personnel Training and Monitoring	80
	E. Problem Reporting	80
	F. Error Correction	82
XIV.	Conclusion	82
	References	83

ISBN 0-12-496720-5

I. INTRODUCTION

In the historically brief life span of screening, much has been learned about the application of screening to target populations. One established principle is that, in most instances, once a person has come in for some form of screening, it is practical, efficient, and provides better service to apply several screening tests at the same visit—an approach originally termed *multiphasic screening* by Breslow in 1949 (Breslow, 1973). Further, we should bear in mind that there is no inherent reason (other than the limitations sometimes set upon activities of, and funding by, agencies dedicated to cancer control) to restrict a combination of screening tests to various forms of cancer. Cancer is itself a heterogeneous collection of diseases and is by no means the only category of illness that might benefit from early detection. Patients, health care providers, and public health workers are, or should be, concerned with overall health, not just with various cancers. Thus, multiphasic screening will usually be targeted both at cancer and at noncancerous conditions such as hypertension or diabetes mellitus.

II. BRIEF HISTORICAL PERSPECTIVE

Screening was first used in the last century to identify infectious diseases in groups of persons of concern, such as immigrants. Such diseases might endanger others or require extensive care if those afflicted were admitted to a jurisdiction. The introduction of simple, inexpensive techniques such as miniature photofluorograms to detect tuberculosis and serological tests for syphilis led to mass screening for specific infectious diseases in the 1930s. As with most screening nowadays, the basic rationale for these large-scale programs aimed at uncovering single diseases was to detect and treat disease at an early stage in order to reduce the chances that death or disability would result. In the late 1940s, batteries of screening tests were administered to detect not only infectious but noninfectious diseases as well, such as heart disease, diabetes mellitus, obesity, and anemia. Some of these programs were community based, and others were directed toward specific occupational or industrial groups.

The next major development, in the early 1950s, was the incorporation of multiphasic screening into prepaid group practice, partly spurred by the need efficiently to fulfill contractual agreements to provide health evaluation and preventive care to subscriber groups. Encouraged by its experience in screening members of the International Longshoremen's and Warehousemen's Union, the Kaiser-Permanente Medical Care Program in 1951 established probably the first long-term, continuous multiphasic screening program within a comprehensive prepaid health plan. About 10 simple screening tests were performed, followed by a breast and pelvic examination and a Papanicolaou test in the gynecology department for women over 35 years of age and a referral for a sigmoidoscopy examination for men and women over age 40. At a later date, a physical examination and a review of laboratory tests and the patient's health status were performed by a physician. Thus, screening for certain cancers was by then being included in multiphasic screening. In the 1960s, automation of screening tests and of information handling, and the use of nonphysician personnel whenever possible, resulted in efficient provision of screening and health testing services at a surprisingly low cost (Breslow, 1973).

The past three decades have seen endorsements of multiphasic screening by prestigious commissions and an expansion of multiphasic screening programs in size, in technological sophistication, and in number; now there is a multiplicity of ongoing multiphasic screening programs in many settings in many countries (Collen, 1978a). Yet this growth has been accompanied by continuing controversy as to the value of multiphasic screening. Even though screening has been clearly defined as simple testing to distinguish the probably sick from the probably well, with definitive evaluation and diagnosis made later by the physician, much resistance and criticism have come from physicians who view multiphasic screening as a threat to their autonomy as practitioners. Also, spurred by experience with multiphasic screening programs that were economically unsound or that lacked effective follow-up of patients with abnormal findings, many have questioned the value of these efforts. Critical evaluation of screening programs led authoritative groups such as the World Health Organization (1971) to specify criteria that must be met for screening activities to prove their merits. These include such requirements as the rigorous demonstration that screening affects health favorably over the long term; that the benefits outweigh the possible detrimental effects of labeling persons as diseased or of adverse results of therapies thereby instituted; and that each screening test used is sufficiently accurate, economical, and appropriate for the population on which it is to be used.

Several comprehensive evaluations of screening and general health examinations have been published (American Cancer Society, 1980; Bayliss, 1981; Breslow and Somers, 1977; Frame and Carlson, 1975; Medical Practice Committee, 1981; Spitzer, 1979; Spitzer and Brown, 1975).

III. SECONDARY ADVANTAGES OF MULTIPHASIC SCREENING

As has been indicated, the primary advantage of multiphasic screening over screening for only one condition at a time is efficiency. Nevertheless, it is often difficult to justify with hard scientific evidence, on a strict cost-versus-benefit basis, every test that might be included in a multiphasic battery for asymptomatic persons. Thus, in setting up a new multiphasic screening program, one may question the addition of each unproven test. There are many multiphasic screening programs, and considerations regarding the discontinuation of unproven tests are somewhat different. Certainly, before dropping tests from an existing multiphasic program, and to some extent before deciding not to include a variety of screening tests in a new program, it is well to take into account some secondary benefits that patients derive from a comprehensive multiphasic program. Consider, for example, the health questionnaire, which is one component of a comprehensive multiphasic screen that is frequently criticized, mostly because of problems with accuracy and reliability of questionnaire responses in general, and because follow-up of positive responses to questions often reveals nothing of clinical significance. The health questionnaire can provide valuable information when a more definitive screening test such as a test for blood in the stool or a chest X ray is supplemented with questions about weight loss, poor appetite, cough, changes in bowel habits, blood in the stool, and so on. Negative or positive responses to these questions help in evaluating the results of the main screening tests. Even if the more definitive screening tests are negative, positive responses to the above questions may lead the health care provider to search further for possible pulmonary or gastrointestinal illness.

Although certain test findings may not be of apparent immediate benefit to the patient, they may be valuable if future health problems develop. This is particularly true of screening or health testing in the context of a medical care program. If, for example, the patient later experiences monoarticular arthritis, a recorded uric acid level may be of great help to a physician in determining the etiology of this condition. Similarly a baseline electrocardiogram recorded when the patient is asymptomatic may assist greatly in evaluating the nature of electrocardiographic abnormalities noted later when chest pain or palpitations develop.

Another value of comprehensive screening is that when many tests are performed, the patient often feels reassured that he/she is receiving a thorough evaluation as part of good medical care. While it is not acceptable to deceive patients by exaggerated claims about a program or, more crudely, by electronic dials, flashing lights, "bells and whistles," or other accouterments of high technology, the real reassurance of comprehensive testing, possibly supplemented by a placebo effect, is not to be ignored. This would seem particularly true when contemplating a reduction of an existing comprehensive program that would provide screening for patients who have used it before.

This brings us to the question of which patients derive benefit from screening. Garfield (1970) proposed an interesting alternative to the usual view that only those who are harboring a disease and who have a positive test result may benefit from screening. This view is exemplified by the typical cost calculations that reduce the total cost of a screen to the cost per positive test or cost per case detected, implying that the only worthwhile end product is the detection of disease. Garfield's concept is that negative test findings are also valuable to patients who receive them in that they supply reassurance, relief of anxiety, and information useful for planning one's affairs. This applies, of course, to individual screening tests as well as to multiphasic screening programs.

IV. HOW TO SELECT A TARGET POPULATION

In a medical care program, there is an overall population consisting of patients or insured subscribers to whom the program is obligated to provide care. Within this universe, there are subgroups differing in characteristics relevant to whether they should be screened. Similarly, a public health agency responsible for a political or geographic jurisdiction can select subgroups for screening or not, or for more or less intensive screening. Several considerations should influence the selection of the target population.

A. Prevalence of Disease

Some identifiable groups are not susceptible to a particular disease at all. There is no point in screening women for prostatic cancer or whites for sickle cell anemia. Less obviously circumscribed is screening for diseases that can occur in all subgroups, but in varying degrees. For any given test, the selection of subgroups with a higher prevalence will yield relatively more persons who screen positive and, among these, a higher proportion of true positives. False positives can be a serious problem. It is costly, time-consuming, and disturbing to physicians to evaluate a substantial proportion of patients referred for a positive test who prove not to have the suspected disease; and, of course, much anxiety may be aroused in the patients. Thus, it may be advisable to provide a particular screening test only for high-risk populations, e.g., to restrict screening for lung cancer to cigarette smokers or to limit screening for colorectal cancer to persons beyond a certain age, such as 50 years. One may also practice selective or discriminate screening with portions of test panels that are tailored to the individual patient's characteristics, some of which may be determined by a questionnaire. An electrocardiogram may be recorded only for those who have certain cardiorespiratory complaints or who have not had a normal one recorded in the past five years.

B. Cooperativeness

There are certain identifiable subgroups that are not oriented to preventive health care. These are sometimes characterized by low educational level or specific cultural backgrounds. If, as is often the case, the screening program is economically feasible or justifiable only when there is a continuing large number of participants, the provider should ascertain that the target population contains an adequate number of persons who are cooperative and interested.

C. Availability of Other Screening and of Follow-Up

There is no point in providing screening that duplicates services that are already available to a population. And it bears repetition that follow-up of abnormal findings must be provided or readily available to the group screened. There is no point in testing persons if little will be done about the results.

V. HOW TO SELECT AN APPROPRIATE SCREENING TEST

In other chapters, individual screening tests are evaluated in detail. To summarize briefly several important considerations in test selection, it is worth repeating that the disease being screened for should be important and prevalent in the target population and that its natural history should be susceptible to favorable alteration if the disease is detected early. The tests should have acceptable levels of sensitivity, specificity, and economy, and should not be unduly hazardous or uncomfortable to the patients.

VI. HOW TO INVITE THE TARGET POPULATION TO BE SCREENED

Depending on the setting, a number of approaches can be employed to invite the target population for screening. In an employment setting, announcements can be made through the usual channels of communication. In a health care program, announcements about screening can be made by posted notices or leaflets at its various clinics or by mail, either separately or included with other mailings to patients. In the community, still other approaches are available, including announcements or advertising in public media. Recruitment of subjects for the cardiovascular screening examinations provided by the Framingham Heart Study had an appealing feature: the use of volunteers living in the community to invite their neighbors who were included in the sample (Dawber *et al.*, 1963). The volunteers themselves had received the examination and were able to describe it and answer questions based on firsthand knowledge. Although the Framingham investigators believed this approach to be helpful, the two-thirds participation rate of members of the selected sample was no better than that of other cardiovascular study examinations of this type (Chapman *et al.*, 1971; Hames, 1971; Kagan *et al.*, 1974).

VII. HOW TO MAINTAIN PATIENT SATISFACTION

There are several considerations involved in maintaining satisfaction of the patients. One, of course, is the behavior of the persons conducting the screening. They must be helpful and friendly, and have a professional demeanor. Tests must be safe, and if they have any potential for harm (such as from X radiation), the risk must be justifiable when weighed against the potential benefits. The personnel who administer such tests should be knowledgeable in these matters and be able to discuss them intelligently with concerned patients, rather than just providing glib reassurances.

Tests should not cause undue discomfort. A venipuncture, while somewhat painful to patients, is a standard procedure and generally acceptable. Procedures producing more physical or mental discomfort than this should probably be excluded from mass or routine screening programs. Even if these tests are accepted by the participants when they receive the screening, word-of-mouth communication may discourage those yet to come.

In a multiphasic program, screenees may have to wait briefly at some stations. Comfortable waiting areas should be provided. The overall content and duration of the examination should not be so great as to produce undue fatigue.

Many screenees are unwilling or unable to attend during weekdays or working hours. Screening services should also be scheduled for evenings and/or weekends to assure maximum attendance. If more than one visit to the facility is required (e.g., laboratory tests at the first session and a nurse practitioner examination and review of findings at the second), the two visits should not be scheduled at too great an interval. If the lapse of time is too great, either the patient or the provider at the second visit may rightly question whether the findings from the first visit are still applicable.

VIII. HOW TO MAINTAIN PROVIDER SATISFACTION

As implied above, the provider will want information that is timely and up-to-date when he/she provides follow-up evaluation and care for the screened patient. In addition, the quality and accuracy of the testing must be acceptable to the provider. Even if just one of several tests is only temporarily inaccurate, dealing with these erroneous results when caring for the patients involved could discredit the entire program in the provider's eyes.

A related problem lies in screening tests with low predictive value of a positive test. As discussed in Chapter 1, this predictive value is determined by both the accuracy of the test and the prevalence of the condition being tested for in the target population. Since the latter is usually low, even screening tests that are highly accurate by most standards yield substantial numbers of false-positive results. While the physician may be willing to put up with some false-positives when convinced that the search for a given disease in a noncomplaining patient is worthwhile, cooperation and morale break down when the great majority of positive findings of a test prove to be false positive. Every effort must be made to keep the proportion of false positives within acceptable limits for the disease being screened. This may involve selective application of the test to high-risk or high-prevalence groups, and sometimes raising the cutoff point for a positive test for a non-life-threatening condition, even at the expense of some test sensitivity. However, for cancers (e.g., mammography for breast cancer or occult blood in stool for colon cancer), a false negative is more serious, so that a higher proportion of false positives is acceptable.

The provider should be given a clearly readable report of findings, free of obscure code numbers and excessive verbiage or print. With quantitative results, the normal limits should be provided. All abnormal results should be starred, underlined, or highlighted in some manner.

The providers should be involved in decisions regarding the content and frequency of screening examinations, since they are ultimately responsible for the care of the screened patients. They should have some say in how the screening is conducted, so that they will feel that the screening procedures are helpful to their efforts.

IX. GENERAL PRINCIPLES FOR IMPLEMENTING MULTIPHASIC SCREENING

Based on the long Kaiser-Permanente experience and observations of other programs, both successful and unsuccessful, Collen (1978b) has advocated several guiding principles for multiphasic screening programs. In the quoted passage that follows, he was referring to multiphasic health testing services (MHTS), which have broader applications than testing that is used only to screen for early disease. Nevertheless, the passages express many valuable ideas that are sometimes neglected in theoretical discussions of screening, yet are worthy of consideration by anyone planning to establish a screening program.

> (1) The MHTS should be an integrated component of a health care program and closely related to its physician services. Such integration is most effective in a formal organized system of care, but it can also function in an informal cooperative relationship, in which case the linkages must be truly operational. Provision for diagnoses, followup, and treatment is essential, for without it MHTS will fall into disrepute. Thus there must be a group of primary care physicians who will support the MHTS by referring to it patients for examination and by accepting patients referred from MHTS for followup care.
>
> (2) A defined or target population of adequate size must agree to support the MHTS. Unless at least several thousand people are willing to travel periodically to the MHTS for examinations, it cannot support itself. A population exceeding 25,000 adults, with an average health examination rate of at least every three years, is advisable.

(3) Population health needs should be clearly defined . . . in terms of medical, psychosocial, occupational, and environmental factors as well as preventive health maintenance. Conditions selected should be important, prevalent, and susceptible to management. A comprehensive battery of appropriate, accurate tests is necessary. A high quality of testing is essential, and a control program of good quality must be maintained.

(4) MHTS should satisfy the specific objectives determined by its sponsoring organization, whether this be personal or public preventive medicine, industry or military.

(5) The user population should be kept informed as to the benefits and limits of MHTS, and health education should be an adjunct to MHTS.

(6) MHTS should have a computerized and/or manual record system adequate to maintain continuing files on each patient and permit comparison of each examination's findings with earlier data on the patient. The record system should satisfy the same requirements for confidentiality of patient data as any hospital record room.

(7) Since MHTS is a systems or ''clinical engineering'' approach, it must be carefully planned and designed, and it must be operated with trained personnel to provide reliable, acceptable service and high-quality patient examinations at sufficient volume to be cost-effective.

(8) The program should be periodically evaluated regarding the extent to which its effectiveness and its efficiency in achieving its objectives can be improved. [Reproduced (and slightly edited) by permission, from Collen, 1978b; copyright by John Wiley & Sons, Inc.]

Collen also emphasized the importance of careful planning of all aspects of the screening program. In addition to all of the considerations already mentioned, close attention to such practical matters as design of the facility and optimum patient flow is needed. If a program is well planned, the entire process will soon function almost automatically. Also essential is that the program be financially sound; it must either be self-supporting or its benefits must be sufficient to be clearly worth subsidizing.

X. PITFALLS TO BE AVOIDED

Many multiphasic screening programs have failed. In reviewing the experience of unsuccessful programs, Collen (1978b) noted several recurring problems. These are as follows:

1. Assuming that a program that is successful in one setting will be equally successful in another.
2. Ignoring the patients' physicians in organizing the program and failing to obtain their support.
3. Assuming that multphasic screening programs can operate separately from a health care delivery system and that health checkups are simply case detection, not requiring physician follow-up.
4. Failure to orient physicians as to the services that multiphasic testing can provide to them and their patients.
5. Assuming that operating a multiphasic testing program is easy.
6. Attempting to implement a multiphasic screening program in too short a time.

7. Failing to analyze population needs, to reassess those needs periodically, and to alter the system when new needs develop and old ones disappear.
8. Failing to obtain continuing financial and professional support.
9. Assuming that MHTS will produce rapid and/or immediately obvious beneficial results in the target population.

XI. MULTIPHASIC HEALTH TESTING SERVICES AS PART OF A HEALTH CARE DELIVERY SYSTEM

When multiphasic screening is viewed as part of a health care delivery system, its use in the early detection of disease in asymptomatic persons can be supplemented by other uses. Physicians often find it useful in monitoring the status of patients with chronic conditions such as diabetes mellitus or hypertension, for which the routine and economical performance of tests such as electrocardiograms and serum creatinine measurements are helpful in detecting target organ damage.

Multiphasic testing can also be used as a setting for health maintenance and health education activities. For example, instructions for breast self-examination can be given at a mammography station or stop-smoking literature can be distributed where pulmonary function tests are performed. It would seem that when obtaining a health examination, patients would be receptive to health promotion literature and instructions.

A multiphasic testing program can also be used as an efficient entry mode into the health care delivery system for patients with nonurgent problems. Traditionally, such patients enter the system by making an appointment with a physician. The doctor, at the first visit, determines each patient's needs and arranges appropriate evaluation and care. A multiphasic testing service with physical examinations by nurse practitioners has been used as an alternative method for evaluation of needs and referral to appropriate care. The latter approach accomplished the triage of patients with nonurgent problems at lower cost and with savings in physician time (Garfield *et al.*, 1976).

XII. SPECIALIZED HEALTH EXAMINATIONS

In addition to the general uses already described, multiphasic testing can be applied to special health examinations that are provided frequently or in large numbers. These include preadmission testing for hospital patients, prenatal examinations for pregnant women, preschool and precamp examinations for children, preemployment examinations when persons must show their fitness to enter certain occupations (including the military), and periodic follow-up examinations to demonstrate continuing fitness. Obviously, each of these uses will dictate the inclusion or omission of particular screening tests. For example, periodic examination of workers in a noisy factory should include an audiogram; routine prenatal examinations should not include tests involving X ray exposure to the fetus.

XIII. QUALITY CONTROL OF SCREENING PROCEDURES

To be useful, acceptable, and ultimately successful, a screening program must produce data that have a high degree of accuracy. It is generally recognized that screening is not definitive or equivalent to a final diagnosis, but this does not allow for a high error rate in the screening tests themselves. Terdiman (1978) has described six essential elements of quality control for screening tests. These are discussed in the following sections.

A. Patient Identification and Linkage of Test Results

Patient identification checking is essential so that results of multiple screening tests at different stations can be linked to the correct patient. In a high-volume screening program, possibilities for mismatch do occur and must be controlled. Accuracy of linkage is usually maintained by assigning each patient a unique identification number. This may be a membership number already assigned by a health care program, a sequential accession number assigned to each patient at the time of screening, or some other standard identifier such as the Social Security number in the United States. (The last is controversial because of implications for protection of privacy but is very useful for ascertaining mortality or other outcomes in epidemiological follow-up studies.)

Secondary identifiers including name, sex, and date of birth are helpful in verifying the primary identification number; and age and sex are often needed in determining cutoff points for positive screening results. Another method of verifying the accuracy of the primary number is to add a check digit to it. This check digit, which can be determined by performing specified calculations on the primary number, permits verification of the primary number by computer and aids in the detection of errors in transcription or data entry, such as transposition of digits.

For screening programs with on-line entry of test results into computer storage, the patient may carry a machine-readable identification badge which can be read by a terminal at each station, along with his or her test finding. Alternatively, the patient may carry a set of preidentified forms for data entry or a pack of data entry keypunch cards, each prepunched with identifying information. While such systems are generally reliable, occasional errors occur due to loss or exchange between family members of identification cards.

B. Test Quality Control

Statistical analysis of test results should be carried out at frequent intervals, daily if possible, to monitor the functioning and calibration of test instruments and the technicians' operation of these instruments. Simple statistical measures are usually employed, such as age- and sex-specific means and standard deviations for quantitative tests, and proportions of tests labeled as abnormal, unsatisfactory, or omitted for both quantitative and qualitative tests. Results are compared from day to day, often by graphic display, in which nonrandom variations such as sudden large shifts or long-term trends can be readily detected. Hoffman and Ward (1965) have described one such method of quality control monitoring.

When suspicions are raised by test quality control monitoring, the source of the problem must be sought and corrected. Sudden shifts may mean instrument malfunction or change in technician performance. Gradual trends in test results may indicate poor stability of the measuring instrument.

Single, nonrepetitive errors in individual test results do not usually come to light by means of statistical quality control procedures. These usually become recognized during follow-up evaluation by the health care provider, who should have a ready means of reporting individual errors, assuring their correction, and, where possible, preventing recurrences.

C. Instrument Calibration and Standardization

Test instruments must be adjusted regularly so that a known input produces the correct output. For example, automatic blood cell counting devices must be tested and adjusted so that operation on reference control standards with known contents, provided by the manufacturer, yield accurate counts. Similarly, mammography equipment must be checked to be sure that the X ray tube voltage and current are at the required levels and that there is no unwanted radiation leakage.

D. Personnel Training and Monitoring

The personnel conducting each screening test must be well trained and periodically monitored. In addition to the quality control monitoring described above, periodic inspection of personnel performance is desirable. A standard procedure manual must be prepared which describes in detail the procedures for calibrating and operating each test instrument and applying it to the patient.

E. Problem Reporting

Effective quality control requires more than error detection. Errors and problems must be communicated to the appropriate personnel. In the quality control

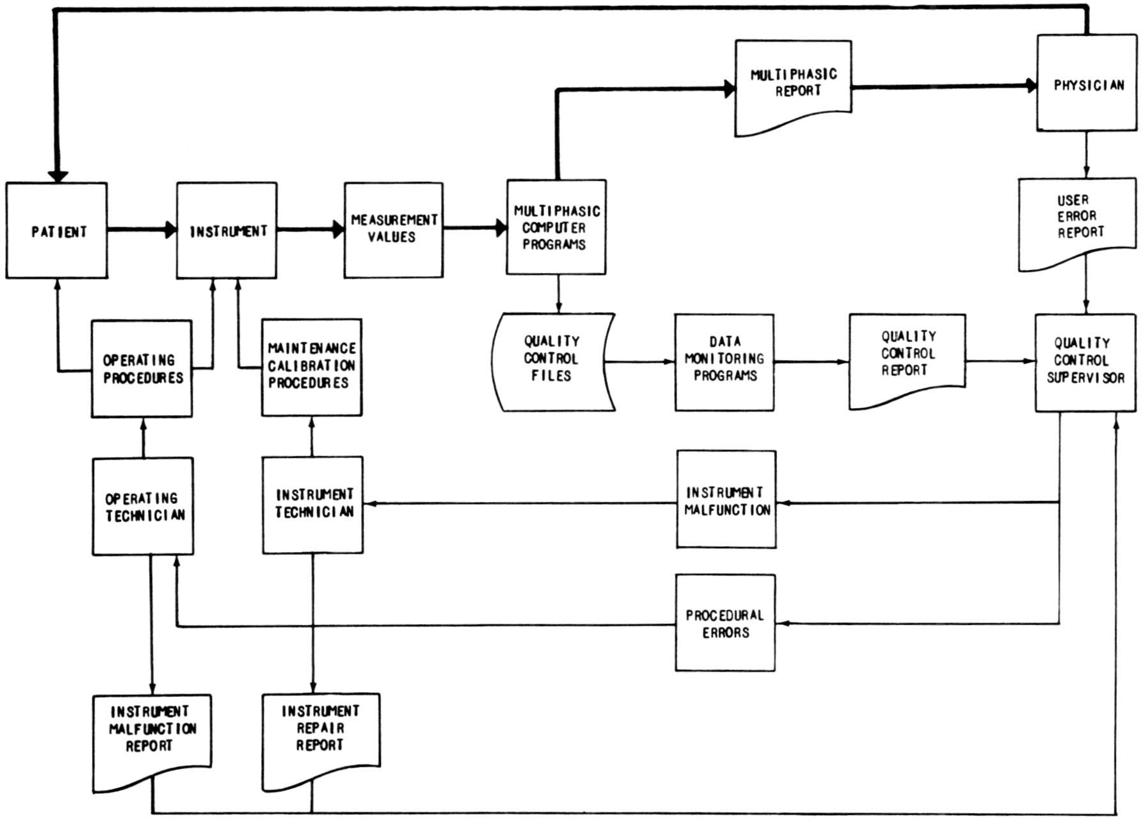

Fig. 1. Quality control system developed by Kaiser-Permanente. Heavy arrows show the primary flow of multiphasic information. Thin arrows show the flow of information for quality control. (Reproduced, by permission, from Terdiman, 1978; copyright by John Wiley & Sons, Inc.)

system developed at Kaiser-Permanente (Fig. 1), the results of statistical test quality monitoring, reports of individual errors detected by the physician, and evidence of malfunctioning instruments noted by technicians are monitored by a quality control supervisor, who initiates appropriate corrective action.

F. Error Correction

Selection of the appropriate error correction methods depends on the location of the patient and the reporting status of the error. If an error in a test result is detected while the patient is still at the screening facility, the test can be repeated and the error corrected. If the patient has left but the screening findings have not been printed, the erroneous test result can be deleted and replaced with a comment such as "unsatisfactory test." If the report has been printed and given to a health care provider and the screening personnel detect an error, an amended report should immediately be sent to the provider, with additional notification of urgent changes by telephone when appropriate. This amended report points out the error and gives the corrected result, if available, or indicates an unsatisfactory test. For medicolegal reasons, the data files and any subsequent reports should contain both the flagged erroneous result and the corrected data. If the provider first detects the error, he or she may write the correction on the printed report and should initiate a procedure whereby the data files are amended to show both the flagged error and the corrected result.

XIV. CONCLUSION

Successful application of screening to target populations requires careful consideration of the goals of the screening program; identification of prevalent and important diseases in, and likely cooperation of, the target population; selection of screening tests with good sensitivity, specificity, and acceptable costs; maintenance of the quality and accuracy of screening methods; adequate medical care and follow-up for abnormal test results; and satisfying the human needs of the patients and providers.

ACKNOWLEDGMENTS

I thank Dr. Morris Collen for reviewing and suggesting improvements in a draft manuscript of this chapter and, more importantly, for his contributions to and leadership in the development of multiphasic health testing.

REFERENCES

American Cancer Society (1980). Report on the cancer-related health checkup. *Ca—Cancer J. Clin.* **30,** 194–240.

Bayliss, R. I. S. (1981). The medical check-up. *Br. Med. J.* **283,** 631–634.

Breslow, L. (1973). An historical review of multiphasic screening. *Prev. Med.* **2,** 177–196.

Breslow, L., and Somers, A. R. (1977). The lifetime health monitoring program: A practical approach to preventive medicine. *N. Engl. J. Med.* **296,** 601–608.

Chapman, J. M., Coulson, A. H., Clark, V. A., and Borun, E. R. (1971). The differential effect of serum cholesterol, blood pressure, and weight on the incidence of myocardial infarction and angina pectoris. *J. Chronic Dis.* **23,** 631–645.

Collen, M. F. (1978a). History of MHTS. *In* "Multiphasic Health Testing Services" (M. F. Collen, ed.), pp. 1–45. Wiley, New York.

Collen, M. F. (1978b). MHTS planning and implementation. *In* "Multiphasic Health Testing Services" (M. F. Collen, ed.), pp. 75–101. Wiley, New York.

Dawber, T. R., Kannel, W. B., and Lyell, L. P. (1963). An approach to longitudinal studies in a community: The Framingham study. *Ann. N. Y. Acad. Sci.* **107,** 539–556.

Frame, P. S., and Carlson, S. J. (1975). A critical review of periodic health screening using specific screening criteria. *J. Family Pract.* **2,** 29–36, 123–129, 189–194, 283–289.

Garfield, S. R. (1970). Multiphasic health testing and medical care as a right. *N. Engl. J. Med.* **283,** 1087–1089.

Garfield, S. R., Collen, M. F., Feldman, R., Soghikian, K., Richart, R. H., and Duncan, J. H. (1976). Evaluation of an ambulatory medical-care delivery system. *N. Engl. J. Med.* **294,** 426–431.

Hames, C. G. (1971). Evans County Cardiovascular and cerebrovascular epidemiology study: Introduction. *Arch. Intern. Med.* **128,** 883–886.

Hoffman, R. G., and Ward, M. E. (1965). The "average-of-normals" method of quality control. *Am. J. Clin. Pathol.* **43,** 134–141.

Kagan, A., Harris, B. R., Winkelstein, W., Jr., Johnson, K. G., Kato, H., Syme, L. L., Rhoads, G. G., Gay, M. L., Nichaman, M. Z., Hamilton, H. B., and Tillotson, J. (1974). Epidemiologic studies of coronary heart disease and stroke in Japanese men living in Japan, Hawaii, and California: Demographic, physical, dietary, and biochemical characteristics. *J. Chronic Dis.* **27,** 345–364.

Medical Practice Committee, American College of Physicians (1981). Periodic health examination: A guide for designing individualized preventive health care in the asymptomatic patient. *Ann. Intern. Med.* **95,** 729–732.

Spitzer, W. O., Chairman (1979). Report of the task force on the periodic health examination. *Can. Med. Assoc. J.* **121,** 1193–1254.

Spitzer, W. O., and Brown, B. P. (1975). Unanswered questions about the periodic health examination. *Ann. Intern. Med.* **83,** 257–263.

Terdiman, J. F. (1978). Quality control. *In* "Multiphasic Health Testing Services" (M. F. Collen, ed.), pp. 241–259. Wiley, New York.

World Health Organization (1971). "Mass Health Examination as a Public Health Tool," Tech. Rep. No. A24, pp. 50–51. World Health Organ., Geneva.

II

Screening Tests

6

Cervical Cytology

GEORGE H. ANDERSON

I. History of the Pap Smear 87
II. Requirements for a Pap Smear Screening Program 88
A. Collecting the Smear 88
B. Processing the Smear 90
C. Screening and Interpreting the Smear 92
D. Reporting the Findings 93
E. Follow-up System 96
F. Quality Control 99
References 102

I. HISTORY OF THE PAP SMEAR

Although it had been recognized since the middle of the nineteenth century that exfoliated malignant cells can be detected in sputum, urine, and pleural and peritoneal exudates, it was not until the work of Dr. George Papanicolaou that the techniques of exfoliative cytology, particularly for the detection of early carcinoma of the cervix, became generally accepted.

In his presidential address, delivered to the tenth annual meeting of the American Society of Cytology in 1963, Dr. Leopold Koss said, "the basic contributions of Papanicolaou have given rise to a new diagnostic science which, in its significance in our fight against cancer, stands unsurpassed in our century" (Koss, 1963). By 1928, Papanicolaou had recognized that it was possible to detect cells from a malignant lesion of the cervix in a vaginal smear. Although these findings were reported in 1928, it was not until 1941, with the publication of his article with Traut, "The Diagnostic Value of Vaginal Smears in Carcinoma of the Uterus" (Papanicolau and Traut, 1941), that interest in this technique became widespread, particularly in North America.

ISBN 0-12-496720-5

Dr. Aurel Babes, also in 1928, published observations similar to those of Papanicolaou regarding the early detection of cancer of the cervix; like Papanicolaou's original observations in North America, Babes' report received little attention in Europe.

While the Pap smear originally was prepared from fluid aspirated from the posterior vaginal fornix, this technique was rapidly superseded by the cervical scrape technique introduced by Ayre (1947, 1952); this technique still remains the most widely used method of preparing a Pap smear.

In 1962, Davis described a self-administered vaginal irrigation technique which, it was thought, might be of value in areas where skilled professional help for obtaining routine Pap smears was not available. Subsequent studies of this technique (Richart and Vaillant, 1965; Anderson and Gunn, 1965) indicated that it was significantly less accurate in detecting early carcinoma of the cervix than the cervical scrape method. Nevertheless, there may still be a place for the irrigation smear, or a similar technique, in underdeveloped countries and in other situations in which cervical scrape smears cannot be obtained.

II. REQUIREMENTS FOR A PAP SMEAR SCREENING PROGRAM

A number of elements are vital for the successful development of a Pap smear screening program:

1. Collecting the smear
2. Processing the smear
3. Screening and interpreting the smear
4. Reporting the findings
5. Follow-up systems
6. Quality control

If the performance in any one of these areas is less than optimal, this will reduce the efficiency and reliability of the whole system. Thus, the proper performance of each element must be considered in some detail.

A. Collecting the Smear

The aim of a cervical smear is to obtain a representative specimen from the squamocolumnar junction or transitional zone of the uterine cervix. Since the majority of precursor lesions of invasive squamous carcinoma of the cervix arise in the region of the squamocolumnar junction, a smear cannot be considered adequate unless this area has been sampled. The cervix should be exposed using a bivalve speculum. Using an Ayre's spatula, as shown in Fig. 1, a circumferen-

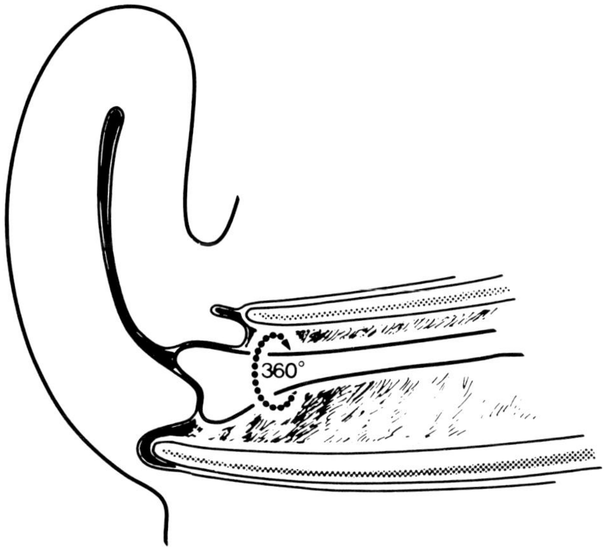

Fig. 1. The use of the Ayre's cervical spatula.

tial sample is obtained by turning the spatula through 360° in order to obtain cells from the entire squamocolumnar junction. At times, difficulty may be experienced if the transformation zone is irregular in shape, and it is important that the collection technique be adapted to ensure that the entire area is sampled. If the squamocolumnar junction cannot be visualized, an additional specimen should be obtained from the endocervical canal, either by using a cotton tip applicator moistened with normal saline or by aspiration of the endocervical canal using a pipette and rubber suction bulb. It has been claimed that the sensitivity of the Pap smear is greatly improved when both the ectocervix and the endocervix are sampled (Richart, 1979; Garite and Feldman, 1978; Gilbert *et al.*, 1973).

Some authors believe that an adequate Pap smear should always contain endocervical cells, their presence indicating that the upper margin of the transformation zone has been sampled. However, experience indicates that as many as 30% of routinely submitted Pap smears do not contain endocervical cells. On the other hand, D. W. Thompson and M. Lickrish (personal communication) state that some lesions of the cervix develop initially in relation to the original squamocolumnar junction, which may, at the time of sampling, be covered by mature squamous epithelium; in this case, the squamocolumnar junction is several millimeters distant to the lesion, so that endocervical cells would almost certainly not be present. Optimally, the smear should be obtained at midcycle, since cell morphology is most easily interpreted at this time, although this is not an essential prerequisite to obtaining an adequate smear.

Factors which may preclude the obtaining of an adequate smear include the use of lubricant jelly on the vaginal speculum and douching by the patient up to 24 hours prior to the examination; both of these procedures should be avoided. If the patient is menstruating, the presence of excessive blood may make the smear unreadable. If there is a large amount of mucus or purulent exudate on the surface of the cervix, this should be gently removed with a cotton wool swab prior to obtaining the sample.

Once the sample or samples have been obtained, they should be placed on a glass slide, marked with the patient's name, and spread smoothly down the length of the slide. The aim is to obtain a uniform monolayer of cells spread over the surface of the slide.

As soon as the cell sample has been spread, it must be fixed; partial air drying, followed by fixation, may make the smear difficult or impossible to interpret. The most commonly used fixative is an aerosol spray fixative, which should be directed at the cellular material on the slide from a distance of approximately 25 cm. If the aerosol nozzle is too close to the slide, it will tend to produce irregular ridging of the cellular material and may even blow it off the slide. Alternatively, fixation may be achieved by using a similar alcohol solution (95% ethyl alcohol), which is dropped onto the surface of the slide or into which the slide is placed for a minimum of 15 minutes. After fixation, the slide is air-dried and sent to the cytology laboratory, together with a requisition containing appropriate clinical information.

While fixation with an aerosol or alcohol fixative, as described above, is the optimum method of cell preservation, it is also possible to air-dry the smear without prior fixation; the smear can then be rehydrated in the laboratory. The rehydration technique produces very acceptable results for squamous epithelial cells, and a number of laboratories find this technique quite acceptable; cells of glandular origin are not well preserved if this method is used.

When the smear is sent to the laboratory, some basic clinical information is of great importance in the adequate interpretation of the Pap smear. The minimum information required is the patient's name, age, and the date of the last menstrual period. Any relevant clinical signs or symptoms, information relating to the use of birth control pills or an intrauterine contraceptive device, and any previous significant illness or surgery, particularly of a gynecological nature, should also be included on the requisition. In addition, if the patient is being treated with estrogen compounds, steroids, or digoxin, this may effect the hormonal pattern and the interpretation of the smear.

B. Processing the Smear

Once received in the laboratory, the slide and requisition should be given an accession number, with appropriate information relating to the specimen being recorded, either in a day book, card file, or computerized file. It is essential that this accession process be performed accurately in order to avoid potential confusion between slides from different patients.

Many variations of the original Papanicolaou staining technique (Papanicolaou, 1942) have been published. Figure 2 outlines a method for processing unfixed, air-dried smears which are first rehydrated using a glycerol/water solution; for fixed smears, the first three steps are omitted. Harris' hematoxylin produces good nuclear detail, while the combination of Orange-G6(OG-6) and Eosin-Alcohol-36(EA-36) will counterstain the cytoplasm and give a transparent appearance to the cytoplasm.

Once staining has been done, mounting medium is placed on each slide, which is then coverslipped in order to protect the cells and prevent fading. A detailed

2 min	2 min	10 dips	2 min	2 min	6 min HARRIS'	10 dips	dip 0.5% AQUEOUS HCL
50% GLY/H_2O	50% GLY/H_2O	TAP WATER; change often	50% ETHYL ALCOHOL	TAP WATER	HEMA-TOXYLIN	TAP WATER	
1	2	3	4	5	6	7	8

1 min	10 dips	10 dips	10 dips	1 min	10 dips	1 min 2% sat. solution	4 min
100% ETHYL ALCOHOL	100% ETHYL ALCOHOL	80% ETHYL ALCOHOL	70% ETHYL ALCOHOL	50% ETHYL ALCOHOL	TAP WATER	LITHIUM CARBONATE	RUNNING TAP WATER
16	15	14	13	12	11	10	9

1.5 min	10 dips	10 dips	1.5 min	10 dips	10 dips	10 dips	10 dips
OG -6	100% ETHYL ALCOHOL	100% ETHYL ALCOHOL	EA-36	95% ETHYL ALCOHOL	95% ETHYL ALCOHOL	100% ETHYL ALCOHOL	100% ETHYL ALCOHOL
17	18	19	20	21	22	23	24

2 min	2 min	2 min	2 min	2 min EQUAL PARTS	2 min EQUAL PARTS	2 min EQUAL PARTS	2 min EQUAL PARTS
XYLOL	XYLOL	XYLOL	XYLOL	100% ETHYL ALCOHOL and XYLOL	100% ETHYL ALCOHOL and XYLOL	100% ETHYL ALCOHOL and XYLOL	100% ETHYL ALCOHOL and XYLOL
32	31	30	29	28	27	26	25

Fig. 2. Pap smear staining procedure. All solutions and stains are changed daily.

account of cytopreparatory techniques by Bales and Durfee is to be found in Koss' "Textbook of Diagnostic Cytology" (1979).

C. Screening and Interpreting the Smear

Each smear must be screened in a systematic manner by a cytotechnologist who has received appropriate training and successfully passed an examination certifying his or her competence. Examinations by the Canadian Society of Laboratory Technologists, the American Society of Cytology, and the International Academy of Cytology may be considered examples of the level of proficiency which should be required of a competent screener. The number of smears which can be safely screened by cytotechnologists will vary according to the number of other duties they may be called upon to perform in the laboratory; for example, in a small laboratory, cytotechnologists may perform all of the tasks—accessioning the cases, staining and mounting the slides, and screening the smears. In larger laboratories, clerical and lab aide staff may perform all of these duties except screening, leaving the cytotechnologists free to screen the smears. It has been recommended, in a symposium on quality control in cytology published by the American Society of Cytology (Frable *et al.*, 1975), that "the average cytotechnologist should screen 20,000 gynecologic slides per year." This recommendation applies to cytoscreeners who perform no other duties in the laboratory and represents a maximum figure.

In a large laboratory which screens in excess of 50,000 to 100,000 smears per year, it is probably more efficient to establish a hierarchical or pyramid system of screening in which the more junior, less experienced screeners pass on to the more experienced screeners those smears with abnormalities beyond a defined range. An example of such a system is outlined in Fig. 3.

The 1976 Canadian Task Force report of cervical cancer screening programs, commonly referred to as the "Walton Report" (Task Force, 1976), recognized that no single model of laboratory applied uniformly to all situations, but recommended that to perform at optimal efficiency, a cytology laboratory should handle a minimum of 25,000 cases per year. The recent update of this report, "Cervical Cancer Screening Programs 1982" (Task Force, 1982) recommends that "to function most efficiently within a mass screening program a laboratory should process a sufficient number of cases annually to require staffing by a minimum of three qualified and experienced cytotechnologists, supervised by a cytopathologist and adequate clerical and technical support staff." Although this recommendation is aimed at achieving maximum efficiency, proficiency is also of concern. Although it is true that many laboratories with fewer staff and a smaller number of cases can perform reliably, one would be concerned about the maintenance of professional skills if a laboratory were seeing fewer than 25 or 30 positive cases per year.

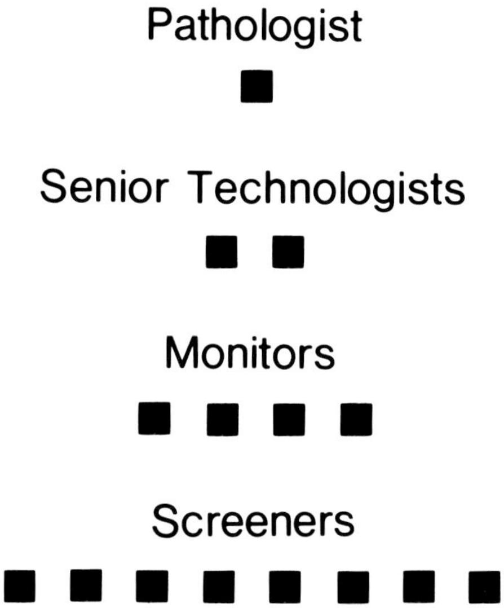

Fig. 3. The screening pyramid.

D. Reporting the Findings

It is strongly recommended that when a report is written on a cytologic smear, the results should be expressed in descriptive terms, whether or not a numerical classification similar to the original Papanicolaou classification is also used. Although some disagreement still exists with regard to the final reporting responsibility for Pap smears, a well-trained, experienced cytotechnologist can be expected to sign out negative Pap smears and Pap smears which show changes related to a benign atypia. Pap smears which show abnormal cells consistent with a significant degree of dysplasia or worse should be referred for the interpretation and recommendations of a medically qualified person with appropriate training and experience, preferably a cytopathologist.

Table I lists the reporting terminology for cervicovaginal cytology as recommended in the recent Canadian Task Force report (Task Force, 1982); this terminology is similar to that recommended by both the Canadian and American Societies of Cytology and by the International Academy of Cytology.

The details of microscopic morphology which apply to the abnormal cells seen in relation to the nondysplastic, benign atypias listed above will not be discussed in this chapter, since they are well described and illustrated in the many textbooks of cytodiagnosis now available. In relation to the histologic entities of dysplasia and carcinoma *in situ,* however, also described by some authors as

TABLE I

Reporting Terminology for Cervical–Vaginal Cytology

Unsatisfactory (reason to be stated)
No abnormal cells
Metaplasia noted
Abnormal cells consistent with benign atypia (nondysplastic)
Inflammatory effect
Trichomonas effect
Viral effect
Yeast effect
Irradiation effect
Keratinization
Atypical metaplasia
Condyloma effect
Other
Abnormal cells consistent with dysplasia
Mild dysplasia
Moderate dysplasia
Severe dysplasia
Abnormal cells consistent with malignancy
Consistent with squamous carcinoma *in situ*
Consistent with invasive squamous carcinoma
Consistent with adenocarcinoma
Type unspecified
Abnormal cells specifically classified
(comments to be attached)

cervical intraepithelial neoplasia (CIN) and illustrated in Fig. 4, the following are the diagnostic criteria which are widely accepted and recommended.

1. Mild dysplasia (CIN 1). Maturation of the squamous epithelial cells is found in the superficial two-thirds of the squamous mucosa, with undifferentiated cells present in the lower one-third. The nuclei of the cells in the superficial two-thirds of the mucosa show some enlargement and hyperchromasia.
2. Moderate dysplasia (CIN 2). The superficial one-third to two-thirds of the squamous mucosa shows maturation of the cytoplasm of the epithelial cells, with undifferentiated neoplastic cells occupying the lower one-third to two-thirds of the mucosa. Loss of polarity of the cells throughout the mucosa is more apparent.
3. Severe dysplasia (CIN 3). Over two-thirds of the thickness of the squamous mucosa is occupied by undifferentiated cells which show loss of polarity and nuclear hyperchromasia; mitotic figures may be found in the lower two-thirds of the mucosa.
4. Carcinoma *in situ* (CIN 3). The entire thickness of the squamous mucosa is occupied by neoplastic cells which show no evidence of differentiation, except

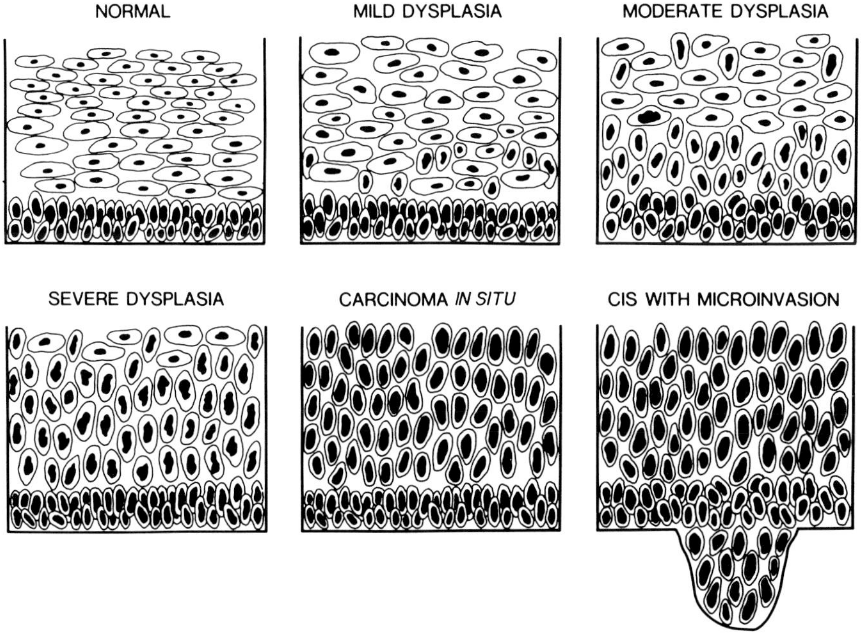

Fig. 4. The pathologic spectrum from normal mucosa to carcinoma *in situ*.

possibly in the most superficial layers. Mitotic figures may be found at all levels of the mucosa.

5. Carcinoma *in situ* (CIN 3) with microinvasion. This lesion is similar to carcnioma *in situ* with, in addition, small discrete foci of invasion extending through the basement membrane to a depth of no greater than 5 mm.

The terminology of CIN, which was originally introduced by Richart (1967) and recently reviewed by Buckley *et al.* (1982), has been the subject of some comment (Walton *et al.*, 1982; Alderson *et al.*, 1983). One objection to the CIN terminology relates to the fact that it eliminates the distinction between severe dysplasia and carcinoma *in situ* by amalgamating these two categories into the single category of CIN 3. While the distinction between these two entities may be subtle and somewhat arbitrary, similar subjective criteria are used to distinguish between mild, moderate, and severe dysplasia, and yet appear acceptable to the supporters of the new terminology. Perhaps even more important, the CIN terminology makes it extremely difficult to correlate data from various cervical cancer screening programs and cancer registries. Finally, it should be pointed out that while the original Papanicolaou numerical classification utilized five categories, ranging from class I to class V, the problems and risks inherent in reporting abnormalities using such a numerical classification alone have long been apparent. Current cytologic practice requires that cellular abnormalities be reported in a descriptive manner in such a way as to predict the type of histologic abnormality which is anticipated.

Three variants of carcinoma *in situ* have been described. The most common is large-cell undifferentiated carcinoma *in situ,* which is generally found in the region of the squamocolumnar junction. The second most common variant is small-cell anaplastic carcinoma *in situ,* which is usually found at the upper end of the transformation zone or within the endocervical canal. The least common variant is large-cell keratinizing squamous carcinoma *in situ,* which usually occurs outside the external os and may be related to the original transformation zone.

E. Follow-Up System

No matter how efficient a cytology laboratory may be, it will fail to provide an optimal service unless adequate follow-up and recall systems exist, whether these are provided by the laboratory itself or by a centralized registry. The most important function of the follow-up system is to determine that appropriate action has been taken once a cytologic abnormality has been reported. In addition, for those patients who have received treatment following the diagnosis of an abnormality at the level of a severe dysplasia or carcinoma *in situ,* long-term follow-up is mandatory, since these patients have a significant risk of developing recurrent or new disease, sometimes many years after the treatment of the original lesion. Even those patients treated for carcinoma *in situ* by hysterectomy, with complete removal of the lesion, may develop new disease in the vagina, usually at the vault; this happens in about 1% of cases.

Over the past decade, the recommended method of investigation for patients with an abnormal Papanicolaou smear has become colposcopy; this technique, which was first described by Hinselman in the 1920s, involves the examination of the cervix by means of a magnifying instrument (Fig. 5) with a range of magnification from 5X to 20X. When the colposcopist identifies an area of abnormality, a small bite biopsy is taken from a representative area of the lesion in order to confirm the colposcopic impression. If no lesion is identified, it is particularly important to perform an endocervical curettage as well.

Over the past decade, in British Columbia as in the rest of the Western world, we have observed a marked increase in number of patients with carcinoma *in situ* of the cervix, as shown in Fig. 6. This may be due in part to the increasing population of the province and in part to increased coverage of the population at risk. However, there now seems to be good evidence that there has been a significant increase in the number of new cases seen in the past few years, particularly in younger women.

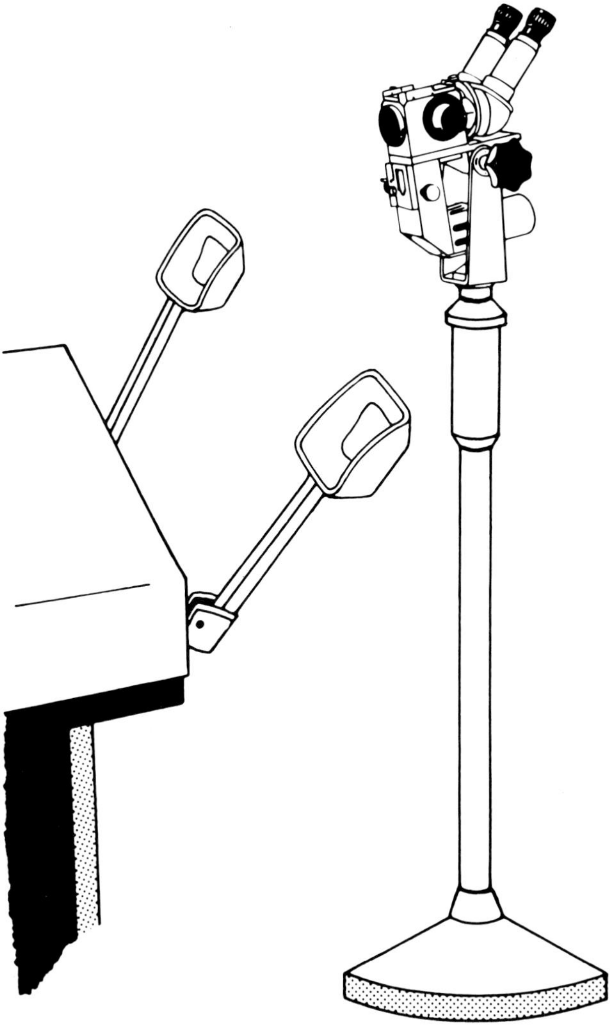

Fig. 5. A modern colposcope.

As reported previously (Benedet *et al.*, 1976), the peak rate of carcinoma *in situ* per 1000 women screened during the 1960s was in the 30- to 34-year age group. The peak rate for this disease in the late 1970s and early 1980s occurred in the 25- to 29-year age group, the disease rate having almost doubled in third-decade women over the past 4 years.

This changing pattern, coincident with the development of colposcopy throughout North America, has resulted in significant changes in the manage-

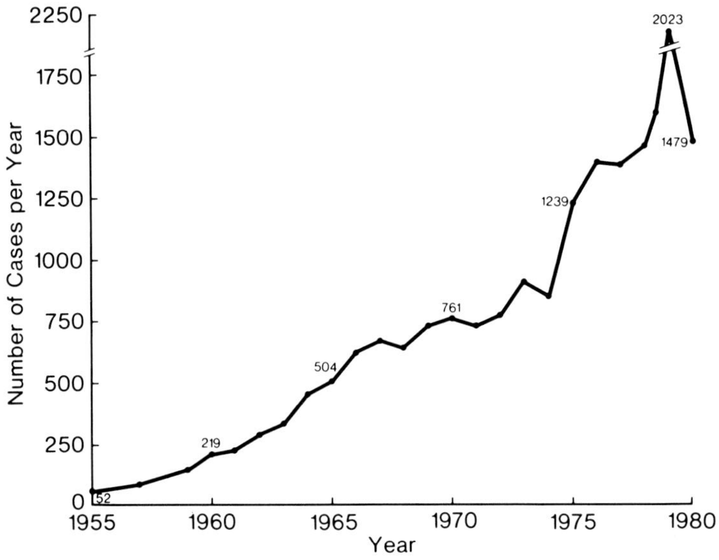

Fig. 6. Carcinoma *in situ*, British Columbia, 1955–1980. Reprinted with permission from The American College of Obstetricians and Gynecologists. (*Obstetrics and Gynecology*, 1982, Vol. 60, No. 5, p. 540.)

ment of the patient with an abnormal Pap smear. Prior to the establishment of colposcopy, many patients with cell changes suggestive of mild or moderate dysplasia were followed for several years by cytology alone; nowadays, these patients are referred for colposcopic examination after only two or three such abnormal smears. If colposcopy confirms the diagnosis, and the full extent of the lesion can be visualized, then local treatment such as cryotherapy or cautery can be utilized, rather than a cone biopsy or hysterectomy, which were the most commonly employed methods of treatment of carcinoma *in situ* prior to the development of colposcopy, with its potential for local ablation of the lesion. In a recent study of the impact of diagnostic colposcopy on conization and hysterectomy practices (Benedet *et al.*, 1982), which involved a review of 2249 patients, a total of 1174 patients were spared a cone biopsy, 856 being treated by cryotherapy or laser surgery and 318 proceeding directly to hysterectomy. Figure 7 illustrates a commonly used schema for the evaluation of patients with an abnormal Pap smear as compared to the traditional method of evaluation.

It is important to be aware that, in inexperienced hands, colposcopy may pose a threat to optimal patient management (Townsend *et al.*, 1981; Nunez and Shapiro, 1981; Sevin *et al.*, 1979). The hazards of underdiagnosis or inappropriate treatment can be avoided only by the establishment of high standards of training and the colposcopist's understanding that in order to maintain expertise,

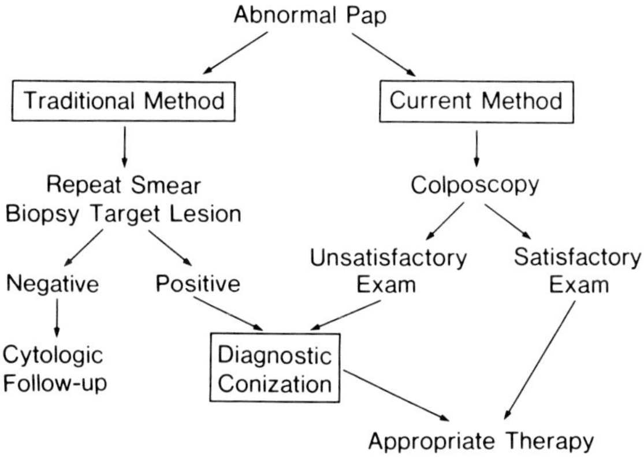

Fig. 7. The investigation of an abnormal Pap test. (From Benedet and Anderson, 1981.)

an adequate number of patients must be seen on a regular basis. It cannot be too strongly emphasized that whenever colposcopy indicates a significantly lesser lesion than was suggested by cytology, the investigation cannot be considered adequate until a cone biopsy has been performed.

F. Quality Control

Much has been written about the importance of quality control in providing an adequate and safe Pap smear screening program (Frable *et al.*, 1975; Melamed, 1976, 1981; Husain *et al.*, 1974; Rodney, 1974). Obviously, an adequate physical facility must be available, including adequate laboratory space, equipment, and good microscopes, the essential daily working tool of the cytologist. Many of the requirements for adequate quality control have been stated specifically or implied in the previous sections of this chapter, including the methods of obtaining the Pap smear; the preparatory procedures in the laboratory; and the screening, interpretation, and reporting of the smears.

The many possible sources of error in a Pap smear screening program have been summarized in the 1982 Canadian Task Force report on cervical cancer screening programs (Task Force, 1982), and are listed below:

I. Errors in documentation
   A. In the physician's office or clinic
   B. In the processing of smears in the laboratory
   C. In the report issued to the clinician
II. Inadequate sampling of lesion
   A. Choice of sampling techniques is not appropriate
   B. Insufficient cellular material
   C. Poor technique in spreading the sample

- D. Transformation zone not well represented
- E. Lesion not amenable to adequate sampling
  - i. Extremely small
  - ii. Unusual location
  - iii. Highly keratinized variant
  - iv. Surface of the lesion is altered by necrosis

III Interfering substances
- A. Cellular material obscured by blood
- B. Cellular material obscured by lubricant
- C. Cellular material obscured by talcum powder granules
- D. Cellular detail altered by bacterial action

IV. Technical problems
- A. Inadequate fixation of smears
  - i. Air drying
  - ii. Incomplete fixation
  - iii. Fixation of air-dried smears prior to rehydration
- B. Overstaining, understaining

V. Errors in screening and reporting
- A. Inadequate screening of a slide
- B. Misinterpretation of cellular abnormalities
  - i. Inadequate training and/or experience
  - ii. Inadequate supervision and quality control

For many years, quality control in cytology laboratories was based on the arbitrary belief that 10% of negative Pap smears should be rescreened in order to detect abnormal cases which were missed at the first screening. In practice, this has proven to be a costly and ineffective method of quality control, particularly in populations which have already been screened once, since the number of abnormal smears will be less than 1% (Melamed, 1981).

In relation to the validity of any screening test, two important parameters are recognized: sensitivity and specificity.

Sensitivity is defined as the ability of a test to detect all members of the diseased population. In relation to a Pap smear screening program, sensitivity is the reciprocal of the false-negative rate.

Specificity is defined as the ability of a test to identify correctly all nondiseased people. In terms of a Pap smear screening program, specificity is the reciprocal of the false-positive rate.

The sensitivity of the Pap smear should be about 75–80% and the specificity at least 95%. A recently published cohort study (Boyes *et al.*, 1982), using the records of the British Columbia cervical cancer screening program between 1949 and 1969, indicated a specificity in excess of 99% for patients reported to have carcinoma *in situ* or worse and a sensitivity of 78%. Further examination of the 22% false-negative cases indicated that 50% of these were due to errors in specimen collection, since, on review of the smears, no abnormal cells were found to be present. The other 50% of this group can be classified as laboratory error, since, on review, abnormal cells were found which had either been missed on the original screening or misinterpreted. The importance of adequate collection techniques in order to reduce the incidence of false-negative smears caused by nonsampling of the lesion was emphasized earlier in this chapter. A number of techniques are available to help reduce the laboratory error component of the false-negative cases.

One of the most useful techniques for detecting false-negative cases in a screening program is the rescreening of previously reported negative smears at the time a positive smear is first reported. This, of course, requires a record- and slide-filing system which will allow easy recall of previously examined material.

Another important quality control technique is the correlation of subsequently obtained biopsy information, either from colposcopic examination, cone biopsy, or hysterectomy specimens from patients, with previously reported abnormal cytology.

A valuable and reliable technique of internal quality control which has been called *positive discrimination performance* has recently been described (Rodney, 1974). This method is particularly valuable, since it does not depend upon input from an external source such as a repeat Pap smear or a biopsy procedure. Positive discrimination performance data are obtained by means of a simple mathematical formula in which the number of abnormal smears reported by a technologist represents the numerator and the number of normal and benign atypia smears is the denominator. Over a defined period of time, during which the number of smears read by each technologist is the same, it will be seen that technologists can be divided into three groups: those who find a higher than average number of significantly abnormal smears, those who find an average number, and those who find a lower than average number. Particular attention can then be paid to the work of those screeners who report a significantly lower than average number of abnormal smears, since it is in this group that one would expect to find a higher than average false-negative screening rate. Once these less effective screeners have been identified, appropriate educational efforts can be directed to improving their screening skills, with a resultant improvement in the overall performance of the laboratory. Since all significantly abnormal Pap smears should be reviewed by a senior technologist and pathologist, it is important to realize that positive discrimination performance must be obtained from the original cytotechnologist's reading and not from the final signout interpretation.

Whatever parameters are used to measure the performance of a cytology laboratory, it is most important that those who work in the program fully understand that quality control is not a punitive technique, but an essential component of any laboratory service. A key element of the quality control program is the effective communication of program results to those working in the laboratory as part of an ongoing educational process.

Continuing education on a regular basis is particularly important in a screening program in which many normal or negative smears are seen, in order to maintain interest in the job and to allow both cytotechnologists and cytopathologists to maintain a state-of-the-art knowledge in their field of expertise.

When abnormal smears are signed out by more senior staff, feedback to technologists at all levels is most important in the maintenance of uniform diagnostic criteria and provides an essential educational experience. In addition, attendance at formal lectures, informal seminars, and at local and national meetings should be encouraged whenever possible.

In the final analysis, the aim of the Pap smear screening program is to provide the physician with the most reliable information available on which further diagnostic procedures and treatment can be based. The end result of the program is improved patient care.

REFERENCES

Alderson, M., Correa, P., Ford, J., Jensen, O. M., Kupka, K., Miller, A. B., Muir, C. S., Nectou, J., Waterhouse, J. A., and Young, J. L. (1983). Letter to the editor. Cervical intra-epithelial neoplasia. *Lancet* **1,** 1166.

Anderson, W. A., and Gunn, S. A. (1965). A comparative study of patient obtained irrigation and physician obtained aspiration and cervical scrape smears in cancer of the cervix. *Ca—Cancer J. Clin.* **15,** 158–160.

Ayre, J. E. (1947). Selective cytology smear for diagnosis of cancer. *Am. J. Obstet. Gynecol.* **53,** 609–617.

Ayre, J. E. (1952). "Cancer Cytology of the Uterus." Churchill, London.

Babes, A. (1982). Diagnostic du cancer du col uterin par les frottis. *Presse Med.* **36,** 451–454.

Benedet, J. L., Boyes, D. A., Nichols, T. M., and Millner, M. (1976). Colposcopic evaluation of patients with abnormal cervical cytology. *Br. J. Obstet. Gynaecol.* **83,** 177–182.

Benedet, J. L., Anderson, G. H., Simpson, M. L., and Shaw, D. (1982). Colposcopy, conization and hysterectomy practices: A current perspective. *Obstet. Gynecol.* **60,** 539–545.

Benedet, J. L., and Anderson, G. H. (1981). Cervical intraepithelial neoplasia in British Columbia. *Gynecol. Oncol.* **12,** 280–291.

Boyes, D. A., Morrison, B., Knox, E. G., Draper, G. J., and Miller, A. B. (1982). A cohort study of cervical cancer screening in British Columbia. *Clin. Invest. Med.* **5,** 1–29.

Buckley, C. H., Butler, E. B., and Fox, H. (1982). Cervical intraepithelial neoplasia. *J. Clin. Pathol.* **35,** 1–13.

Davis, H. J. (1962). The irrigation smear: Accuracy in detection of cervical cancer. *Acta Cytol.* **6,** 459–467.

Frable, W. J., Gilbert, F. E., Inhorn, S. L., Kern, W. H., King, E. B., Melamed, M. R., Worth, A., and Feldman, M. (1975). Quality control in the cytology laboratory. *Cytotechnol. Bull.* **12,** Nos. 2 and 3.

Garite, T. J., and Feldman, M. J. (1978). An evaluation of cytologic sampling techniques: A comparative study. *Acta Cytol.* **22,** 83–85.

Gilbert, F. E., Hicklin, M. D., Inhorn, S. L., Koss, L. G., Naib, Z. M., Patten, S. F., Schwinn, C. P., Toll, M. W., and Wied, G. L. (1973). Standards of adequacy of cytologic examination of the female genital tract. *Am. J. Clin. Pathol.* **61,** 285–286.

Husain, O. A. L., Butler, E. B., Evans, D. M. D., Macgregor, J. E., and Yule, R. (1974). Quality control in cervical cytology. *J. Clin. Pathol.* **27,** 935–944.

Koss, L. G. (1963). Presidential address delivered at the 10th annual meeting of the American Society of Cytology. *Acta Cytol.* **7,** 143–145.

Koss, L. G. (1979). "Diagnostic Cytology and It's Histopathologic Bases," 3rd ed. Lippincott, Philadelphia, Pennsylvania.

Melamed, M. R. (1976). Quality control in the cytology laboratory. *Acta Cytol.* **20,** 203–206.

Melamed, M. R. (1981). Quality control in cytology laboratories. *Gynecol. Oncol.* **12,** 206–211.

Nunez, C., and Shapiro, S. P. (1981). Invasive carcinoma of the cervix after cryosurgery. *J. Reprod. Med.* **26,** 29–34.

Papanicolaou, G. M. (1942). A new procedure for staining vaginal smears. *Science* **95,** 438–439.

Papanicolaou, G. M., and Traut, H. F. (1941). The diagnostic value of vaginal smears in carcinoma of the uterus. *Am. J. Obstet. Gynecol.* **42,** 193–206.

Richart, R. M. (1967). Natural history of cervical intraepithelial neoplasia. *Clin. Obstet. Gynecol.* **10,** 748–784.

Richart, R. M. (1979). Screening techniques for cervical neoplasia. *Clin. Obstet. Gynecol.* **22,** 701–712.

Richart, R. M., and Vaillant, H. W. (1965). The irrigation smears false negative rates in a population with cervical neoplasia. *JAMA, J. Am. Med. Assoc.* **192,** 199–202.

Rodney, M. B. (1974). A new way to review cytology performance. *Lab. Manage.* **12,** 56–59.

Sevin, B., Ford, J. H., Girtanner, R. D., Hoskins, W. J., Ng, A. B. P., Nordquist, S. R. B., and Averette, E. A. (1979). Invasive cancer of the cervix after cryosurgery. *Obstet. Gynecol.* **53,** 465–471.

Task Force (1976). Cervical cancer screening programs. (Dept. of National Health and Welfare Task Force Report.) *Can. Med. Assoc. J.* **114,** 1003–1033.

Task Force (1982). "Cervical Cancer Screening Programs 1982." Minister of National Health and Welfare, Ottawa, Canada.

Townsend, D. E., Richart, R. M., Marks, E., and Nielsen, J. (1981). Invasive cancer following out patient evaluation and therapy for cervical disease. *Obstet. Gynecol.* **57,** 145–149.

7

Pulmonary Cytology in Lung Cancer Screening

LEWIS B. WOOLNER AND ROBERT S. FONTANA

I.	Introduction	105
II.	Sputum Cytology Test: Technical Aspects	106
III.	Processing of the Sputum Specimen	107
IV.	Morning "Pooled" Spontaneous-Cough Sputum	108
V.	Adequacy of the Specimen	108
VI.	Preparation of Slides	109
VII.	Microscopic Screening	109
VIII.	Cytologic Reports	110
	A. Negative Results on Examination and Squamous Metaplasia	110
	B. Abnormal Cytologic Findings	111
IX.	Management of Subjects with an Abnormal Sputum Specimen	112
X.	Discussion	114
XI.	Sensitivity and Specificity	117
XII.	To Test or Not to Test?	118
	References	119

I. INTRODUCTION

The detection of presymptomatic lung cancer is currently feasible with only two tests: pulmonary cytology and chest roentgenography. A program to assess the usefulness of these tests in screening for early lung cancer was established in 1969 by the National Cancer Institute (NCI). An NCI Cooperative Early Lung Cancer Group was formally established in 1972 (NCI, 1979). The three participating institutions are the Johns Hopkins Medical Institutions, the Mayo Foundation, and the Memorial Sloan-Kettering Cancer Center. All three institutions are conducting long-term, randomized clinical trials designed to determine

ISBN 0-12-496720-5

whether screening of high-risk populations by 4-monthly cytologic examinations of sputum and either yearly or 4-monthly chest roentgenography can reduce mortality from lung cancer in comparison with that in a control population tested less intensively. In the Mayo screening program, known as the *Mayo Lung Project,* the subjects were scheduled to have the two tests every 4 months for 6 years (Fontana *et al.*, 1975).

This chapter on pulmonary cytology as a screening test is based on data derived during a 10-year period of participation by the authors in the Mayo Lung Project. Technical procedures relating to the use of the test will be described, and problems in microscopic interpretation and reporting will be presented. Finally, an assessment of the test as a screening device will be attempted.

II. SPUTUM CYTOLOGY TEST: TECHNICAL ASPECTS

Success in pulmonary cytology testing, either for large-scale screening programs or for routine diagnostic workups, depends largely on the quality of specimens examined and on the excellence of preparation and staining techniques. Careful initial instructions to subjects participating in a screening program are therefore mandatory. It should not be assumed that the subjects know what sputum is, what amount of sputum is required, or what may be the best time for collection of the specimen.

At the time of initial screening, each subject in the Mayo Lung Project had the sputum cytology test explained, with emphasis on the necessity of obtaining material from deep within the bronchial tree. The following written instructions for collection of a "pooled" specimen of spontaneously expectorated sputum were also provided.

Instructions for Collecting Three-Day
"Pooled" Specimen of Sputum

1. The desired material for testing is called *sputum.* (Sputum is secretion coughed up from the bronchial tubes and lungs, in contrast to saliva, or "spit," which accumulates in the mouth.)

2. The best time for collecting sputum is probably early in the morning just after waking. A deep cough effort at this time is often very productive. Before coughing up sputum, first clear the mouth by spitting out or washing out saliva and food particles. Then cough deeply and vigorously to raise sputum from the lungs. All that can be raised at this time should be put into the collection bottle. This procedure is repeated each morning for 3 days using the same container.

3. *For those with scanty sputum,* it may take 15–30 minutes of intermittent coughing attempts in the morning to produce enough material. If you have difficulty, sputum coughed up at any time of the day may also be used. Try to collect as much of this sputum raised during the day as you can. Avoid the natural tendency to swallow it. Keep your sputum container in a convenient place, if possible, to aid in this collection.

4. Always keep the cap screwed on tightly when not coughing and when you mail in your specimen. Shake the bottle occasionally to mix the sputum with the preservative. [From NCI, 1979.]

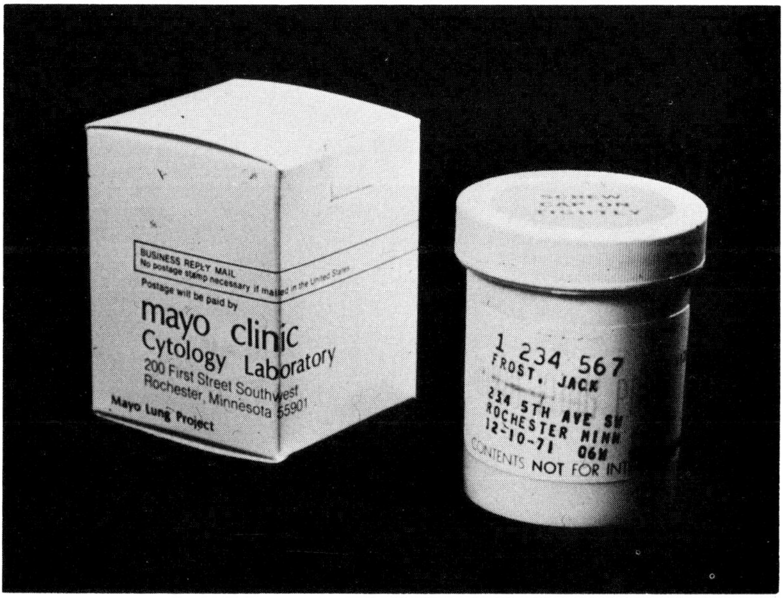

Fig. 1. Mayo Lung Project: screw-top plastic bottle for collecting a specimen of sputum and preaddressed mailing carton for returning the specimen.

A wide-mouthed, opaque, screw-top plastic bottle with a volume of 120 ml proved to be best for collecting the specimen. The bottle, which contained a small amount of alcohol solution as preservative, was mailed to the subject before each scheduled test (Fig. 1).

III. PROCESSING OF THE SPUTUM SPECIMEN

After the acquisition of a satisfactory specimen of sputum, the next step involves the preparation of slides from the sputum prior to staining. Two techniques are available (Miller and Woolner, 1981).

The older technique, which was used in the early days (1940s) of sputum cytology testing, involves simple smearing of multiple samplings of discolored areas of the sputum specimen. Four slides are routinely prepared from each specimen. This technique is still satisfactory for laboratories that process relatively few specimens. Some laboratories have used it in combination with a process of paraffin embedding and sectioning of formalin-fixed sputum.

In the 1960s, a homogenization or blending technique for processing sputum was introduced by Saccomanno *et al.* (1963). In this technique, sputum is collected in a special fixative (50% alcohol and 2% Carbowax), and is then homogenized in a commercial blender and centrifuged. After centrifugation, slides are prepared from the concentrated, resuspended sediment. The waxy fixative permits the slides to be air-dried before staining and prevents significant loss of cellular detail.

The Saccomanno technique is the preferred method of processing specimens in a program of screening for lung cancer. It provides slides with an even distribution of cells, the concentration of which can be controlled by the initial amount of sediment used. The uniformity of processing facilitates the comparison of slides prepared from additional sputum samples obtained from the same subject. It also enables one to compare sputum specimens from other laboratories. The adequacy of a given sputum specimen, which is based on the number of pigmented macrophages observed, is readily determined on homogenized specimens. Abnormal squamous cells, which are the essential diagnostic elements in screening for roentgenographically inapparent (occult) lung cancer, stand out vividly and colorfully in Papanicolaou-stained smears prepared from the concentrated, homogenized material.

IV. MORNING "POOLED" SPONTANEOUS-COUGH SPUTUM

For routine diagnostic pulmonary cytology, it has been demonstrated that multiple samples of sputum are more valuable than a single specimen (Miller and Woolner, 1976). Historically, an adequate sputum cytologic examination was one performed on three or more specimens of sputum collected on consecutive mornings.

In the Mayo Lung Project screening program, a homogenized "pooled" collection of sputum was used instead of numerous single specimens. Vigorous coughing and expectoration were carried out by the subject on 3 successive mornings, and the sputum collected each day was deposited in the same bottle. This method provided results that were comparable to those obtained by examination of three separate specimens, and it significantly reduced the cost of the procedure.

V. ADEQUACY OF THE SPECIMEN

A sputum specimen is considered satisfactory or unsatisfactory by the number of pigmented macrophages observed on the stained slides. The presence of these intra-alveolar "dust cells" indicates that the material has come from the lower bronchial tree.

Experience in the Mayo Lung Project has indicated that, among cigarette-smoking men 45 years of age or older, a satisfactory sputum specimen will be obtained from slightly more than 90% (Fontana *et al.*, 1972). In the initial screening of nearly 11,000 subjects, 5.8% either could not or did not submit an initial sputum specimen. Among those who did submit a specimen, the first specimen was satisfactory in 96.8%; this was equivalent to 91.2% of the subjects in the initial screening. In an additional 1.6%, specimens were found to be satisfactory on repeated testing. Thus, 98.4% of the subjects who submitted a sputum specimen, or 92.7% of all subjects screened, had satisfactory specimens after one or more tests were attempted.

When little or no sputum can be produced spontaneously or when microscopic examination of the slides indicates that the specimen is unsatisfactory, an induced sputum specimen may be obtained. Sputum induction involves inhalation of ultrasonic or heated, hypertonic aerosols. A variety of nebulizers and aerosol solutions may be used. The patient is instructed to breathe the aerosolized solution for 10 to 20 minutes and periodically attempt to cough. The sputum is collected during the test. At the conclusion of the procedure, the patient is given a collection bottle and is instructed to deposit in it all material coughed up during the remainder of the day and during the following morning (NCI, 1979).

VI. PREPARATION OF SLIDES

Careful preparation and staining of the sputum specimen is the second prerequisite of a successful cytologic screening test. The mailed-in 3-morning pooled sputum specimen is processed according to the homogenization technique by a specially trained cytopreparatory technician. Six slides are made from each specimen. Staining is performed according to the Papanicolaou technique, with careful attention to quality control of the staining process (Miller and Woolner, 1976). It is recommended that each day the supervisor of the cytology laboratory check the quality of the stains being used and the microscopic appearance of the finished product.

VII. MICROSCOPIC SCREENING

Any laboratory in which a sputum cytology screening program is conducted should be staffed by a cytopathologist who has special expertise in pulmonary cytology, by a supervisor who has experience with cytology procedures, and by certified cytotechnologists in sufficient number to perform the routine scanning of slides and marking of any suspicious areas. Microscopic screening and marking of abnormal areas with dots of ink are carried out on four of the six slides prepared from each specimen of sputum. The remaining two slides are held in reserve and are used to provide additional information on specimens in which a significant abnormality is noted. Internal quality control is facilitated by having numerous cytotechnologists examine each specimen; ideally, each of the four slides from a single specimen should be screened by a different cytotechnologist.

All specimens for which there are dotted slides representing abnormalities and at least 10% of all specimens for which results are negative should be reviewed by a senior cytotechnologist or supervisor. All marked slides should be further studied by the cytology supervisor, who has a key role in the diagnostic procedure. He or she makes a preliminary judgment on the severity of any abnormality noted and refers all specimens showing more than a slight degree of atypia to the cytopathologist for final diagnosis. Special attention is given to specimens from any subject for whom prior cytologic abnormalities have been reported.

VIII. CYTOLOGIC REPORTS

The cytologic classification used in the Mayo Lung Project is shown in Table I. Certain comments on problems encountered in the microscopic examination and the classification of sputum are pertinent.

A. Negative Results on Examination and Squamous Metaplasia

In a lung cancer screening program involving middle-aged and older men who are heavy cigarette smokers, the great majority of sputum specimens will be satisfactory and the results will be negative on microscopic examination. As noted, a satisfactory specimen is one that contains alveolar macrophages, and their presence is an indication that the specimen originated from the lower bronchial tree. An unsatisfactory specimen usually consists of watery saliva in which macrophages are absent. A specimen may also be unsatisfactory because it contains purulent material or extraneous matter such as food and vegetable cells. Repeated efforts to obtain specimens after appropriate corrective measures are indicated in such instances.

TABLE I

Mayo Lung Project: Cytologic Classification

Specimen unsatisfactory
Negative result
Negative result and squamous metaplasia
Atypical squamous metaplasia
Slight atypia
Moderate atypia
Marked atypia
Carcinoma cells present (World Health Organization classification)

In addition to alveolar macrophages, a normal sputum specimen may contain desquamated bronchial epithelial cells in various stages of degeneration. Occasionally, it may contain metaplastic squamous cells, which are most easily recognized in bronchial brush specimens or bronchial secretions, where their presence provides clear proof of a metaplastic process within the bronchial tree. Metaplastic squamous cells may also be detected in sputum specimens, although identification is more difficult because these cells tend to resemble squamous cells from the upper respiratory tract. However, residual cytologic evidence of columnar bronchial epithelial cells within or at the margin of clumps of squamous cells is indicative of metaplasia. Squamous metaplasia, whether detected in sputum or in bronchial material (brushings, secretions, or biopsies), should not be regarded as a significant cytologic observation, and its presence has neither neoplastic nor prognostic significance.

B. Abnormal Cytologic Findings

In screening for early lung cancer, cytology makes its contribution largely in the detection of roentgenographically occult cancers. These cancers are almost always intrabronchial carcinomas of the squamous cell type, arising in the subsegmental or more proximal "hilar" bronchi (Woolner *et al.*, 1981). In contrast, roentgenographically visible early lung cancers tend to appear as small peripheral tumors, which are usually associated with negative results on sputum cytologic examinations. It follows that with sputum specimens in a screening program for detection of early lung cancer, the microscopic findings of diagnostic importance are largely limited to cells of the squamous type—either frankly cancerous cells or cells showing varying degrees of squamous cell "atypia."

Since its development, the specialty of cytology has had to deal with the problem of "atypical" versus "frankly cancerous" cells in material submitted from various organs in the body, the lung being no exception. In the cervix, abnormal squamous cells lacking some of the necessary cytologic criteria for cancer have been referred to as *dysplastic,* and the abnormal, supposedly precancerous condition has been designated *dysplasia.* In the lung, the term *squamous cell atypia* has been used to describe squamous cells with varying degrees of abnormality that fail to fulfill all the criteria for carcinoma. In such instances, the precise pathologic change in the bronchial epithelium is difficult to determine because of the complexity and relative inaccessibility of the bronchial tree. It is unfortunate, but true, that unlike the uterine cervix, one cannot "cone" the lung.

Frankly cancerous squamous cells in the sputum can be diagnosed readily. Although much variation in the number and quality of abnormal cells may be encountered, classic squamous cancer cells are large and have enlarged, hyperchromatic nuclei and an altered nucleocytoplasmic ratio. In addition, well-preserved cells may show a nuclear pattern consisting of coarse chromatin, irregularity of shape, and wrinkling of the membrane. With the Papanicolaou stain, cytoplasmic orangophilia, the hallmark of this type of cancer cell, is usually a striking feature.

In a sputum specimen that contains diagnostic cancer cells, there are usually additional abnormal cells showing atypia—that is, cells demonstrating some of the above-mentioned abnormalities, but to a lesser degree. Because there is a spectrum of cellular alteration, and because the number of abnormal cells varies from specimen to specimen, accurate diagnosis requires experience and judgment.

In our practice, the term *marked atypia* is used for specimens suggestive of cancer, but in which either the number of abnormal cells or the degree of nuclear change is not considered fully diagnostic of cancer. Specimens showing lesser degrees of cellular change are diagnosed as showing moderate or slight atypia. *Slight atypia,* representing minimal cellular or nuclear alteration, is commonly diagnosed in specimens from heavy smokers but, as with squamous metaplasia, the changes are not considered of diagnostic or prognostic importance.

Moderate atypia denotes an intermediate degree of suspicion of cancer on the part of the cytologist. It is the equivalent of the Papanicolaou class III in cervical cytologic terminology. Such a diagnosis, especially when encountered repeatedly, can become a particularly difficult and frustrating problem in management.

IX. MANAGEMENT OF SUBJECTS WITH AN ABNORMAL SPUTUM SPECIMEN

The action that is taken after detection of an abnormality on the sputum specimen depends on the cytologist's acuity of suspicion. In general, abnormalities at both extremes of the spectrum are most easily managed. Abnormalities other than squamous metaplasia or slight atypia should be confirmed by repeated cytologic examination. This is true whether the initial abnormality is moderate atypia, marked atypia, or frank squamous cancer. Because of the importance of repeated examination in problem cases, we have routinely requested two additional 3-morning pooled specimens rather than just one. Requests for additional sputum specimens are made in such a way as to avoid alarming the patient—simply by a communication indicating that more material is needed before the examination can be considered complete.

Mayo Lung Project subjects who submitted specimens that were reported as normal or as showing slight atypia were continued on the regular screening protocol. If a sputum specimen was unsatisfactory for any reason (insufficient alveolar phagocytes or excessive inflammatory cells), additional specimens were requested until a satisfactory one was submitted. If a satisfactory sputum specimen could not be produced spontaneously, an aerosol-induced specimen was requested whenever facilities for obtaining such specimens were available.

Any subject whose sputum specimen shows a significant cytologic abnormality, such as moderate atypia, marked atypia, or cancer cells, requires careful management. The crucial problem for the cytologist is to define the point at which there is sufficient cytologic evidence of cancer to justify initiation of localization procedures, which include examination of the upper respiratory tract and flexible fiberoptic bronchoscopy (Sanderson *et al.*, 1974).

In practice, localization has been recommended in cases showing cancer cells or marked atypia on initial and subsequent specimens. It should be emphasized that if there is convincing cytologic evidence of cancer, a negative result on a single bronchoscopic examination does not preclude the presence of an occult carcinoma. In such situations, a meticulous repeat bronchoscopic evaluation with the use of general anesthesia is indicated (Sanderson *et al.*, 1974).

Among the somewhat less impressive cytologic abnormalities, there are various combinations of moderate and marked atypia which may be deemed sufficient for a recommendation for localization. For subjects who have more than one sputum specimen exhibiting moderate atypia but in whom cytologic evidence alone is insufficient for recommending localization, careful follow-up is essential and should include frequently repeated sputum examinations. If the evidence for cancer is equivocal, clinical judgment may dictate routine inspection of the larynx and bronchial tree rather than a detailed fiberoptic bronchoscopic examination with general anesthesia.

As might have been expected, the cytologic detection of occult lung cancer in the Mayo screening program has resulted in a number of variations and unexpected findings. Experience with proven roentgenographically occult cancers that were detected during the course of rescreening of a population previously considered to be free of cancer has shown that cytologic abnormalities may develop either abruptly or gradually. Some cases, after a series of negative results, show a sudden transformation to marked atypia or frank carcinoma. On the other hand, it is also possible for a case to evolve more slowly from a moderate level of suspicion to one showing marked atypia or frank carcinoma.

Yet, not all reports of moderate atypia are significant. Such a finding on a single specimen may represent an isolated, unexplained episode in a series of otherwise negative results. If further test results remain negative, one may assume an inflammatory or other nonneoplastic basis for the single episode of atypia observed.

In general, some variation is to be expected with regard to subsequent specimens. Those specimens showing cancer cells or marked atypia tend to be confirmed on repeated examinations. However, not all specimens are of equal diagnostic value, particularly with regard to the number of abnormal cells per specimen. Subsequent specimens in cases of moderate atypia may vary greatly.

X. DISCUSSION

As a result of experience with the Mayo Lung Project over a 10-year period, several impressions have evolved concerning the use of sputum cytology as a screening test for early lung cancer (Woolner *et al.*, 1981). The test itself, involving the collection of a 3-morning pooled sputum specimen in an alcohol fixative, is relatively simple and inexpensive. It is a test without pain or discomfort. It is safe, and it can be repeated whenever additional information is required. Testing has been conducted successfully on a mail-in basis throughout the United States and Canada. Accurate results depend on the adequacy of the sputum collection and the quality control of the processing and microscopic examination of the specimens.

The Saccomanno homogenization technique with Papanicolaou staining is the most satisfactory examination for use in screening for occult lung cancer. The uniformity of preparation and staining so obtained facilitates comparison of one specimen with another from the same patient and comparison of slides from one laboratory with those of another.

A sputum cytologic screening program is best conducted in a clinical setting where there is close cooperation among the cytologist, chest physician, bronchoscopist, and surgeon. The problems involved in microscopic diagnosis from sputum specimens and the management of subjects with abnormal or atypical findings require special expertise on the part of the cytopathologist, who should be skilled in both pulmonary cytology and pulmonary pathology. Because of the many and varied problems associated with interpretation of sputum specimens and bronchoscopic localization, it is more efficient for the smaller laboratory to refer its sporadic cases of suspected occult lung cancer to a center with established routines and expertise.

The effectiveness of sputum cytology as a screening test for early lung cancer compared with that of chest roentgenography was evaluated in a preliminary report on the Mayo Lung Project (Woolner *et al.*, 1981). That study established that both chest roentgenography and sputum cytology are effective in the detection of early-stage lung cancer, that is, cancer categorized as stage I according to the classification of the American Joint Committee on Cancer (1983). The two tests are complementary, however, in that peripheral stage I cancer is detected with chest roentgenography, and intrabronchial squamous carcinoma involving the larger, centrally located bronchi is detected with sputum cytology. There is little overlap between the two tests.

The Mayo Lung Project also demonstrated a surprising distribution of the cell types of bronchogenic carcinoma within a high-risk group of cigarette-smoking men 45 years of age or older. Squamous cancer constituted 30% of the incidence cases—those cases of lung cancer detected in subjects whose initial screening results had been considered satisfactory and negative and who were offered 4-

monthly radiologic and cytologic rescreening. This figure was almost matched by a 26% incidence for small-cell carcinoma. The remaining cases were distributed between adenocarcinoma and large-cell carcinoma (Table II).

When one considers the various cell types of lung cancer, cytology contributes most to the early diagnosis of squamous cell carcinoma but is of little or no value in the early detection of adenocarcinoma or large-cell carcinoma. Cancers of these two cell types tend to be peripherally located, and stage I cancers of these cell types are usually positive roentgenographically but negative cytologically. Small-cell cancers, which tend to metastasize early and widely, are not amenable to screening by either modality.

Stage I squamous carcinoma of the lung appears to be equally distributed between occult intrabronchial cancers and radiographically visible peripheral tumors. The detection of the occult squamous cancer is the contribution of cytology to lung cancer screening (Table III).

Pathologic study of a large series of resected occult squamous bronchogenic carcinomas suggested that these tumors evolve through *in situ* and invasive stages, the latter passing from minimally invasive to progressively deeper penetration of the bronchial wall and extrabronchial tissues. On serial block sectioning, approximately a third of the occult cancers proved to be entirely *in situ*, a third showed minimal invasion into the mucosa up to the inner aspect of the bronchial cartilages, and a third showed deeper invasion through the entire thickness of the bronchial wall or into the extrabronchial tissues (Woolner and Farrow, 1982).

What proportion of lung cancer is occult, as defined herein? The evidence, based on the initial (prevalence) screen of the Mayo Lung Project and the subsequent 4-monthly (incidence) rescreening of those with presumably negative results on the initial screen, suggests that occult lung cancer makes up a rather small proportion of lung cancer as a whole (Woolner *et al.*, 1981).

TABLE II

Mayo Lung Project: Cell Types in 109 Incidence Cases[a]

	Patients	
Cell type	Number	Percentage
Squamous	33	30
Adenocarcinoma	26	24
Large cell	21	19
Small cell	28	26
Bronchial carcinoid	1	1
Total	109	100

[a] Modified from Woolner *et al.* (1981).

TABLE III

Mayo Lung Project: Squamous Carcinoma (31 Incidence Cases) by Stage and Location[a]

			Central (by size, cm)		Peripheral (by size, cm)	
Stage (AJCC)	Number of cases	Occult	< 2.5	> 3.0	1.4–2.5	3.0–5.5
I	24 (15)[b]	11 (11)	2		7 (2)	4 (2)
II	2 (1)			1 (1)		1
III	5[c] (2)			1		1

[a] Modified from Woolner *et al*. (1981).
[b] Numbers in parentheses are the number of cases with positive results on sputum cytology.
[c] Three cases were inoperable.

In the Mayo Lung Project group of cigarette-smoking men 45 years of age or older, squamous carcinoma (roentgenographically visible or occult) constituted no more than a third of the total number of incidence cancers. Approximately half of the cancers were central, occult, and intrabronchial, and the remainder were peripheral, radiologically visible, and parenchymal. Some of the peripheral cancers were also positive cytologically, but these peripheral squamous cancers were detected and localized more efficiently with chest roentgenography than with sputum cytology.

The best estimate of the frequency of occult lung cancer, based on the Mayo Lung Project data, is that it constitutes no more than half of all squamous cancers; therefore, less than 20% of all cases of bronchogenic carcinoma are occult.

XI. SENSITIVITY AND SPECIFICITY

There are two ways of addressing the sensitivity and specificity of the sputum cytology test as a screening device for presymptomatic lung cancer. The first way is to evaluate the test as a part of a *screening program* that also includes chest roentgenography. Considered in this context, cytology should be related to the *totality* of lung cancer detected by *both* screening procedures. This aspect of the sensitivity and specificity of sputum cytology is discussed in Chapter 20.

However, as has been noted previously, sputum cytology contributes to screening for early lung cancer primarily by detecting *roentgenographically occult squamous cancer* located in the subsegmental or larger central bronchi (Woolner *et al.*, 1981). The earliest manifestations of peripheral squamous cancers are detectable roentgenographically. Considered from this perspective, it might be argued that it is more appropriate to ask, how sensitive is the sputum test in detecting central, occult intrabronchial squamous cell cancer?

This restricted application of the term *sensitivity* creates significant problems. Sensitivity, which would then be defined as the ratio of detected occult cancers to the total number of occult cancers, is difficult to determine in this context. There is no way of accurately measuring the denominator—that is, of determining how many such cases are present but undetected in a screened population. How does one determine that a cytology report is falsely negative when the chest roentgenogram is normal? Centrally located, roentgenographically visible lung cancers for which sputum findings are negative (presumably a genuine false-negative result) have been observed in the Mayo screening program, but uncommonly. Failure to recommend localization procedures when there are sputum findings of moderate atypia on cytologic examination followed by the development of a roentgenographically visible cancer might also be regarded as a falsely negative sputum test result. The various diagnostic implications of the term *moderate atypia* have already been described, and this category represents an inherently difficult area in cytologic diagnosis.

Specificity, defined as the extent to which a test will correctly distinguish persons free of disease, is also difficult to apply to screening for roentgenographically occult lung cancer by sputum cytology alone. Here, the problem lies both in the definition of a *disease-free* individual and in the definition of a *negative* test result. If one considers only a report of cancer cells as nonnegative, a very high specificity is achieved. This specificity decreases when reports of marked atypia, and especially moderate atypia, are included in the nonnegative category. The diagnosis of moderate atypia, in particular, varies greatly from laboratory to laboratory and is hardly subject to precise and readily reproducible criteria.

XII. TO TEST OR NOT TO TEST?

Has sputum cytology a place in a program of screening for early lung cancer? Should the test be included in a physician's examination of an individual patient believed to be at high risk for lung cancer?

In answering the first question, one balances the relatively small number of occult lung cancers that can be detected by means of sputum cytology against the high probability of curing such cancers after surgical resection. If large-scale screening of high-risk groups is found to be beneficial, it would appear advisable to include both chest roentgenography and sputum cytology, although admittedly, the majority of early cases will be detected with roentgenography.

In considering the application of sputum cytology to the detection of asymptomatic lung cancer in the individual high-risk patient, the physician is addressing another matter. In such cases, it should be remembered that when subjected to careful pathologic scrutiny, two-thirds of all diagnosed and resected occult lung cancers have already begun to invade the bronchial wall. Among those cancers with deeper extrabronchial invasion, two-thirds are already associated with involvement of the peribronchial lymph nodes in the region of the tumor. Allowing such cases to progress to a roentgenographically visible stage, as would be likely in the absence of cytologic testing, would tend to lessen the chances of success of resection for cure.

ACKNOWLEDGMENTS

This investigation was supported in part by Research Grant CN-53886 from the National Cancer Institute, National Institutes of Health, Public Health Service.

REFERENCES

American Joint Committee on Cancer (1983). Lung. *In* "Manual for Staging of Cancer" (O. H. Beahrs and M. H. Myers, eds.), 2nd ed., pp. 99–105. Lippincott, Philadelphia, Pennsylvania.

Fontana, R. S., Sanderson, D. R., Miller, W. E., Woolner, L. B., Taylor, W. F., and Uhlenhopp, M. A. (1972). The Mayo Lung Project: Preliminary report of "early cancer detection" phase. *Cancer* **30,** 1373–1382.

Fontana, R. S., and Sanderson, D. R., Woolner, L. B., Miller, W. E., Bernatz, P. E., Payne, W. S., and Taylor, W. F. (1975). The Mayo Lung Project for early detection and localization of bronchogenic carcinoma: A status report. *Chest* **67,** 511–522.

Miller, F., and Woolner, L. B. (1976). Specimen preparation for material from the respiratory tract. *In* "Compendium on Diagnostic Cytology" (G. L. Wied, L. G. Koss, and J. W. Reagan, eds.), 4th ed., pp. 275–298. Tutorials of Cytology, Chicago, Illinois.

National Cancer Institute, Cooperative Early Lung Cancer Group (NCI) (1979). "Manual of Procedures," 2nd ed. (NIH Publ. No. 79–1972). U.S. Govt. Printing Office, Washington, D.C.

Saccomanno, G., Saunders, R. P., Ellis, H., Archer, V. E., Wood, B. G., and Beckler, P. A. (1963). Concentration of carcinoma or atypical cells in sputum. *Acta Cytol.* **7,** 305–310.

Sanderson, D. R., Fontana, R. S., Woolner, L. B., Bernatz, P. E., and Payne, W. S. (1974). Bronchoscopic localization of radiographically occult lung cancer. *Chest* **65,** 608–612.

Woolner, L. B., and Farrow, G. M. (1982). Mayo Lung Project: Pathological findings in occult bronchogenic carcinoma detected through lung cancer screening. *Clin. Oncol.* **1,** 513–526.

Woolner, L. B., Fontana, R. S., Sanderson, D. R., Miller, W. E., Muhm, J. R., Taylor, W. F., and Uhlenhopp, M. A. (1981). Mayo Lung Project: Evaluation of lung cancer screening through December 1979. *Mayo Clin. Proc.* **56,** 544–555.

8

Screening Tests for Bladder Cancer

WILLIAM H. KERN

I. Introduction 121
II. Cytologic Screening 122
A. Methodology 122
B. Cytologic Examination 123
C. Classification and Nomenclature 129
D. Accuracy 131
E. Screening Programs 133
III. Other Screening Procedures 134
A. Occult Blood 134
B. Flow Cytometry 135
C. Tumor Markers 136
III. Summary 137
References 138

I. INTRODUCTION

The American Cancer Society estimates that there will be 40,000 new cases of bladder cancer in the United States in 1985 and 10,800 deaths from this disease (Silverberg, 1985). Since the prognosis of low-grade bladder carcinomas is good with conservative therapy (Hellsten *et al.*, 1981), and since even high-grade and invasive tumors have an improved survival rate after radical cystectomy (Skinner, 1980), early diagnosis in a presymptomatic state of this disease should be associated with improved survival rates. A number of possible screening procedures for this purpose have been evaluated and reviewed (Lent, 1975; Lessing, 1978; Betkerur *et al.*, 1980). Of these, urinary cytology remains the primary test for bladder cancer (Betkerur *et al.*, 1980; de Voogt, 1980). The currently available methods will be reviewed in this chapter.

ISBN 0-12-496720-5

II. CYTOLOGIC SCREENING

A. Methodology

For a screening program, voided rather than catheterized urine should be used. In order to preserve the cells, the urine is best collected in an equal amount of fixative. A solution of 50% alcohol is suitable. At our institution, the patient is asked to void directly into a plastic 200 milliliter specimen container that is half filled with 50% alcohol. Ethyl alcohol is preferable, but isopropyl or denatured alcohol is acceptable. Urothelial cells remain well preserved for processing for several days, regardless of whether the urine is collected after hydration or not, or during the morning hours or later during the day. First-morning voided specimens appear to have poorer cellular preservation and should not be used. Urine osmolality does not significantly influence cell preservation (Kern and Bales, 1969), but a low pH is desirable and the ingestion of 1 gram of vitamin C at bedtime before the examination has been recommended (Pearson *et al.*, 1981). This is not practical for screening purposes.

Filter preparations provide greater cellularity than sediment smears (Kern *et al.*, 1966) and are therefore preferred. Our own procedure for urine specimen preparation is as follows:

Specimens are collected in 200-milliliter cups containing 100 milliliters of 50% isopropyl alcohol. An equal volume of urine should be added.

Three filters are prepared, two Nuclepore and one Millipore. Eight-micron filters are used. They allow red blood cells and bacteria to pass through in order not to obscure cellular detail.

A. Nuclepore filter preparation

1. Wet glass grid with saline.
2. Place filter on grid.
3. Place funnel on grid with clamp.
4. Mix specimen well and pour into funnel. Use approximately one-third of specimen per filter; stop when filtration slows.
5. Break suction before entire specimen has run the through filter so that the filter is not permitted to dry.
6. Remove filter and clip to glass slide which has been identified with specimen accession number, and immediately place in 95% ethyl alcohol. Fix for 20–30 minutes.
7. Stain by Papanicolaou method (Koss, 1979a).
8. After staining, remove filter from slide, turn cell side down on slide, and blot dry. (Filter will be slightly opaque when completely dry.)
9. With slide on a flat, even surface, rapidly flood filter with chloroform and cover with a *glass* Petri dish to allow the filter to evaporate slowly.

10. When filter is completely dry, dip the slide into xylene and coverslip. If filter dries cloudy, reflood it and allow it to dry again. This should remove the cloudiness.

B. Millipore filter preparation

1. Identify the filter with the specimen accession number written clearly at one end of the filter.
2. Expand the filter by submerging it in a Petri dish of 95% ethyl alcohol for at least 10 seconds. Unexpanded filters will cause a hill-and-valley effect when screening.
3. Filter in the same manner as with Nuclepore filters, starting with step 1.
4. Stain according to Millipore staining procedure (Danos and Keebler, 1977).

Two Nuclepore or Millipore filter preparations should be examined. At our laboratory, we currently prepare and examine two Nuclepore and one Millipore filter because, using the described cytopreparatory process, the Nuclepore filters have a clear background which facilitates the examination, but the Millipore filters are often slightly more cellular. Their background, however, is granular and darker. Either preparation is perfectly adequate, and the choice is one of individual preference.

B. Cytologic Examination

Transitional epithelial cells are present in at least small numbers in all urine specimens, and squamous cells are present in many (Kern, 1983a). Normal urine is often sparsely cellular, but at least 100 urothelial cells can be found on two filter slides in practically all cases. Screening can be performed rapidly, although there may be considerable variation in nuclear and cell size. The average nuclear diameter of urothelial cells is 7.6 μm, and the average cell diameter is 19.6 μm, as determined by measurements of 4340 cells. The range in cell diameter is from 9 to 40 μm (Kern and Bales, 1969). In spite of this marked variation in cell size, the nuclei are fairly uniform, round, or slightly irregular (Fig. 1). The cells are occasionally arranged in clusters. The cytoplasm may be opaque but is often vacuolated, even in cells that are well preserved. Such presumably artifactual vacuolization of transitional cells is also evident in biopsy specimens that were promptly fixed after they were obtained (Kern, 1971). Planimetric measurements of 500 nuclei of normal transitional cells showed a mean nuclear area of 36 μm^2, with a range of 11 to 89 μm^2 (Table I) (Kern, 1975). Other cellular elements in urine from patients without significant urinary tract disease include readily recognizable superficial or intermediate-type squamous cells, found more commonly in women than in men, and columnar cells that may originate from areas of the bladder that occasionally are lined by columnar epithelium, or from the

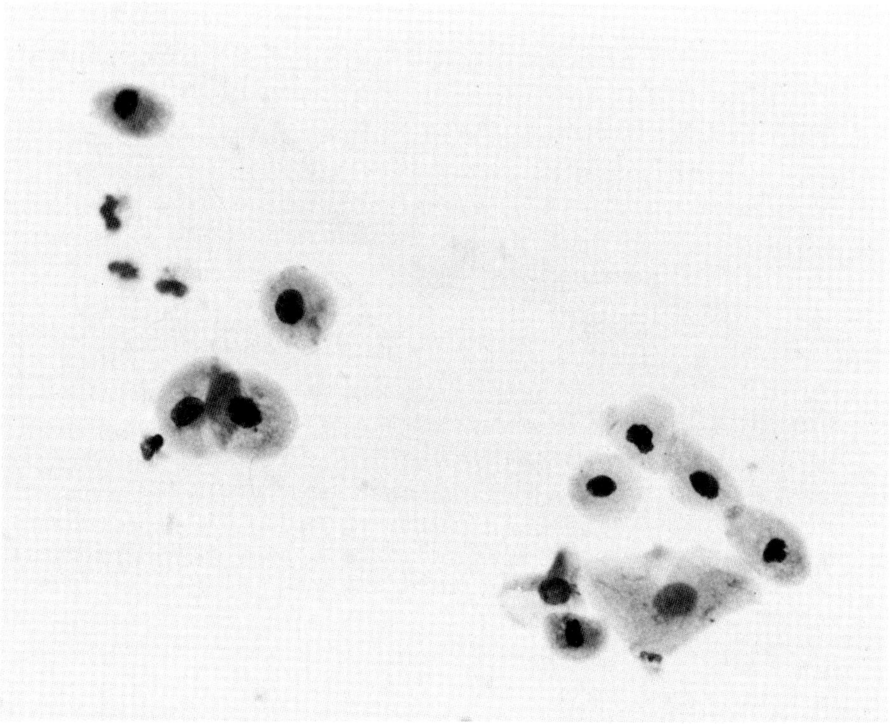

Fig. 1. Urine with normal transitional epithelial cells, a squamous cell, and few leukocytes. Nuclepore filter, Papanicolaou stain. 300X.

urethra, prostate, or, rarely, the seminal vesicles. Histiocytes are found in inflammatory conditions and resemble histiocytes in other cytologic specimens. They have indistinct cell borders, a foamy cytoplasm, and eccentric, lobed, or bean-shaped nuclei, and may be difficult to differentiate from degenerated transitional epithelial cells. They should not be confused with malignant cells.

The cytologic appearance of cells that are exfoliated from poorly and moderately differentiated transitional cell carcinomas is strikingly different from that of normal or even reactive cells. Most importantly, there is considerable nuclear enlargement. The average nuclear diameter of carcinoma cells from grade III or IV tumors is 12–15 μm, as compared to 7.6 μm for normal cells and 10 μm for reactive or well-differentiated tumor cells (Kern *et al.*, 1968). Based on planimetric measurements, the mean nuclear area of papillary transitional cell carcinomas, grade II, is 78 μm^2 and that of grade III and IV carcinomas is 90 μm^2 (Table 1).

TABLE I

Cell and Nuclear Size Determined by Planimetry

Cytopathologic classification	Mean cell area/range	Mean nuclear area/range	N/C ratio
Normal (501 cells and nuclei)	341 μm^2 (75–1434)	36 μm^2 (11–89)	12
Benign-reactive (908 cells, 1328 nuclei)	181 μm^2 (56–1554)	52 μm^2 (11–311)	34
Papillary transitional cell carcinoma, grade I (2148 cells, 3272 nuclei)	169 μm^2 (45–2663)	54 μm^2 (11–534)	37
Papillary transitional cell carcinoma, grade II (1352 cells, 1965 nuclei)	217 μm^2 (42–4693)	78 μm^2 (11–726)	42
Transitional cell carcinoma, grades III and IV (1061 cells, 1389 nuclei)	235 μm^2 (56–1070)	90 μm^2 (17–450)	42

The qualitative nuclear characteristics of malignant cells also include a greater irregularity of the nuclei, characterized by considerable variation in nuclear size as compared to normal cells. The nuclei are more hyperchromatic than normal or reactive cells, and the nucleoli are large, multiple, and generally more prominent. Sixty percent of moderately differentiated and three-fourths of poorly differentiated carcinoma cells have a coarsely granular nucleoplasm, without the clear zones often seen in reactive cells (Fig. 2). The nuclear/cytoplasmic ratio is increased (Table I). Many of these moderately or poorly differentiated carcinomas are ulcerated, and necrotic debris and inflammatory cells are therefore seen. This material may somewhat obscure the cytologic pattern, but in most cases numerous malignant cells are present. We found 1000 or more neoplastic cells in 60% of moderately or poorly differentiated carcinomas on two Nuclepore filter preparations in our own case material (Kern, 1975). This means that urine preparations need not be meticulously screened, unlike smears from the uterine

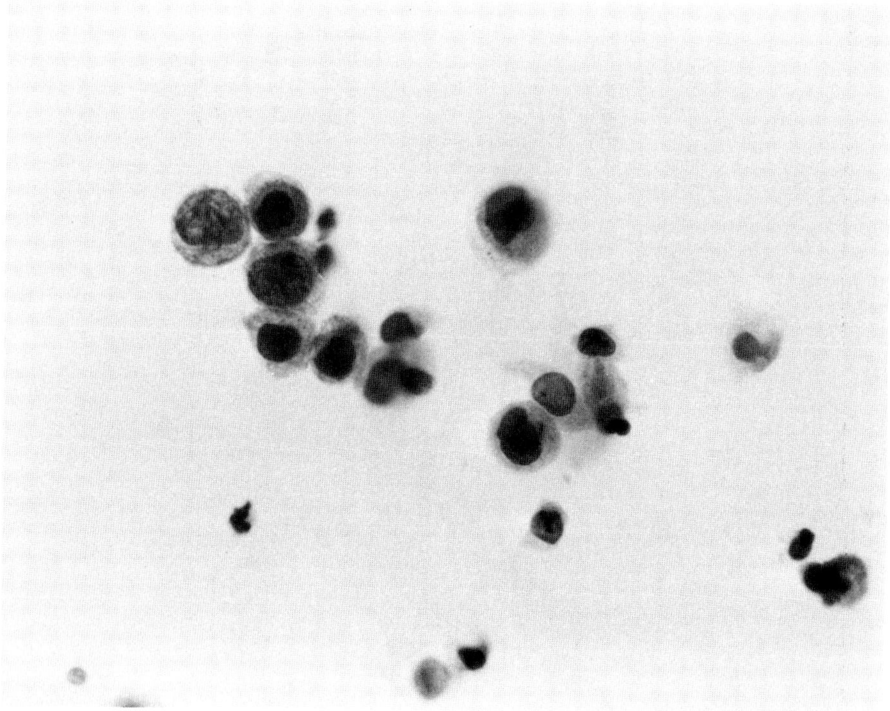

Fig. 2. Urine with cells exfoliated from poorly differentiated (grade III) transitional cell carcinoma. The nuclei are enlarged and coarsely granular, and the N/C ratio is high. Nuclepore filter, Papanicolaou stain. 300X.

cervix or sputum specimens, in which frequently only a few malignant cells are present among numerous nonmalignant cells and may be diagnostic. Most bladder cancers that can be diagnosed cytologically are high-grade tumors, and malignant cells are present in large numbers. The problem is that of identifying these cells as malignant, not of finding them in a large nonneoplastic cell population. One should be reluctant to suggest a diagnosis of bladder cancer on cytologic grounds if a specimen is sparsely cellular or if, in a cellular specimen, only a few cells are abnormal.

It is important to recognize that well-differentiated papillary tumors (papillomas and grade I papillary carcinomas) cannot be detected cytologically with any degree of certainty (El-Bolkainy, 1980). The urine cytology is, however, rarely normal. Unless the papillary tumors are very small, there are often increased numbers of papillary clusters, averaging 15 per 1000 cells found (Kern,

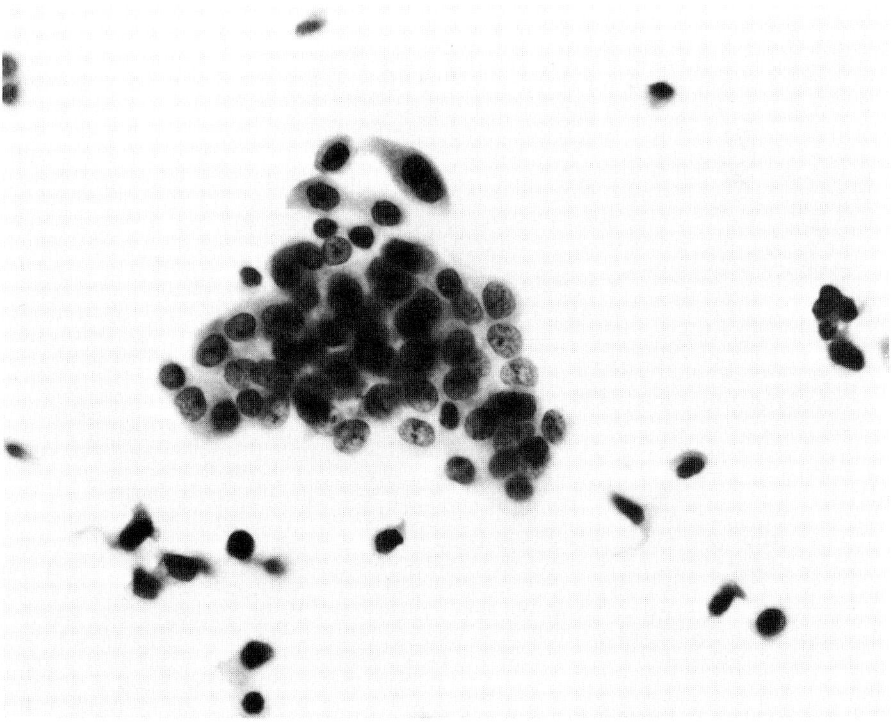

Fig. 3. Well-differentiated (grade I) papillary transitional cell carcinoma. Increased numbers of transitional cells, with slightly enlarged but regular nuclei, often arranged in clusters present in urine. Considered consistent with but not diagnostic of well-differentiated papillary carcinoma. Nuclepore filter, Papanicolaou stain. 300X.

1975). These clusters rarely, if ever, contain a central fibrous core that would definitely identify the structure as a papillary projection. Cytologically, the cells may be slightly abnormal, with moderately enlarged nuclei, but they cannot objectively be identified as malignant. As shown in Table I, the range of the nuclear enlargement is identical to that of nonneoplastic abnormal or reactive cells or, according to some reports, resembles that of normal cells (Boon *et al.*, 1981). Based on increased cellularity, slight nuclear enlargement, and the presence of increased numbers of clusters, a diagnosis of "suggestive of well-differentiated papillary tumor" but not a definitive diagnosis of cancer can often be made (Fig. 3). This, however, is no major drawback for screening programs, because it is more significant to detect *in situ* transitional cell carcinomas that have a greater tendency to become invasive cancers rather than the clinically less significant papillary tumors.

Transitional cell carcinoma *in situ* is a flat, neoplastic, nonpapillary lesion that precedes invasive carcinoma, sometimes by several years. Malignant transfor-

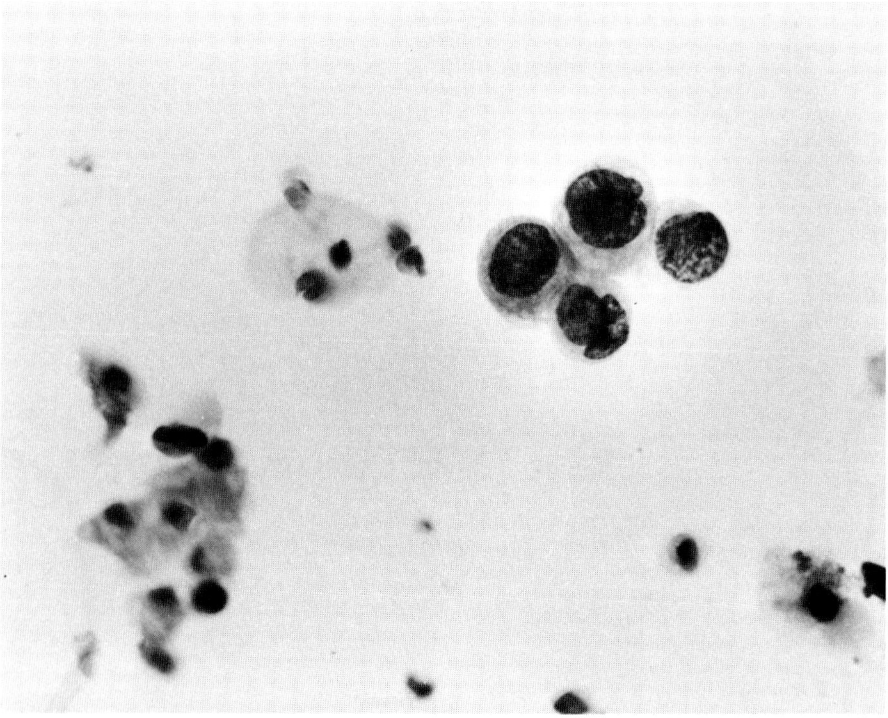

Fig. 4. Neoplastic cells with large nuclei with coarsely clumped chromatin. The N/C ratio is high, and most cells are isodiametric. The patient had extensive transitional cell carcinoma *in situ*. Nuclepore filter, Papanicolaou stain. 300X.

mation frequently takes place, and these lesions are therefore of considerably greater importance than well-differentiated papillary tumors (Koss, 1979b; Utz *et al.*, 1980; Brawn, 1982). These flat neoplasms, in contrast to many papillary tumors, are poorly differentiated cytologically. The exfoliated cells are larger than normal transitional cells, and have hyperchromatic, irregularly outlined nuclei, frequently with a coarsely clumped chromatin and sometimes with prominent nucleoli. Most cells are isodiametric, and bizarre, very large, or strikingly pleomorphic cells are unusual. The cells occur singly or in small groups. Since there is no ulceration or inflammation, the background is usually clean, but some leukocytes or red blood cells may be present (Fig. 4). Properly collected and interpreted cytologic specimens are the most accurate screening test for this important variety of bladder cancer (Utz *et al.*, 1980).

Degenerative and reactive changes are seen in association with inflammation, in patients with calculi, or after instrumentation. Marked reactive changes also follow chemotherapy and radiotherapy. Patients with this history are unlikely to be included in a screening program, but if reactive changes of this type are found, the specimens usually contain fewer abnormal cells than specimens in cases of bladder cancer, and there are associated degenerative changes. Neither the nuclear size nor the coarse granularity, prominent nucleoli, and pleomorphism characteristic of cancer are evident (Table 1). Nuclei with irregular clumps of chromatin often also contain large clear zones.

C. Classification and Nomenclature

The pathologic classification of bladder tumors and the results of cytologic studies correlate well, as will be seen in the next section and as illustrated in Table 2. Several studies have also shown that, based on the cytologic findings, the grade as well as the histologic type of the bladder tumor can be predicted (Eposti and Zajicek, 1972; Suprun and Bitterman, 1975), and that there is a relationship between the cytologic findings, grade, and pathologic stage (Kern, 1984). Because of this correlation between cytology and tumor type, the cytologist must be familiar with the current classifications of bladder tumors and, most importantly, must report the findings in a cytopathologic classification that is understandable to and consistent with the classification used by the surgical pathologists and clinicians with whom he or she collaborates. The classification of bladder tumors that is now generally in use divides urothelial tumors into papillary and nonpapillary and into noninvasive or *in situ* and invasive neoplasms (Koss, 1975; Friedell *et al.*, 1980; Prout, 1980). They are further graded by differentiation, either on a scale of I to III or I to IV. Papillomas are recognized in most classifications as relatively uncommon small tumors with delicate, frond-like projections, covered by no more than seven layers of well-differentiated urothelial cells and without stromal invasion (Koss, 1975; Friedell *et al.*, 1980).

These tumors make up approximately 2% of urothelial neoplasms and cannot be diagnosed cytologically. The grade I papillary carcinomas are also rarely diagnosable cytologically for the reasons stated above. They are usually noninvasive. Grade II papillary carcinomas are characterized by greater cytologic abnormalities but are still fairly orderly. They usually invade the lamina propria but rarely muscle. High-grade (grade III) papillary carcinomas frequently invade the muscle (Kern, 1984). Well-differentiated nonpapillary carcinomas are virtually nonexistent. The flat *in situ* carcinomas are cytologically of a high grade; otherwise they could not be categorized as carcinomas, since they show no other morphologic, architectural evidence of malignancy. Invasive nonpapillary tumors invariably are of a high grade (Kern, 1984). All systems of classification recognize the occurrence of adenocarcinomas and of squamous cell or epidermoid carcinomas, either in a pure form or associated or mixed with transitional cell carcinomas, and of various sarcomas.

Staging systems can be correlated with the grade of the tumor and, to some extent, with the cytology (Kern, 1984), and indicate the depth of infiltration. All pathologic staging systems indicate whether the tumor extends into the lamina propria (P1), superficially into muscle (P2), deeply into muscle (P3A), into perivesical fatty tissue (P3B), or into adjacent structures and organs (P4).

In a screening program, the most important cytologic distinction is between those patients with normal findings who require no further follow-up and those with abnormalities that mandate further diagnostic evaluation. Even if malignant cells are present, and if the tumor can be cytopathologically classified as moderately or poorly differentiated urothelial carcinoma, tissue evaluation is invariably required for further assessment, if only to determine the extent of invasion. If a definite cytologic diagnosis can be made, this should, of course, be indicated in the report, worded, for example, as follows: "positive, malignant cells present; consistent with poorly differentiated transitional cell carcinoma." If the findings are less definite but still suggest that a neoplastic process may exist, the cytopathologist may only be able to state, in a given case, "abnormal cells present; suggestive of well-differentiated papillary tumor; cannot exclude reactive process; recommend cystoscopic examination and biopsy." A carcinoma *in situ* can usually be diagnosed as positive, but it may not be possible to differentiate it from invasive lesions. Whether a definite cytopathologic diagnosis can be made or whether the findings are such that a neoplasm cannot be excluded, the effect in a screening program will be identical, namely, to cause further prompt evaluation of a patient with such findings.

The greatest problem is presented by patients with abnormal findings that are considered to be probably reactive but nevertheless have a degree of atypia that causes concern. Depending upon the experience and best judgment of the examiner, a cytologic follow-up examination or, on occasion, cystoscopic examination should be recommended. This type of case has to be evaluated with great care, since obviously it is undesirable to have many individuals undergo cystoscopic examination unnecessarily in order to find one case of carcinoma. In utilizing urine cytology for screening and applying the criteria of malignancy that are described, this should rarely present a major problem.

Whether terms such as *positive, suspicious,* and *negative* or brief, concise cytopathologic terms are utilized in the report is less important than communication between the cytologist and the clinician to make it perfectly clear which individuals need to undergo further diagnostic evaluation. A system of numbering such as the old Papanicolaou classification, without further elaboration on the precise meaning of the terminology, can be misleading and should be avoided.

D. Accuracy

The combined tabulated results of cytologic diagnoses in bladder cancer (El-Bolkainy, 1980) and our own results are given in Table II.

There is considerable variation in the reported results because of differences in the patient population, in the method of examination, and in the diagnostic criteria and nomenclature employed. If papillomas or well-differentiated papillary carcinomas are included, the results will differ significantly from series in which these are excluded. Generally, the probability that an individual with abnormal test results has disease varies with the sensitivity and specificity of the test and the prevalence of the disease. The overall sensitivity of cytology for cases of primary carcinoma of the bladder, meaning the ability to identify correctly patients with malignant disease as measured by the rate of positive cytologic diagnoses in cases of cancer, ranges from 47 to 97%, with a mean of 74%; the specificity of cytology, namely, the ability to identify patients who do not have malignant disease or the rate of negative cytology in nonneoplastic conditions, varies from 88 to 99%, with a mean of 97%. In nonneoplastic conditions, the cytologic diagnosis was inconclusive in 1.4% and falsely positive in 1.5% of the cases (El-Bolkainy, 1980). In our own laboratory, during the 24-year period from 1961 through 1984, 6378 urine specimens were obtained from 3876 patients, including many with urologic symptoms. A total of 679 of these patients had subsequently proven primary bladder cancer, and 121 had carcinomas of the kidneys or prostate. The urine examination in the bladder cancer cases resulted in 344 positive, 215 suspicious, and 120 negative cytologic diagnoses, for a sensitivity of 82%. Predictably, the sensitivity is low for grade I papillary carcinomas, but 98% of transitional cell carcinomas *in situ* and 94% of all grade III and grade IV transitional cell carcinomas were cytologically positive or suspicious, as were 78% of grade II carcinomas.

The best and most essential quality control procedure for urine cytology is that of correlation and comparison of cytologic findings with the subsequently established tissue diagnosis or other follow-up. This follow-up must be obtained for

TABLE II

Cytologic Diagnosis in Primary Carcinoma of the Bladder

Tumor type	Cases	Urine cytology		
		Negative	Suspicious/ inconclusive	Positive
Hospital of the Good Samaritan, 1961–1984				
Transitional cell carcinoma *in situ* (75–84)	56	1 (2%)	19 (34%)	36 (64%)
Papillary transitional cell carcinoma, grade I	140	51 (36%)	50 (36%)	39 (28%)
Papillary transitional cell carcinoma, grade II	233	51 (22%)	88 (38%)	94 (40%)
Transitional cell carcinoma, grades III and IV	217	14 (6%)	50 (23%)	153 (71%)
Squamous cell carcinoma	18	1 (6%)	4 (22%)	13 (72%)
Adenocarcinoma	15	2 (13%)	4 (27%)	9 (60%)
Series compiled from the literature (El-Bolkainy, 1980)				
Primary carcinomas, nonbilharzial	1920	384 (20%)	97 (4%)	1439 (76%)
Total	2599	504 (19%)	312 (12%)	1783 (69%)

all cases reported as positive or suspicious. In most hospitals, but not necessarily in screening programs, the slides are first screened by a cytotechnologist and then reviewed by a cytopathologist. All abnormal cases must be examined by a cytopathologist. In addition, rescreening of a certain number of negative cases (10%), such as is done for cervical smears in many institution, may be employed.

The described results obtainable in the diagnosis of significant flat *in situ* transitional cell carcinomas and of higher-grade tumors compare favorably with those reported in cytologic screening of other body sites, including the uterine cervix. These results, and the ease with which specimens can be obtained and normal urines can be rapidly and efficiently eliminated by quick microscopic examination, make this procedure a feasible test for bladder cancer screening.

E. Screening Programs

Screening programs for bladder cancer by cytologic examination have been undertaken and reported sparingly. Such programs are used for individuals who are considered to be at high risk for this disease, such as industrial workers exposed to aromatic amines (El-Bolkainy, 1980; Cartwright *et al.*, 1981; Glashan *et al.*, 1981; Davies and Parkes, 1982), bilharzial populations (El-Bolkainy, 1980; El-Bolkainy and Chu, 1980), phenacetin abusers (Dalquen *et al.*, 1980), and urologic and nonurologic patients admitted to hospitals or seen in clinics as part of a routine workup (Holmquist, 1977; Moffat, 1978; de Voogt, 1979; Hausermann *et al.*, 1979; Nemoto *et al.*, 1981, 1982; Hradec *et al.*, 1982; Huland and Kruger, 1982). In most screening programs, particularly for high-risk groups, voided urine prepared as outlined in this chapter or as Papanicolaou-stained sediment smears are used (Keebler and Reagan, 1977; Koss, 1979a; Huland and Kruger, 1982). Particularly in screening programs for hospitalized or clinic patients, when the examination may be performed in conjunction with a urinalysis, the sediment may be stained with 1% toluidine blue (Holmquist, 1977; Nemoto *et al.*, 1981, 1982). Phase contrast microscopy has also been advocated for rapid screening (de Voogt *et al.*, 1975; de Voogt, 1979). If this procedure reveals even slight abnormalities, it must be supplemented by examination of stained slides. For hospitalized patients, the procedure is generally a one-time examination, but some authors recommend examination of several specimens taken on 3 successive days (Hradec *et al.*, 1982). The procedure for the screening of high-risk groups requires a repeat examination once or twice yearly (Utz *et al.*, 1980; Glashan *et al.*, 1981).

Based on the known anticipated rate of detection of bladder cancer by cytologic examination (see Table II), the results of these screening examinations, if done with adequate cytopreparatory techniques and conducted by experienced cytotechnologists and cytopathologists, should closely correspond to the incidence of bladder cancer in the population examined. Since it is usually nonpapillary carcinoma *in situ* that develops in individuals exposed to carcinogens and precedes invasive carcinoma (Koss, 1979a), and since this important lesion can be detected readily by cytologic examination, screening programs should yield significant results in a carefully chosen high-risk population. This is indeed the case, and the positive yield in screening programs for such high-risk groups ranges from 10 to 70 per 1000 persons screened (El-Bolkainy, 1980) and is approximately 10 per 1000 in phenacetin users (Dalquen *et al.*, 1980). The reported yield is considerably lower, only 2 per 1000 (El-Bolkainy and Chu, 1980), in a bilharzial population, and is very low in routinely screened clinic or hospital patients where no attention is paid to selection of high-risk groups. In this category, only 1 in 700 to 1 in 5000 patients examined is found to have bladder cancer (Holmquist, 1977; Moffat, 1978; Nemoto *et al.*, 1981, 1982).

In the development of bladder cancer, an unpredictably long period of slight, nonspecific cytologic abnormalities is followed by a period of clearly positive cytologic findings (Koss, 1979a). This may be associated with papillary or often nonpapillary clinically obvious bladder cancer or with nonpapillary sessile carcinoma *in situ*. The cytologic detection of cancer during this asymptomatic period is possible and is of the greatest use. The selection of a population at risk and the experience and interpretive skills of the cytologist are more important than the use of sediment smears versus filter preparations and Papanicolaou, toluidine blue, or other stains, although we prefer filter preparations and Papanicolaou stains. Repeat, periodic examinations are essential in such evaluations.

III. OTHER SCREENING PROCEDURES

A. Occult Blood

Gross hematuria is a common presenting complaint in bladder cancer; 80% of patients with bladder tumors have gross or microscopic hematuria (Rowland and Garrett, 1980). In adults with hematuria, an intravenous pyelogram is mandatory because of the possibility of renal adenocarcinoma, but bladder tumors must also be ruled out by cystoscopy (Benson and Brewer, 1981). In every adult with microscopic as well as gross hematuria, found in routinely performed urinalyses, a cytologic examination of the urine should be performed (Freni and Freni-Titulaer, 1977). This essential, noninvasive, and harmless procedure will demonstrate *in situ* or invasive carcinoma in most instances, and the failure to apply this test often results in delays in the diagnosis of bladder cancer (Koss, 1982). If a routine urinalysis or, more specifically, examination of urine for the presence of occult blood by hemoccult or other highly sensitive procedures is performed and further follow-up studies are done as indicated, these simple and inexpensive tests may be considered a screening examination for bladder cancer, although they are not as sensitive or specific as urine cytology.

B. Flow Cytometry

Automated analytical cytology currently uses two basic techniques: high-resolution image analysis or cytometry (ICM) of biologic objects that have been fixed and deposited on glass microscope slides or delivered as photonegatives; and low-resolution flow cytometry (FCM) of biologic particles in liquid equilibrium suspensions (Goerttler and Stohr, 1982). Of these two procedures, FCM is being increasingly used for the diagnosis and evaluation of bladder cancers. The method evaluates cells as they rapidly pass, one by one, stations at which their properties are measured. It is an outgrowth of the discovery of nucleic acids, the description of DNA as a double helical molecule, and the methodology for measuring the amount of nucleic acids in single cells and nuclei.

In preparing the specimens—so far usually bladder washings rather than voided urine—the cells are stained with a fluorescent dye, most commonly acridine orange. This allows quantitation of DNA and RNA in each cell and the measurement of nuclear and cell diameters (Klein *et al.*, 1982). The centrifuged cell suspension is stained with acridine orange, which binds to the double helical DNA by intercalation and fluoresces green in blue light, and to single-stranded RNA by electrostasis and fluoresces red. The fluorescence emission at two different wavelength bands is separated optically and quantified for each cell per sample in a flow cytometer. The measurements are stored in a computer and can be recalled for analysis. The magnitudes of green (DNA) and red (RNA) fluorescence and green fluorescence pulse width (nuclear diameter) for each cell are transposed to two-dimensional scattergrams of DNA versus RNA or DNA versus pulse width. The principal difference of FCM and a cytologic-morphologic evaluation of abnormal cells is that FCM not only segregates out the abnormal cells, that but the computer can sort out cells based on their ploidy and provide a graphic display of the number of cells that are other than normal diploid. The percentage of cells in the S (DNA synthesis), G2 (postsynthetic gap), and M (mitotic division) stages correlates, to some degree, with the type and grade of the tumors (Tribukait *et al.*, 1982) and is of great interest and importance in following patients with known, previously treated bladder cancer. The diagnostic results obtained are comparable to those of conventional cytology if the latter is performed by expert cytotechnologists and cytopathologists, but appears to be somewhat more sensitive (Devonec *et al.*, 1982). A recent study of 100 untreated cases showed 40% of T1 tumors and the tumors in most other categories to be aneuploid. With few exceptions, grade I tumors and many grade II tumors were diploid and most grade III tumors were aneuploid. In the aneuploid tumors, tetraploid cases were the least malignant. Increasing malignancy paralleled an increasing deviation from the tetraploid stage (Tribukait *et al.*, 1982).

Modifications of the procedure to provide for the examination of voided urine samples may make it possible to use it in the screening of individuals at high risk. A recent report of a modified technique using an anticoincidence discrimination device permitted a biparametric DNA/protein measurement of urine samples, bladder washings, and tumor tissues. There was a high degree of correlation, so that, for tumor diagnosis from DNA histograms, voided urine specimens can indeed be used rather than bladder washings. The diagnostic sensitivity of this study was 91% and the specificity was 75% (Schwabe, 1982).

The current state of the art and, in particular, the needed technical support for the systems described still limit the use of FCM at this time to a few centers where the procedures can be closely monitored, but wider applications can be anticipated.

C. Tumor Markers

1. Carcinoembryonic Antigen (CEA)

The ideal test for cancer is a simple laboratory procedure that indicates the presence of cancer with a high degree of specificity and sensitivity before metastases occur. Such a simple test is not generally available, and specifically not for the diagnosis of bladder cancer (Berlin, 1981). Oncofetal antigens and, in particular, carcinoembryonic antigen (CEA) and enzymes, however, have been utilized in the diagnosis and monitoring of bladder cancer, and their potential use in screening may be considered.

CEA was first described as a tumor marker for cancer of the colon but is found in varying concentrations in many other tumors as well. It is at this time the clinically most widely used tumor marker (Kern, 1983b). Exfoliated urothelial tumor cells were found to contain CEA in 18 of 40 specimens, including 61% of well-differentiated and 24% of poorly differentiated carcinomas (Wahren *et al.*, 1977). A wide range of the CEA antigen content in the exfoliated cells is generally found. More recently, the urine of 425 patients treated for bladder cancer at the Radiumhemmet Institute was examined, and CEA levels of greater than 30 μg/ml were associated with decreased relative and symptom-free survival. These findings were especially significant in high-grade and high-stage tumors and suggest that urinary CEA may be an independent variable in prognostic evaluation (Wahren *et al.*, 1982; Kern, 1983b). Corresponding serum CEA levels are found to be increased in approximately 50% of patients with bladder cancer in advanced stages, but usually not to high levels (Kern, 1983b). The presence of CEA has been correlated with the deletion of ABH blood group antigen in bladder cancer cells (Wiley *et al.*, 1982), but while the latter finding importantly correlates with invasiveness and prognosis of the tumor, its determination is even more complex than that of CEA. The potential value of urinary CEA lies in the screening of men without urinary tract infections and an especially high risk of bladder tumors (Korsten and Persijn, 1977), but because of the high cost and low sensitivity of this procedure, it is not considered a practical test for this purpose.

2. Enzymes

The levels of a number of enzymes are raised in the urine of patients with bladder cancer. Included are lactic dehydrogenase (Kern and Webster, 1964), alkaline phosphatase, and β-glucoronidase. Bladder carcinoma cells have also been found to contain more galactosyl transferase isoenzymes than normal bladder epithelium, and lysozymes have been shown to be elevated in most patients with bladder carcinomas (Siracusano *et al.*, 1982). None of these enzymes are specific for neoplastic disease, and their measurements are not suitable screening examinations.

3. Other Tests

Many other sophisticated tests have been studied in connection with the diagnosis and monitoring of bladder cancer. These include cytogenetic studies; plasma membrane alterations determined by electron microscopy; immunofluorescent probes; the deletion of urothelial organ antigen in tumor cells; and increased amounts of metabolites such as tryptophan, cotinine, and polypeptide antigens (TPA), as well as herpes simplex virus (HSV)-specific markers (Siracusano *et al.*, 1982; Wahren and Perlmann, 1982; Kern, 1983b). Many of these procedures are of interest and may prove to be useful in the diagnosis and management of bladder cancer, but their complexity and lack of sensitivity and specificity make them unsuitable for purposes of screening.

III. SUMMARY

The methodologies available today for screening for bladder cancer are principally these:

1. Cytologic examination of voided urine is simple, noninvasive, and inexpensive, and will detect most cases of flat carcinoma *in situ* and poorly differentiated invasive carcinoma. It does require skilled, experienced cytotechnologists and cytopathologists for good results, and is incapable of diagnosing most well-differentiated papillary tumors.
2. Flow cytometry of voided urine can quantitate DNA and RNA in numerous cells, measure nuclear diameters, and display these findings graphically. With

further refinement of the technical aspects of this procedure, it will probably be an important tool in screening for bladder cancer.

3. Routinely performed urinalyses, and especially tests for occult blood, are not screening examinations for bladder cancer per se, but are simple procedures and are frequently preformed. More bladder cancers will be detected in their early stages if the presence of microscopic or occult hematuria, as well as gross hematuria, will be promptly followed by cytologic examination of the urine or other urologic examinations.

Some of the other procedures discussed in this chapter may be developed into screening tests in the future but are not practical at this time.

REFERENCES

Benson, G. S., and Brewer, E. D. (1981). Hematuria: Algorithms for diagnosis. *JAMA, J. Am. Med. Assoc.* **246,** 993–995.

Berlin, N. I. (1981). Tumor markers in cancer prevention and detection. *Cancer* **47,** 1151–1153.

Betkerur, V., Hlaing, V., Baumgartner, G., Rao, R., Rhee, H., and Guinan, P. (1980). Screening tests for detection of bladder cancer. *Urology* **16,** 16–19.

Boon, M. E., Kurver, P. H. J., Baak, J. P. A., and Ooms, E. C. M. (1981). Morphometric differences between urothelial cells in voided urine of patients with grade I and grade II bladder tumours. *J. Clin. Pathol.* **34,** 612–615.

Brawn, P. M. (1982). The origin of invasive carcinoma of the bladder. *Cancer* **50,** 515–519.

Cartwright, R. A., Gadian, T., Garland, J. B., and Bernard, S. M. (1981). The influence of malignant cell cytology screening on the survival of industrial bladder cancer cases. *J. Epidemiol. Commun. Health* **35,** 35–38.

Dalquen, P., Fasel, J., Mihatsch, M. H., Rist, M., and Rutishauser, G. (1980). Phenacetin abuse: IV. Are cytological urine studies successful and usable in the prevention of tumors in phenacetin abusers? *Schweiz. Med. Wochenschr.* **110,** 302–306.

Danos, M., and Keebler, C. M. (1977). Cytopreparatory techniques. *In* "A Manual of Cytotechnology" (C. M. Keebler and J. W. Reagan, eds.), 5th ed., pp. 264–317. Am. Soc. Clin. Pathol., Chicago, Illinois.

Davies, J. M., and Parkes, H. G. (1982). Benefits of cytologic screening for bladder cancer. *Acta Cytol.* **26,** 98.

Devonec, M., Darzynkiewicz, Z., Kostyrka-Claps, M. L., Collste, L., Whitmore, W. F., and Melamed, M. R. (1982). Flow cytometry of low stage bladder tumors: Correlation with cytologic and cystoscopic diagnosis. *Cancer* **49,** 109–118.

De Voogt, H. J. (1979). The significance of urinary cytology for the early diagnosis of urothelial tumors. *Therapiewoche* **29,** 2242–2245.

de Voogt, H. J. (1980). Urinary cytology as a screening test for diagnosis of urinary bladder cancer. *Onkologie* **3,** 233–237.

de Voogt, H. J., Beyer-Boon, M. E., and Brussee, J. M. (1975). The value of phase contrast microscopy for urinary cytology, reliability and pitfalls. *Acta Cytol.* **19,** 542–546.

El-Bolkainy, M. N. (1980). Cytology of bladder carcinoma. *J. Urol.* **124,** 20–22.

El-Bolkainy, M. N., and Chu, E. W. (1980). Cytologic detection of bladder carcinoma in a rural Egyptian population infested with schistosomiasis. Abstr. Medit. Cancer Conf., Fed. Middle East Cancer Organ., Meeting abstract, p. 106.

Eposti, P., and Zajicek, J. (1972). Grading of transitional cell neoplasms of the urinary bladder from smears of bladder washings. A critical review of 326 tumors. *Acta Cytol.* **16,** 529–537.

Freni, S. C., and Freni-Titulaer, L. W. J. (1977). Microhematuria found by mass screening of apparently healthy males. *Acta Cytol.* **21,** 421–423.

Friedell, G. H., Parija, G. C., Nagy, G. K., and Soto, E. A. (1980). The pathology of human bladder cancer. *Cancer* **45,** 1823–1831.

Glashan, R. W., Wijesinghe, D. P., and Riley, A. (1981). The early changes in the development of bladder cancer in patients exposed to known industrial carcinogens. *Br. J. Urol.* **53,** 571–577.

Goerttler, K., and Stohr, M. (1982). Automated cytology. The state of the art. *Arch. Pathol. Lab. Med.* **106,** 657–661.

Hausermann, M., Sommer, E., and Blumberg, A. (1979). Urinary cytology in tumors in the lower part of the urinary tract. *Schweiz. Med. Wochenschr.* **109,** 304–308.

Hellsten, S., Glifberg, I., Lindholm, C. E., and Telhammar, E. (1981). Therapy of bladder carcinoma. *Scand. J. Urol. Nephrol.* **15,** 115–120.

Holmquist, N. D. (1977). Screening a hospital population for urinary tract cancer. *Acta Cytol.* **21,** 682–684.

Hradec, E., Svoboda, P., and Smolova, H. (1982). Significance of routine cytology for detection of urothelial carcinoma and other malignancies. *Eur. Congr. Cytol., Eur. Fed. Cytol. Soc., 11th, 1982,* Meeting Abstract, p. 171.

Huland, H., and Kruger, A. (1982). Critical evaluation of urine cytology as a screening method with the example of 1535 consecutive findings. *Therapiewoche* **32,** 490–492.

Kern, W. H. (1971). Epithelial cells in urine sediments. *Am. J. Clin. Pathol.* **56,** 67–72.

Kern, W. H. (1975). The cytology of transitional cell carcinoma of the urinary bladder. *Acta Cytol.* **19,** 420–428.

Kern, W. H. (1983a). Urinary tract. *In* "A Manual of Cytotechnology" (C. M. Keebler and J. W. Reagan, eds.), 6th ed., pp. 191–203. Am. Soc. Clin. Pathol., Chicago, Illinois.

Kern, W. H. (1983b). Bladder cancer. *In* "Urological Cancer" (D. G. Skinner, ed.), pp. 137–148. Grune & Stratton, New York.

Kern, W. H. (1984). The grade and pathologic stage of bladder cancer. *Cancer* **53,** 1185–1189.

Kern, W. H., and Bales, C. E. (1969). Quantitative studies of urine cytology. *Am. J. Clin. Pathol.* **51,** 225–228.

Kern, W. H., and Webster, W. W. (1964). Combined lactic acid dehydrogenase and cytologic examinations of urine in the diagnosis of cancer of the urinary tract. *Acta Cytol.* **8,** 302–305.

Kern, W. H., Webster, W. W., and Bales, C. E. (1966). Heat fractionation of urine lactic acid dehydrogenase and combined cytopathologic evaluation in the diagnosis of cancer of the urinary tract. *J. Urol.* **96,** 551–558.

Kern, W. H., Bales, C. E., and Webster, W. W. (1968). Cytologic evaluation of transitional cell carcinoma of the bladder. *J. Urol.* **100,** 616–622.

Klein, F. A., Herr, H. W., Sogani, P. C., Whitmore, W. F., and Melamed, M. R. (1982). Detection and follow-up of carcinoma of the urinary bladder by flow cytometry. *Cancer* **50,** 389–395.

Korsten, C. B., and Persijn, J. P. (1977). Immunochemical and clinical aspects of CEA (carcinoembryonic antigen) in the urine (meeting abstract). *Ned. Tijdschr. Geneeskd.* **121,** 1408–1977.

Koss, L. G. (1975). Tumors of the urinary bladder. *In* "Atlas of Tumor Pathology" (M. O. Dayhoff, ed.), 2nd ser., Fasc. II, pp. 36–38. Armed Forces Inst. Pathol., Washington, D.C.

Koss, L. G. (1979a). "Diagnostic Cytology and Its Histopathologic Bases," 3rd ed., pp. 750–753, 1211–1214. Lippincott, Philadelphia, Pennsylvania.

Koss, L. G. (1979b). Mapping of the urinary bladder: Its impact on the concepts of bladder cancer. *Hum. Pathol.* **10,** 533–548.

Koss, L. G. (1982). Evaluation of hematuria (letter). *JAMA, J. Am. Med. Assoc.* **247,** 1274.

Lent, V. (1975). Possibilities of prophylactic screening for malignant tumors of the urogenital tract. *Dtsch. Med. Wochenschr,* **100,** 2452–2454.
Lessing, J. A. (1978). Bladder cancer: Early diagnosis and evaluation of biological potential. A review of newer methods. *J. Urol.* **120,** 1–5.
Moffat, N. A. (1978). Urinary cytology as a screening study to detect urinary milagnancies. *Wis. Med. J.* **77,** 537–538.
Nemoto, R., Kato, T., Shibata, K., and Kano, M. (1981). Urinary cytology as a test in mass screening. *Tohoku J. Exp. Med.* **135,** 115–116.
Nemoto, R., Kato, T., Harada, M., Shibata, K., and Kano, M. (1982). Mass screening for urinary tract cancer with urine cytology. *J. Cancer Res. Clin. Oncol.* **104,** 155–159.
Pearson, J. C., Kromhout, L., and King, E. B. (1981). Evaluation of collection and preservation techniques for urinary cytology. *Acta Cytol.* **25,** 327–333.
Prout, G. R. (1980). Classification and staging of bladder carcinoma. *Cancer* **45,** 1832–1841.
Rowland, R. G., and Garrett, R. A. (1980). Tumors of the urinary bladder. *In* "Current Diagnosis" (H. F. Conn and R. B. Conn, eds.), p. 824. Saunders, Philadelphia, Pennsylvania.
Schwabe, H. W. (1982). Improved application of impulse cytophotometry for the diagnosis of urinary bladder carcinoma. *Urol. Res.* **10,** 61–66.
Silverberg, E. (1985). Cancer statistics. *Ca—Cancer J. Clin.* **35,** 26–27.
Siracusano, F., Tarro, G., Biviano, D., Flaminio, G., Saladino, J., and Piccolo, A. (1982). TAF test: A tumor diagnosis device in oncologic urology. *Cancer* **50,** 2215–2217.
Skinner, D. G. (1980). Current perspectives in the management of high-grade invasive bladder cancer. *Cancer (Amsterdam)* **45,** 1866–1874.
Suprun, H., and Bitterman, W. (1975). A correlative cytohistologic study on the interrelationship between exfoliated urinary bladder carcinoma cell types and the staging and grading of these tumors. *Acta Cytol.* **19,** 265–273.
Tribukait, B., Gustafson, H., and Eposti, P. L. (1982). The significance of ploidy and proliferation in the clinical and biological evaluation of bladder tumours: A study of 100 untreated cases. *Br. J. Urol.* **54,** 130–135.
Utz, D. C., Farrow, G. M., Rife, C. C., Segura, J. W., and Zincke, H. (1980). Carcinoma *in situ* of the bladder. *Cancer (Amsterdam)* **45,** 1842–1848.
Wahren, B., and Perlmann, P. (1982). Bladder and renal tumor markers. *In* "Human Cancer Markers" (S. Sell and B. Wahren, eds.), pp. 303–319. Humana Press, Clifton, New Jersey.
Wahren, B., Eposti, P., and Zimmerman, R. (1977). Characterization of urothelial carcinoma with respect to the content of carcinoembryonic antigen in exfoliated cells. *Cancer (Amsterdam)* **40,** 1511–1518.
Wahren, B., Nilsson, B., and Zimmerman, R. (1982). Urinary CEA for prediction of survival time and recurrent in bladder cancer. *Cancer (Amsterdam)* **50,** 139–145.
Wiley, E. L., Mendelsohn, G., Droller, M., and Eggleston, J. C. (1982). Immunoperoxidase detection of carcinoembryonic antigen and blood group substances in papillary transitional cell carcinoma of the bladder. *J. Urol.* **128,** 276–280.

9

Mammography

PHILIP STRAX

I. Introduction 141
II. Rationale 142
III. Historical Review 143
IV. Technical Factors 144
V. Radiation Risk 147
VI. Interpretation 148
A. Benign Changes 149
B. Malignant Changes 152
C. Breast Calcifications 155
D. Mammography in Screening 157
VII. Conclusions 159
References 160

I. INTRODUCTION

Mammography is a radiological procedure that uses soft tissue X rays to visualize breast structure. It is generally agreed that the mammogram is the most reliable method for imaging breast lesions.

In recent years, it has become increasingly apparent that clinical examination of the breast, including inspection and palpation, is not fully adequate to detect breast pathology. It is also becoming obvious that breast cancer exists in a nonpalpable stage for a varying length of time, and that detection of a lesion during that time may lead to long survival and increased curability. A radiological study of the breast can improve the specificity of diagnosis by helping to differentiate a benign from a malignant process and can improve the sensitivity of the examination by identifying a malignancy before it becomes palpable—when it is most curable. Mammography still remains the most effective—if not the only—imaging method that can detect nonpalpable cancer. Modern mam-

ISBN 0-12-496720-5

mography does not usually involve injections or painful manipulation of the organ. It is comfortable, easily performed, and uses small amounts of radiation that are considered negligible, particularly in light of the great potential benefit.

II. RATIONALE

Mammography has made a substantial contribution to breast cancer for the following reasons:

1. It can make a clinical diagnosis more definite and move the clinician to effective treatment without unnecessary delay. Because the breast is normally multinodular, the dominant mass that suggests pathology may not be clearly evident on palpation. This is particularly true of an early cancer. The mammogram can be a useful diagnostic modality in that it often, although not always, gives the physician the extra assurance that the lesion noted may be malignant and may need prompt exploration. Also, physicians, particularly primary practitioners exposed to clinical examination of the breast, have expertise that varies greatly with their training, inclination, and experience. The woman who sees her primary physician with the problem of a vague breast mass, localized pain, or a nipple discharge often presents the even greater problem of determining whether exploration is indicated. A mammogram under such conditions can be lifesaving in avoiding delay.
2. It can yield additional information about the remainder of the breast in question or about the opposite breast. A nonpalpable cancer may be present elsewhere in either breast; that other lesion, not the suspected mass, may be cancerous.
3. It can be particularly useful in differentiating the benign from the malignant lesion. As such, it can aid in avoiding unnecessary exploration. Even more importantly, however, it can expedite exploration when indicated.
4. It can prevent the error of tapping a cyst and missing a cancer in close proximity.
5. It can detect nonpalpable cancer that is occult and totally unsuspected by even the most expert physician, but that is in the early stages of serious disease. Breast cancer screening activities, using mammography in addition to clinical examination, that have been in use for over 20 years have turned up hundreds of such lesions. It is patients with these nonpalpable cancers, who have a high degree of no nodal involvement and a substantially greater survival than those normally noted in general medical practice, who have emphasized the importance of X ray examination of the breast.

It must be emphasized that mammography, even under the best circumstances, will not detect 100% of the cancers present. Depending on the age of the patient, type of breast, parity, techniques used, and expertise of the radiologist, some 10–20% of cancers will not be visualized on a mammogram. Some of these may be detected on palpation alone. Some may be detected by the woman herself within months of a supposedly negative examination—the so-called interval cancer. Therefore, it is imperative that if a lesion is palpable and clinical judgment dictates exploration, a negative mammogram should never delay biopsy. At the same time, it is also most important to realize that negative palpation in the light of a positive finding on a mammogram should be disregarded and prompt exploration considered. Clinical examination and mammography are truly complementary and should never be considered competitive.

III. HISTORICAL REVIEW

The first recorded use of radiography to visualize breast structure was by Salomon (1913), a German pathologist, who used the method on amputated breasts. He described the irregular mass density and calcifications we still consider the important signs of malignancy on the mammogram. The procedure has had a varied career since that time. Over the years, it has been taken up by various radiologists in various countries with various modifications, but never found general acceptance until recently. In the United States, the first real impetus to mammography was given by Warren (1930), who published his results on stereoradiography of the breast.

Leborgne (1953) presented an exhaustive study of mammography with and without instillation of contrast material. He placed the subject on a firm scientific basis and delineated the changes associated with cancer and with noncancerous conditions; this work is the basis of modern mammography.

Over the years, European radiologists have been the strongest proponents of the method. Gros (1963) in Strasbourg, Von Ronnen (1956) in Amsterdam, Desprez-Curely *et al.* (1959) in Paris, and Buttenberg and Werner (1962) in Heidelberg all praised this procedure. In the United States, Gershon-Cohen (1963) in Philadelphia was virtually alone in espousing the technique.

A new era of acceptance of the procedure was ushered in with the presentation of a new technique of mammography by Egan (1960). He reported that a high degree of accuracy was achieved in a group of 1000 patients from the M.D. Anderson Hospital. In a special study conducted by the U.S. Public Health Service (Clark *et al.*, 1965), Egan's technique was found to be highly reproducible. Egan's use of fine-grain film and improved radiologic equipment made possible improved visualization of breast detail and great diagnostic accuracy.

It was, however, difficult to produce mammograms of good quality. The Egan technique produced much wear and tear on radiographic equipment and required a great deal of experience in technique and interpretation. Because of these difficulties, xeromammography, an electrophoretic method, which had been neglected for many years, was revived, renewed, and perfected by Wolfe (1972) as an improved method of mammography. Finally, it was the support of the U.S. Public Health Service and the development of teaching centers for mammography that stimulated increased interest in this procedure. The big push came with the report from the Health Insurance Plan of Greater New York (HIP) study that the use of mammography combined with palpation under mass screening conditions led to a decrease in mortality from breast cancer (Shapiro *et al.*, 1974). Mammography, with somewhat varying techniques, is now in widespread use in most areas of the world. It is being increasingly realized that the procedure is indeed very useful and potentially lifesaving.

IV. TECHNICAL FACTORS

Until recently, the most widely used technique for mammography was the one developed by Egan (1964). In his original technique, three views are made of each breast: craniocaudal, mediolateral, and axillary. The axillary view has been discarded by most radiologists, because it contributes least to diagnosis and because its elimination reduces wear and tear on equipment and lowers the radiation dose delivered to the breast. The essential elements of Egan's techniques are fine-grain film (type M Eastman or its equivalent), a low kilovoltage (below 30 kV), a high milliamperage (1800 mA), close coning, a target–film distance that varies with the size of the breast, added filtration to the tube, close collimation without compression, and hand development of the films. The mediolateral view is made with the patient lying down; the craniocaudal view is taken with the patient comfortable so as to avoid motion for the long exposure times needed. The film must be exposed in a cardboard holder; no cassettes or intensifying screens are used. The mediolateral view especially requires much care on the part of the technician to encompass the entire breast on the film. The radiation dose to the breast with this technique is usually 8–12 R to the skin per exposure.

In recent years, improvements in technique for mammography have involved the use of special screens and new films, as well as the reintroduction of the Xerox process by Wolfe (1972) to display the image. Both methods have added compression to increase resolution. Both have improved detail and contrast in the mammographic image. Many film techniques now use a molybdenum anode tube, following the lead of the Senograph, introduced by Gros (1963) and associates in Strasbourg. Machines with this type of tube are now produced by several manufacturers, both in the United States and abroad, with notable enhancement of detail. These devices, dedicated to mammography, have been constructed to make the examination more efficient and to place less strain on the equipment, patient, and technician. Xeromammography, in which the image is recorded on a selenium plate and then transferred to special paper, results in a marked edge enhancement effect that serves to sharpen images, especially the microcalcifications of cancer. The Xerox process, however, is especially effective with the tungsten anode tubes used in general radiography. There is a difference of opinion as to the relative value of improved film techniques versus xeromammography. Strong preferences are expressed by advocates of both methods.

Most importantly, a dramatic improvement has been noted in both the quality of the mammogram produced and the radiation dose used. The change has been due to the introduction of new faster film–screen combinations in vacuum cassettes. Under the leadership of British radiologists (Price and Nathan, 1975) and others in the United States (Ostrum *et al.*, 1973), mammograms are being produced with remarkable improvements in contrast and resolution, as well as with reductions in radiation dosage to 0.2–0.3 R to the skin per exposure. Measurements by Miller and associates (1977) of the Northeastern Physics Center in New York City indicate that such skin radiation (with low kilovoltages used in combination with the molybdenum-anode tubes and compression techniques) should approximate 0.02–0.03 rad to the midbreast for a right-angle pair of films. These techniques are readily available and are being used by an increasing number of radiologists. The revision of xeromammography techniques, with the introduction of the negative mode and increased kilovoltage, has resulted in a reduction of radiation, although not to the low levels attainable by the newer film–screen techniques.

The most important ingredient in mammography is the interest and conscientiousness of the radiologist, who must be willing to devote the time and effort needed to evaluate the procedure in light of the equipment used and to become experienced in interpreting the manifold variations of mammograms.

Different film–screen combinations have been developed by film manufacturers in an ongoing attempt to reduce radiation in mammography while improving detail and contrast (Table I).

An interesting and valuable approach has been introduced by Lundgren and Jakobsson (1976), who advocate the use of one oblique view in mammography when used in screening. This view appears to cover even more breast surface than the usual craniocaudal and mediolateral views together. If a positive finding is noted, the right-angle pair is needed for delineation of the lesion to a breast quadrant.

Surveys of modern techniques in mammography, as well as evaluations of xeromammography versus film–screen techniques, have been made by Hoeffken and Lanyi (1973), Logan (1977), Bjurstam and Noch Quiding (1975), and Snyder *et al.* (1977). In general, there has been agreement that overall similar diagnostic information is obtained with all modern systems, provided the procedure is done with care and close attention is paid to detail. Film–screen

TABLE I

Films and Screens for Use in Mammography

Technique	Surface Dose (roentgens)
Egan: type M, tungsten tube, no screen	8–12
Xeromammography	
Tungsten tube	2–3 or 1–2 with more filtration
Molybdenum tube	3–4
Senograph-type machine (molybdenum)	
Kodak SO 146, no screen	5–6
AFGA Osray M, no screen	2–3
DuPont Lo-Dose, screen No. 1	1–1.5
DuPont Lo-Dose, screen No. 2	0.8–0.9 or less to 0.6–0.7
Kodak Min-R (rare earth screen)	0.8–0.9
AFGA (rare earth screen)	0.8–0.9
Fuji Rx-m (rare earth screen)	0.8–0.9
3M (special alpha rare earth screen)	0.2
Kodak 105 mm No. RF-FC 874 with Min-R screen	0.3
Kodak 105 mm No. RF-FC 874 with US Radium special screen	0.2
DuPont 105 SF2 with Min-R screen	0.3
Sakura with Min-R screen	0.3

techniques require the use of a molybdenum anode with a molybdenum filter in a machine dedicated to mammography, while xeromammography is best performed on a tungsten anode X ray unit, which may be the same apparatus used by the radiologist for general radiography. Of course, the Xerox processor must be used.

It is generally agreed that the Xerox process provides better evaluation of microcalcifications but is less accurate in visualizing mass densities than film–screen techniques (Sickles, 1982). Also, the radiation dose to the midbreast is 6–10 times higher with xeromammography. However, there are ardent enthusiasts of both systems. The main ingredient still remains the dedication of the radiologist and his or her close attention to technical details.

A special soft tissue grid system has been described by Friedrich and Weskamp (1978) for use in thick breasts. It can enhance the image by reducing scattered radiation. Under special conditions, improved images can be obtained at the expense of an increased radiation dose.

The actual radiation dose absorbed by the breast depends on a number of factors, including the type of recording medium, the target material in the tube, the kilovoltage applied, the radiation filtration, the thickness of the breast, compression techniques, density of the film, and film-processing techniques. The dose absorbed by the midbreast varies with modern techniques from 0.5 to 0.02

rad, depending on the above factors. All techniques today should be delivering less than 1 rad to the body of the breast for an examination using the usual right-angle pair of views.

Details of the physical characteristics of film–screen combinations have been described by Webster and Kalisher (1977), and the physical factors in xeroradiography have been evaluated by Wolfe (1976).

A more recent electrostatic imaging technique has been introduced as Xonics electron mammography. This system uses a bromine-freon imaging gas and produces a latent image on a thin polyester sheet that is developed with a liquid toner. Ionography results in improved edge enhancement and contrast compared to xeroradiography. The radiation dose used is considerably less than that of xeroradiography and is in the range of that used in film–screen combinations (Muntz, 1978).

Magnification techniques have been suggested to improve image quality. With a very small focal spot, image sharpness comparable to that of conventional techniques can be obtained with a magnification above 1.5X, leading to improved visibility, particularly of microcalcifications (Sickles, 1977).

More recently, techniques of computed tomography (CT) have been applied to breast examination by Chang (1979) and by Gisvold *et al.* (1977). For proper results, contrast material is infused prior to the study. The method seems to be useful for examining dense breasts. Some cancers have been visualized on the basis of increased CT numbers that were not seen on conventional mammograms. The expense of the equipment, the need for contrast injections, and technical difficulties have prevented the method from becoming popular.

In general, success in mammography depends on the type of breast being examined. Interpretation of images in the usual fatty breast of the postmenopausal woman is far more accurate than in the dense, fibroglandular breast of the younger woman in her twenties or thirties, particularly if she is nulliparous. Also, accuracy of interpretation depends on good imaging techniques.

However, it should be emphasized that regardless of which technique is used or how much close attention is paid to detail, all of the radiological characteristics of malignancy can be mimicked by benign conditions, and vice versa. The mammogram provides additional diagnostic information that leads to the determination of the need for histological study. Mammography, of necessity, will lead to biopsy recommendations that produce benign results. This is the price that must be paid for detection of cancer in an earlier, more curable stage than was the case in the premammography period. Improved techniques and attention to detail are used to keep biopsies down to reasonable levels.

V. RADIATION RISK

By the mid-1970s, mammography had achieved increasing popularity as a modality for imaging breast structure and pathology. At that time, increasing awareness was developing that diagnostic X radiation could be carcinogenic to the breast. This concept was emphasized by Bailar (1976), who sounded a note of caution after reviewing the evidence of increased incidence of breast cancer after exposure to the atomic bomb, multiple fluorescopies in the course of treatment for tuberculosis, and following radiation therapy for breast abscess. His conclusion was that periodic exposure of the breast to the dose (about 1 rad) of radiation being used in mammography could produce cancers and their sequelae in as many or more women than could benefit from early detection.

Subsequent careful evaluation of all factors related to X-radiation carcinogenicity of the breast has led most investigators to the conclusion that radiation hazard is dependent on the radiation dose to the breast and to the age of the woman exposed. Modern techniques of mammography that deliver doses of 0.2–0.3 R to the skin per exposure, which is equivalent to doses of 0.02–0.03 rad for two views to the midbreast of average size, are considered acceptable by most authorities. The radiation hazard under such conditions, even with periodic studies, is probably unmeasurable. For example, at least one investigator has calculated that if 1 million women aged 40 were to receive a dose to the midbreast of a size readily available today on a periodic basis, during the lifetime of these women 2 or 3 cancers might develop as a result of radiation exposure, while over 70,000 breast cancers would occur naturally (Berlin, 1979).

It is also generally accepted that the radiation risk to the breast of a woman over the age of 30 is minimal, if any. Obviously, we have been exaggerating the risks of mammography and minimizing the benefits. Perhaps we should agree with Holleb (1976) when he wrote in an editorial in *CA* at a time when only 1 woman in 15 developed breast cancer compared to 1 in 11 at present:

> The risk of mammography in expert hands may well have been overstated, sensationalized and misunderstood by not emphasizing the lack of concrete information. We can only hope that not too much damage has been done to those women who, in fear, are neglecting to have examinations which diagnose breast cancers in a readily curable stage.
>
> We cannot easily lay aside the knowledge that in the United States today one of every 15 women will get cancer of the breast, or that every 15 minutes three women develop breast cancer and one woman dies of this disease, or that breast cancer is the number one cancer killer of American women. We are just beginning to demonstrate at the community level that mammography is capable of detecting extremely early, nonpalpable breast cancer in older women, and even in those under 50 years of age. The use of mammography in conjunction with other methods now offers the promise of significantly improving what has been a relatively constant mortality rate.
>
> Surely we all agree that it is important to avoid needless risks. Let us also agree to avoid needless deaths due to delayed diagnosis.

VI. INTERPRETATION

A mammogram is a compressed, two-dimensional, gross anatomical visualization of the breast. Breast structure, normal and abnormal, can be delineated with a potential for accurate localization of a lesion. It cannot and should not replace inspection and palpation, which remain sources of vital information. It can make a clinical diagnosis more definite and, even more importantly, it can visualize a nonpalpable cancer. The clinician should use the report of the radiologist as additional information in caring for the patient.

Since the female breast is a target gland of the endocrine system, it reflects the interplay of secretions from that system throughout the life of the woman. It is a dynamic structure that undergoes continuous change with age, menstrual state, parity, and bodily status. Just as clinical appearance varies greatly from woman to woman (and in the same woman at different periods of her life), so the mammogram presents markedly different appearances at different times.

Gross radiological appearances can be classified according to the amount and distribution of glandular, fibrous, and fatty elements present. Although the proportion of these elements varies considerably with age, it is most probable that the greatest variation is tied to the endocrine pattern in any particular woman. Thus, although it is likely that a young, nulliparous woman will have a dense breast with many fibrous and glandular elements and that a postmenopausal, multiparous women will have a predominantly fatty breast, there are many exceptions to the rule, and the mammographic appearance may be the reverse of what is expected. It seems more helpful to classify normal breasts on the basis of type as seen on a mammogram, e.g., glandular or fatty, with subdivisions relating to the amount and appearance of the fibrous, glandular, and fatty elements present. Mammography makes it possible to follow breast changes in serial studies during the life of a woman and to visualize the changes associated with development and involution. It may be possible to correlate such changes with endocrine patterns at different stages and to associate unusual breast patterns with hormonal aberrations.

A. Benign Changes

Terms such as *cystic mastitis, fibrocystic mastopathy, mazoplasia,* or *dysplasia* are used by clinicians to describe the many clinical appearances of the lumpiness of a breast with various degrees of pain or tenderness. They are used to describe the vast majority of breasts considered benign, normal, or without clinical suspicion of malignancy. The mammogram is, for the most part, a collection of black and white densities that represent different facets of nonmalignant breast tissue. Such histologic terms as *fibrocystic disease* or *adenosis,* in addition to those mentioned above, usually do not correlate with radiological appearance. It might be more expedient to classify these nonmalignant variations radiologically on the basis of the three main identifiable structural elements—ductal, lobular, and stromal changes. This has been done by Strax and Pomeranz (1968). Such a classification can serve as a framework within which to evaluate malignant variations. The reader is referred to the original article for further

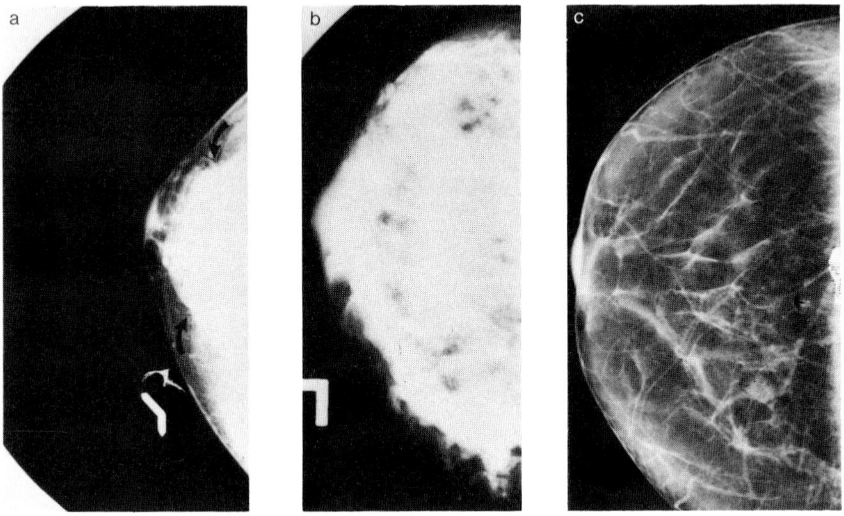

Fig. 1. Breast structure types: (a) fibrous, (b) glandular, (c) fatty.

details. However, because a discrete mass is of particular importance to the clinician, special attention must be given to nonmalignant masses, such as a papilloma, fibroadenoma, cyst, or lipoma, which present as clinical masses. Just as cancer can masquerade as a benign lesion clinically, it may assume the appearance of a benign mass on a mammogram. Every type of benign growth has

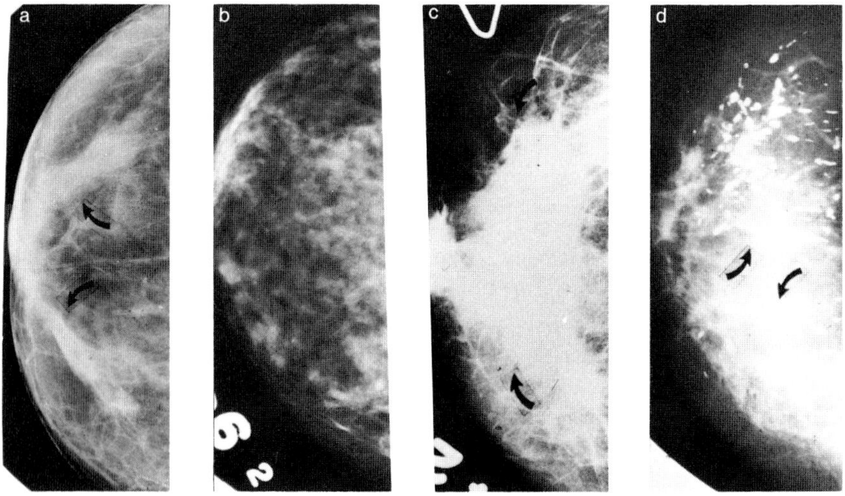

Fig. 2. Nonmalignant variations (no mass): (a) ductal changes, (b) glandular changes, (c) stromal changes, (d) benign calcifications.

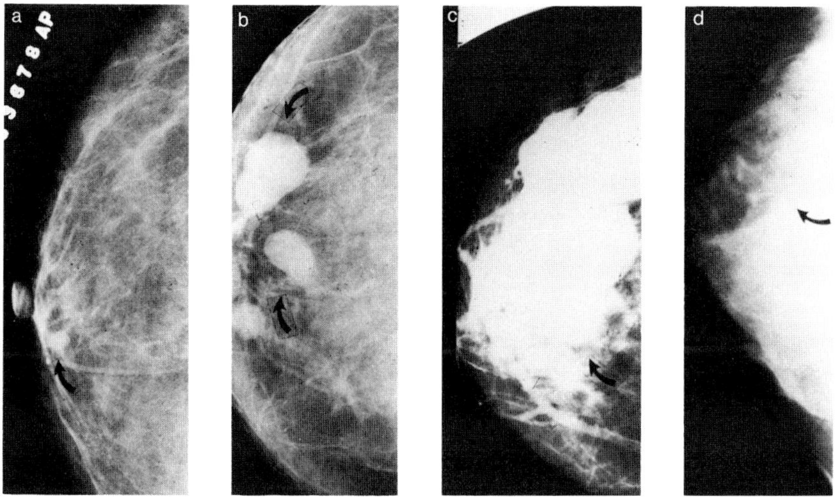

Fig. 3. Nonmalignant variations (mass): (a) papilloma, (b) fibroadenoma, (c) cyst, (d) lipoma.

been mimicked radiologically by a malignancy. The X ray findings in such cases must be correlated with the clinical findings, and differentiation must be made clinically, e.g., by aspiration or exploration. Benign masses or other tissue changes may assume malignant characteristics on the mammogram, just as they may clinically. For that reason, mastectomy should always be preceded by biopsy and should never be performed on the basis of a mammogram alone, no matter how suspicious or characteristic of malignancy the X ray picture may be.

Benign masses usually are well circumscribed, round or oval, and lobulated. They extend into their milieu, displacing the breast elements but not invading them. These masses are homogeneous in density, occasionally containing large, regular, scattered calcifications—in the mass in fibroadenomas or in the periphery in cysts. They are usually the same size to palpation as on the mammogram. Papillomas are seen in the line of the ducts in the subareolar region. Fibroadenomas are usually found in women under 35 and are often present in nulliparous women with dense fibroglandular breasts on the mammogram, where they may be obvious to the clinician but undetectable by the radiologist. Occasionally, calcified fibroadenomas containing an amorphous, dense type of calcification are seen in older women.

Probably the most common palpable mass in women over 35 years of age is the so-called fibrocystic, nonmalignant process, which may have the clinical appearance of a malignancy and probably accounts for most biopsies with a benign result. Recommendations for exploration in such cases vary with the type and size of the breast and the expertise of the clinician. The mammogram can be useful in supplying peripheral information.

At the same time, definite benign cysts are also common in women from 35 years of age up to the time of involution. They may, and often are, multiple and bilateral. They may present with thickened walls due to inflammatory change and irregular margins on the mammogram, suggestive of malignancy. Many cysts are visible on the mammogram but are not palpable. The opposite is also true. A malignancy occasionally may be present in close proximity to a benign cyst or may even lie in the wall of the cyst.

Aspirations of cysts, as is widely practiced, should be followed by clinical observation as well as by mammography. Lipomas may also present clinically as discrete, firm masses, and many are removed on suspicion of malignancy; mammography can be helpful in the differential diagnosis. Less frequently, a galactocele may be found, which is diagnosed by its translucency and its well-demarcated periphery.

B. Malignant Changes

The two most important reasons for the use of mammography are its ability to help differentiate a malignant change from nonmalignant variations and its ability to detect a cancer in a nonpalpable stage.

1. Primary Signs

The primary signs of malignancy are:

1. A more or less infiltrative mass
2. Sand-like, numerous, irregular grouped microcalcifications
3. A localized area of trabecular distortion

A malignant mass usually invades its surrounding milieu, with distortion of the structure of the breast, increased areas of fibrosis, and a clouding and increased density of the stroma caused by what French workers call *edema*. The mass is usually ragged or spiculated, with a poorly circumscribed border. It is often smaller on the mammogram than it appears on palpation. In many cases, it contains the fine, punctate, grouped calcifications associated with malignancy. There are, however, circumscribed carcinomas, such as the medullary or colloid types, which resemble benign masses both clinically and radiologically. Both the clinician and the radiologist must be on guard in such cases, especially since the prognosis for patients with such cancers is better after removal of the cancerous lesion than is the case with the usual infiltrative ductal lesion.

The microcalcifications that appear in a group, like grains of sand or salt, often are small and uncountable, and may be present on the mammogram without evidence of a mass. They represent necrotic, intraductal material and may be present in nonpalpable or preclinical cancer. The importance of such microcalcifications is that when they are found in the absence of a mass density, they

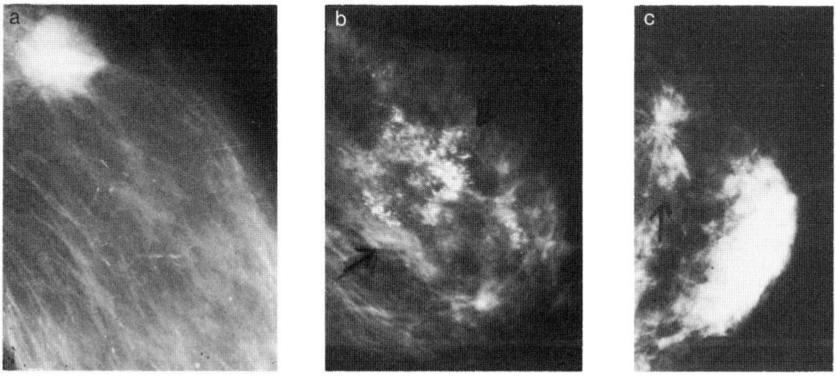

Fig. 4. Malignant changes (primary): (a) mass, (b) microcalcifications, (c) trabecular distortion.

are usually detected without axillary node involvement in a noninvasive stage, resulting in a better prognosis. After a variable interval, such cancers do become detected as masses, palpable densities with glandular involvement, as in other infiltrating carcinomas. Cancers diagnosed on the basis of microcalcifications alone present a problem in management, because most of these cancers are not palpable and often are not grossly visible at surgery. Since the cancer can be localized to a breast quadrant by the radiologist, the entire quadrant may be removed for biopsy, if feasible. If the breast is very large, other localizing procedures can be employed. The specimen removed must be divided into portions, which are radiographed prior to frozen section analysis. Multiple slides are made of the portion that contains the microcalcifications. Otherwise, the danger of making sections only through nonmalignant areas is great, and an incorrect diagnosis may result.

Mammography has been of particular value in detecting malignancies on the basis of these microcalcifications, which are present in approximately one-third of the cases. It can also detect small, infiltrative densities in the large fatty breasts so common in the postmenopausal patient, in whom clinical examination is difficult.

Altered architecture may be the only clue to malignant change. Fine changes of trabecular distortion or localized areas of fibrosis, especially when associated with haziness due to edema, may be the earliest signs of cancer even in the absence of a mass density. Diagnosis on the basis of such changes is difficult. Serial changes may be the clue in such cases.

Dilated or prominent ducts, particularly when localized, or diffuse areas of density in one breast when compared to the other, may be the only sign of a malignant or even a premalignant process, especially when correlated with the age of the woman and her parity status.

Radiologists have always noted the marked variability in the parenchymal patterns visualized on mammography. Most have felt, like the author, that they reflected in large part hormonal effects on the breast. Wolfe (1976) developed a classification of these patterns that he considers to be related to the degree of risk for the development of breast cancer. There are four categories, termed N1, P1, P2, and DY. In brief, N1 signifies an essentially normal breast, P1 a breast involved with a prominent duct pattern to a minimal degree, P2 a breast involved with a prominent duct pattern to a moderate to severe degree, and DY an extremely dense parenchyma, which Wolfe felt usually denoted connective tissue hyperplasia. It is women with the P2 and DY patterns who Wolfe reported had the highest risk of breast cancer. Some authors, like Krook *et al.* (1978), agree completely; some, like Egan and McSweeney (1979), disagree completely; and others, like Peyster *et al.* (1977), agree only partially. It should be emphasized that examination of prevalent cancers for risk patterns will not tally with the concepts of Wolfe, who insists that the patterns indicate only a degree of risk and thus apply only to incident cancers. The author agrees with this concept but feels that the degree of risk as indicated by Wolfe has been exaggerated. The risk patterns are useful only as an additional indicator of risk up to twice the normal and are probably closely tied to other risk factors, like parity status.

2. *Secondary Signs*

Secondary signs of malignancy include skin changes, nipple retraction, and increased vascularity. Diffuse skin thickening is associated with diffuse cancer, as in advanced infiltrative cancer or inflammatory malignancy. The skin may become considerably thickened because of cancer infiltrating skin lymphatics. Localized skin thickening or dimpling may be associated with a comparatively superficial cancer through duct infiltration and periductal and collagenous thickening. Nipple changes are associated with a subareolar carcinoma, and result in marked nipple retraction with thickening of the areola. Nipple retraction per se in the absence of other findings is usually due to congenital factors or old secretory duct changes with duct fibrosis. Paget's disease is a special type of cancer associated with clinically apparent nipple erosion. Mammograms are particularly useful in such cases. The breast cancer in such instances may betray its presence by a linear group of microcalcifications, often leading from the nipple area to an infiltrating, nonpalpable density deep in the breast.

Increased vascularity is a reflection of the increased metabolism associated with the malignant process. Many malignant masses have enlarged veins leading to their vicinity. Usually only the veins are visualized on a mammogram. Arteries are seen only in older women when calcium is deposited in the artery walls. A dilated vein in the vicinity of a well-demarcated density increases the suspicion of malignancy. As the malignant process advances, these veins may show a progressive increase in caliber on serial mammograms. Some observers state that if the veins in a breast are 1.4 times or more the size of the contralateral

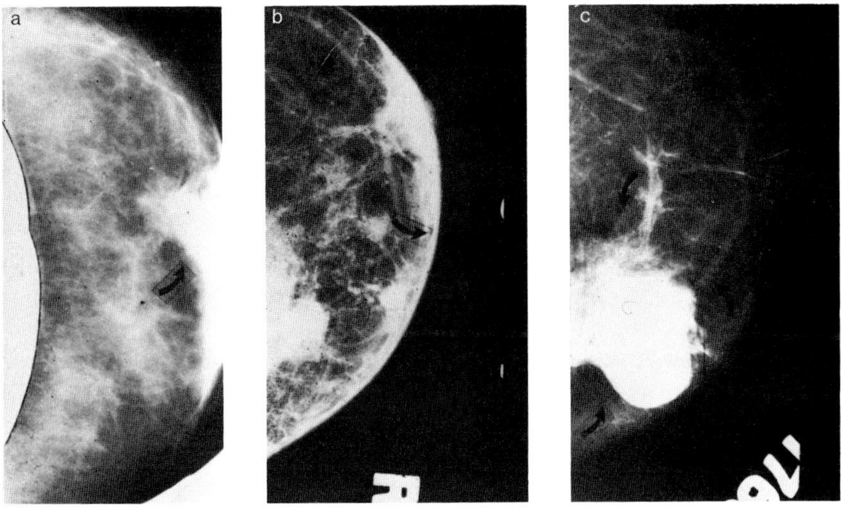

Fig. 5. Malignant changes (secondary): (a) nipple changes, (b) skin changes, (c) enlarged vein.

veins, that breast should be searched carefully or observed for the development of malignancy. Many cancers, however, do not seem to be associated with increased vein caliber.

Estimates of accuracy in mammography vary from 65% to 95% or higher. Results vary markedly with the type of patient or breast being examined, the quality of the technique, and the experience of the observer. It is well known that mammography, in conjunction with clinical examination done by the radiologist, can achieve a high degree of accuracy in the diffusely fatty breast of the postmenopausal woman. However, in the small, dense, glandular breast of the premenopausal woman, especially without a clinical examination, diagnostic accuracy is markedly reduced. A small carcinoma may be obscured completely on X ray in a dense, fibrotic breast, although it may be readily apparent to the clinician. In a clinical setting, the radiologist should have the opportunity to examine the breast physically, if at all possible, or at least to have all the clinical findings available when the mammogram is interpreted.

C. Breast Calcifications

Calcifications within the breast parenchyma have always been important because they are commonly found histologically in relation to breast cancer. However, it should be emphasized that most calcifications seen on a mammogram are not associated with cancer. They do deserve special consideration because certain types of calcifications may be the only manifestation of a nonpalpable cancer and are conscientiously sought by radiologists and clinicians alike, often too zealously. They represent an important source of biopsies that, in the majority of instances, turn out to be benign. It is important, therefore, to consider their general characteristics in order to help differentiate the benign from the malignant type. There are three main types of calcifications, considered in terms of their appearance and distribution in the breast:

1. Diffuse, scattered deposits of calcium that do not form groups. These are usually rounded (although they may be elongated), are often bilateral, and have a consistent density, so that they are easily visualized. They are often associated with duct ectasia where they are seen in the lines of the ducts. They are benign and rarely cause difficulty in the differential diagnosis. More rounded, scattered calcifications are associated with nonmalignant conditions such as adenosis. However, in such cases, the type of calcification is very similar to malignant calcifications and leads to biopsies for definite diagnosis. Calcifications are also seen in the walls of breast arteries. These usually present as parallel streaks in the walls of branching arteries and seldom cause difficulty in diagnosis.

2. Grouped or clustered calcifications not associated with a mass. These often vary in polarity, density, and size. They are usually irregular. Their size is expressed in millimeters. Good radiological technique and careful examination, often with the use of a magnifying lens, are often needed for detection. Their importance is underlined by the fact that they may be present without a mass density, are not palpable, and yet may be in the early stages of a killing cancer. They are sometimes difficult to localize, are not visible at exploration, and may require specimen radiography before pathological study to make sure that the proper section is being given to the pathologist for study. This type of calcification may be the only sign of a potentially localized and curable cancer. Under screening auspices, cancers presenting with this type of calcification represent one of the goals of study and one of its important rewards. It should be noted, however, that even in the most expert hands, not more than one in three or four biopsies performed under such conditions actually results in a malignant diagnosis. It is, however, considered a worthwhile price to pay for the potential salvage. These calcifications are considered an indication for exploration when they are at least five in number. Occasionally, two or three small calcifications are considered subject to follow-up but not exploration.

3. Calcifications associated with a mass. These are, in general, usually found as small masses of amorphous calcifications within a well-demarcated mass and, as a rule, represent a calcified fibroadenoma. The mass of calcification may remain even after the soft mass is absorbed into the general breast structure. This type of calcification is benign and does not change with repeated examinations. It is usually found in older women.

A more ominous type of calcification is seen within the irregular, spiculated mass suspicious of malignancy. Here the characteristics of the calcifications are those in group 2 mentioned above. These calcifications no longer represent a localized, preinfiltrative stage, but are merely an extension of the malignant process represented by the mass itself.

All in all, it should be emphasized that microcalcifications as a manifestation of cancer suffer from the same problem as do the other malignant signs. Benign disease can mimic cancer, and malignancy can be very similar in its signs to a nonmalignant process. The responsibility of the radiologist is to make a reasonable judgment, based on experience and on the mammogram, as to whether or not the breast requires exploration. Often the decision is like sailing between Scylla and Charybdis, with pitfalls on either side.

D. Mammography in Screening

The above discussion of malignant versus benign changes in the breast is most appropriate in considering mammography as a diagnostic tool of help in solving the problem of the woman who presents to her physician with a potential breast abnormality. Mammography with modern techniques is a most useful and necessary addition to clinical examination for differential diagnosis.

However, there is increasing awareness of a great need to detect breast cancer even before the woman is aware of a change in her breasts that motivates a physician examination. The presumably well woman may be harboring an occult, symptomless, sign-free cancer that may have to be detected at such a stage to reduce mortality. To find a cancer in the asymptomatic or minimally symptomatic woman requires periodic screening. Mammography, with its ability to detect the nonpalpable cancer, has become an increasingly important modality in the screening process. This concept is pointed up by the substantial contribution made by mammography in the large-scale screening program for breast cancer detection conducted by HIP under contract with the National Cancer Institute of the U.S. Public Health Service. In this study, one-third of the cancers were detected only on mammography and were not noted on clinical examination. In 79% of these cases, there was no axillary node involvement. Of 44 women with such cancers in an 8-year follow-up, only 3 died of breast cancer; six of these nonpalpable cancers were present in women under 50 years of age, none of whom died of the disease (Shapiro *et al.*, 1974).

The Guttman Breast Diagnostic Institute in New York City, operating in cooperation with the American Cancer Society, has been functioning as a mass screening center for breast cancer since 1968. Here, too, substantial numbers of cancers have been detected in a nonpalpable, localized stage (Strax, 1971).

With the Guttman Institute as a prototype, 28 other screening centers for breast cancer were funded by the National Cancer Institute and the American Cancer Society for a 5-year period. In all of the centers, substantial numbers of breast cancers were found to have no axillary node involvement—up to 48%.

It is of interest to compare data from this program with those from HIP. Overall, 42% of the cancers were found by mammography alone, with 77% negative nodes in the Breast Cancer Detection Demonstration Project (BCDDP), versus 33% with 79% negative nodes in HIP. However, in the under-50 age group, 35% of the cancers were found by mammography alone in BCDDP with 73% negative nodes, versus 19% in the HIP study with 68% negative nodes. Also—and this may be particularly important—13.8% of the cancers found in BCDDP were minimal cancers under 1 cm in size; 58.6% of these were found on mammography alone, versus only 3.5% of this type found in the HIP study (Table II). Thus, the improved mammographic techniques used in the BCDDP program have resulted in a substantially increased percentage of early cancers found on the X ray alone, particularly in women under 50, as compared to the findings in the HIP study.

Because of the concern in some quarters over X-radiation hazard to the breast, other modalities such as thermography with various techniques, ultrasonography, and diaphanography have been suggested, not only for differential diagnosis but also in mass screening. These newer modalities have shown value in differentiating benign from malignant lesions and have been of help in possibly delineating a high-risk woman or even offering prognostic information. These modalities, unfortunately, have been of little if any value in detecting the nonpalpable, occult lesion and, therefore, have not been of any practical importance in mass screening. Thermography has, however, been suggested as an indicator of high risk. Ultrasonography (see Chapter 12) and diaphanography have not yet been fully evaluated for mass screening.

TABLE II

Percentage of Breast Cancers Found by Mammography

	HIP (132 cancers) Percentage	BCDDP (2379 cancers) Percentage
Mammography alone (all ages)	33	48
Negative nodes	79	77
Mammography alone (under age 50)	19	45
Negative nodes	68	73
Minimal cancers under 1 cm in size (mammography and clinical exam)	4	14[a]

[a] A total of 59% found on mammography alone.

At present, mammography in mass screening appears indicated in the following situations:

1. There is definite proof that mass screening, using mammography in combination with clinical examination, leads to substantial mortality reduction in women over 50.
2. All women with a positive family history or a previous breast cancer should have periodic examinations, including mammography.
3. All women who are symptomatic with a dominant mass, persistent pain, or nipple discharge may have an underlying cancer and should receive periodic study, including mammography.
4. All women between 35 and 40 should have a baseline mammogram, not only to detect unsuspected disease but to be of value for future studies. Subsequent examinations, including mammography, should be carried out at the discretion of the physician.

It should be noted here that because there is no consensus on the value of mass screening in women under 50 (since the HIP study showed only a mortality improvement that was not statistically significant), a new study to clarify this point is needed before mammography can be generally recommended in screening women under 50. Such a study has been initiated by Miller in Canada (see Chapter 17). Nevertheless, the American Cancer Society and the American College of Radiology have recently advocated an annual or, at most, a biennial mammogram, in addition to palpation, in women between 40 and 50 years of age.

VII. CONCLUSIONS

A few principles to bear in mind in breast cancer diagnosis, and especially in mass screening, follow.

1. The clinician bears the ultimate responsibility for the decision on treatment for breast cancer. The radiologist has an important input in providing a service to the clinician, especially in the case of doubtful and nonpalpable lesions. Because up to 15% of palpable cancers are not visualized on X ray, the radiologist must never dissuade the clinician from exploration.
2. The vast majority of radiological masses are benign. In those that are palpable and radiologically benign, the decision to intervene should be left to the clinician, without prodding by the radiologist. In those masses that appear benign on X ray but are not palpable, it is often safe and proper to temporize, but with frequent observation. In those masses that are suspicious to the radiologist with

expertise, it is proper for the radiologist to urge his or her clinical colleague to explore, even when the lesion is not palpable.

3. Detection of microcalcifications as a sign of cancer represents the greatest potential of success for the radiologist in the search for the curable cancer. However, emphasis on this fact has led to many an elusive hunt. There has been a proliferation of surgical procedures to remove minimal groups of calcifications that turn out to be noncancerous. The problem is compounded by the fact that a nonpalpable lesion requires a substantial biopsy specimen with attendant specimen radiography. It takes considerable experience and expertise to achieve success in the gray area of breast calcifications. Cooperation between the clinician and the radiologist is the key to success in these cases.

4. The mammographic technique used under all circumstances should be the one that produces the greatest detail and resolution with the lowest amount of radiation needed to produce high-quality films. Such techniques should be subject to change as new knowledge and technology provide improvement in these areas. Techniques are readily available that deliver doses down to 0.02 rad to the midbreast. This low dosage can be considered negligible in comparison with the acknowledged benefit from mammography.

5. Clinicians should be aware of the limitations of mammography and should remember that, after all, the X ray study of the breast is an ancillary, although most valuable, ally when the clinician is confronted with a patient's breast problem.

6. It can be said categorically that mammography has turned out to be the best single modality for detecting potentially curable breast cancer.

REFERENCES

Bailar, J. C., III (1976). Mammography, a contrary view. *Ann. Intern. Med.* **84,** 77–84.

Bjurstam, N. G. (1978). Radiography of the female breast and axilla. *Acta Radiol., Suppl.* **357.**

Bjurstam, N. G., and Noch Quiding, L. (1975). ''Provning Av Ultrustning for Mjukdelsrontgen Av. Brostkorteln, Sjukvards for Valtningen.'' Gothenburg.

Buttenberg, D., and Werner, K. (1962). ''Die Mammographie.'' Schattauer, Stuttgart.

Chang, C. H. J. (1979). Computed tomographic mammography. Experiences with 1000 patients. *In* ''Reduced Dose Mammography'' (W. W. Logan, ed.), pp. 495–499. Masson, Paris.

Clark, R. L.. Copeland, M. M., Egan, R. L. *et al.* (1965). Reproducibility of the technic of mammography (Egan) for cancer of the breast. *Am. J. Surg.* **109,** 127–133.

Desprez-Curely, J. P., Picard, J. D., and Markovits, P. (1959). Lexamen Radiologique Due Sein. *Gaz. Med. Fr.* **66,** 249.

Egan, R. L. (1960). Experience with mammography in a tumor institution; evaluation of 1000 studies. *Radiology* **75,** 894–900.

Egan, R. L. (1964). ''Mammography.'' Thomas, Springfield, Illinois.

Egan, R. L., and McSweeney, M. B. (1979). Mammographic parenchymal patterns and risk of breast cancer. *Radiology* **133,** 65–70.

Friedrich, M., and Weskamp, P. (1978). Newere Entwicklungstendenzen Der Mammographie-Technik. *Medicamundi* **23,** 29–46.

Gershon-Cohen, J., and Berger, S. N. (1963). Mastography. *Radiol. Clin. North Am.* **1,** 115–143.

Gisvold, J. J., Karsell, P. R., and Reese, D. F. (1977). Computerized tomographic mammography. *In* "Breast Carcinoma" (W. W. Logan, ed.), pp. 219–238. Wiley, New York.

Gros, C. (1963). "Les maladies du sein." Masson, Paris.

Hoeffken, W., and Lanyi, M. (1973). "Rontgenuntersuchung der Brust." Thieme, Stuttgart.

Holleb, A. I. (1976). Risk vs benefit in breast cancer diagnosis. *Ca—Cancer J. Clin.* **26,** 63–64.

Krook, P. M., Carlile, T., Bush, W., and Hall, M. H. (1978). Mammographic parenchymal patterns as a risk indicator for prevalent and incident cancer. *Cancer* **41,** 1093–1097.

Leborgne, R. A. (1953). "The Breast in Roentgen Diagnosis." Impresora Uruguaya, Montevideo, S. A.

Logan, W. W. (1977). Overview of the radiologist's role in breast cancer. *In* "Breast Carcinoma" (W. W. Logan, ed.), pp. 343–365. Wiley, New York.

Lundgren, B., and Jakobsson, S. (1976). Single-view mammography. *Cancer (Amsterdam)* **38,** 1124–1129.

Miller, D. W., Hammerstein, G. R., White, D. R., Masterson, M. E., and Laughlin, J. S. (1977). Radiation absorbed dose in mammography. *Annu. Meet. Am. Assoc. Physicists Med.*

Muntz, E. P., Welkowsky, M., Kaegi, E., Morsell, L., Wilkinson, E., and Jacobson, G. (1978). Optimization of electrostatic imaging systems for minimum patient dose or minimum exposure in mammography. *Radiology* **127,** 517–523.

Ostrum, B. J., Becker, W., and Isard, H. J. (1973). Low-dose mammography. *Radiology* **109,** 323–376.

Peyster, R. G., Kalisher, L., and Cole, P. (1977). Mammographic parenchmal patterns and the prevalence of breast cancer. *Radiology* **125,** 387–391.

Price, J. L., and Nathan, B. E. (1975). Radiological aspects of the West London screening programme for breast neoplasms. *Proc. R. Soc. Med.* **68,** 438–440.

Salomon, A. (1913). Beitrage Zur Pathologie und Klinik der Mammakarzinome. *Arch. Klin. Chir.* **101,** 573–668.

Shapiro, S., Strax, P., Venet, L., and Venet, W. (1974). Changes in 5 year breast cancer mortality in a breast cancer screening program. *Proc., Natl. Cancer Conf., 7th, 1974,* pp. 663–678.

Sickles, E. A. (1977). Magnification mammography. *In* "Breast Carcinoma" (W. W. Logan, ed.), pp. 177–184. Wiley, New York.

Sickles, E. A. (1982). Mammographic detectability of breast microcalcifications. *AJR, Am. J. Roentgenol.* **139,** 913–918.

Snyder, R. E., Masterson, M. D., Miller, D. W., Kirch, R. L., Rothenberg, L. N., Hammerstein, G. R., and Laughlin, J. S. (1977). Image quality control and radiation exposure in mammography. *In* "Breast Carcinoma" (W. W. Logan, ed.), pp. 167–176. Wiley, New York.

Strax, P. (1971). New techniques in mass screening for breast cancer. *Cancer (Amsterdam)* **28,** 1563–1568.

Strax, P., and Pomeranz, M. M. (1968). Non-malignant variations in mammography. *Am. J. Roentgenol., Radium Ther. Nucl. Med.* **92,** 21–28.

Von Ronnen, J. F. (1956). "Plain Roentgenography of the Breast." Academic Press, New York.

Warren, S. L. (1930). A roentgenologic study of the breast. *Am. J. Roentgenol. Radium Ther.* **21,** 113–124.

Webster, E. W., and Kalisher, L. (1977). Minimal exposure film-screen techniques for mammography. *In* "Breast Carcinoma" (W. W. Logan, ed.), pp. 197–206. Wiley, New York.

Wolfe, J. N. (1972). "Xeroradiography of the Breast." Thomas, Springfield, Illinois.

Wolfe, J. N. (1976). Risk for breast cancer development determined by mammographic parenchymal pattern. *Cancer (Philadelphia)* **37,** 2486–2492.

10

Chest Radiology

FREDERICK P. STITIK, MELVYN S. TOCKMAN, AND NAGI F. KHOURI

I.	Introduction	163
II.	Radiographic Techniques	164
	A. Previous Chest Radiographic Screening Techniques	164
	B. Current Chest Radiographic Techniques	164
	C. Future Chest Radiographic Techniques	172
III.	Quality Control	173
IV.	The Value of Screening Radiography in Detecting Lung Cancer	174
	A. Introduction	174
	B. Results	175
V.	Conclusions	182
	References	189

I. INTRODUCTION

Radiographic examination of the chest is the most common radiographic procedure, comprising up to 50% of examinations performed in a radiology department (Lindheim, 1971). Despite this frequency, there is no uniform agreement on the optimal chest radiographic technique. This lack of agreement is largely due to the wide range of radiographic densities that must be visualized on a chest radiograph. Besides relatively dense structures such as the thoracic spine that must be seen through the mediastinum, they include structures of medium density such as the heart and extend to the low-density small blood vessels in the lungs. Visualization of all of these structures on one image implies a compromise. Optimization of chest radiographic technique has been the subject of numerous scientific investigations and symposia (U.S. Department of Health and Human Services, 1980).

ISBN 0-12-496720-5

Most of the research on improvement of technique or of observer performance has used the solitary pulmonary mass as a test object. The solitary pulmonary mass, whether present on original radiographs (Breckenridge and Bird, 1977; Kelsey *et al.*, 1982a; Kundel, 1981; Revesz and Kundel, 1977; Stitik and Tockman, 1978), photographically simulated (Brogdon *et al.*, 1978; Kelsey *et al.*, 1977; Kundel *et al.*, 1978; Kundel and Revesz, 1976) or created within a phantom (Christensen *et al.*, 1977a, Gray *et al.*, 1978; Kelsey *et al.*, 1982b), is much simpler and easier to reproduce than other forms of pulmonary pathology, i.e., diffuse interstitial disease. This choice is fortuitous, because information obtained by these studies can be advantageously applied to screening for lung cancer, the solitary pulmonary mass being the most common radiographic presentation of lung cancer (Muhm *et al.*, 1983; Stitik and Tockman, 1978; Theros, 1977).

II. RADIOGRAPHIC TECHNIQUES

A. Previous Chest Radiographic Screening Techniques

Most previous projects—the Philadelphia Pulmonary Neoplasm Research Project (Boucot *et al.*, 1961, the South London Lung Study (Nash *et al.*, 1968), and the North London Cancer Study (Brett, 1969)—have used photofluorography of the chest. This photographic representation of the fluoroscopic appearance of a chest is no longer employed in the United States because of the poor resolution obtained and the unacceptably high radiation exposure (U.S. Department of Health Education and Welfare, 1978). Consequently, observations pertaining to the quality and efficiency of radiographic screening for lung cancer cannot be extrapolated to modern-day techniques, described below.

B. Current Chest Radiographic Techniques

In most facilities that perform more than 40 chest radiographic examinations per day, a unit designed only for chest radiography is considered cost effective. Normally, these units have phototiming (automatic exposure control). Once a devoted chest unit is obtained, the practicing radiologist still has a number of parameters to choose from. These include:

1. Beam energy (kVp)
2. Focal spot size
3. Filtration
4. Antiscatter methods
5. Film–screen combinations
6. Number and type of views of the chest

1. Beam Energy (kVp)

Considerable controversy has developed over kVp selection. The kVp values for chest radiography can be divided into three ranges: (1) standard, 80–125 kVp; (2) high, 125–150 kVp; and (3) very high, 300–350 kVp. The trend in recent years has been toward higher kVp values. The reasons include (1) better penetration of the mediastinal and subdiaphragmatic structures, (2) decreased bonc contrast enabling us to "see through" ribs, (3) a decrease in the radiation exposure to the patient, and (4) wider latitude; thus, repeat examinations are less common using higher-kVp techniques. Fewer repeats is a second way of decreasing radiation exposure. High-kVp films with wide latitude also look remarkably similar from one examination to another, thus enabling subtle changes to be more easily detected than with other techniques, in which they may be ignored or wrongly attributed to differences in radiographic technique.

The energy of the beam has a marked effect on image quality. With increasing kVp there is increased penetration, and as the kVp is increased, there is a decrease in contrast between bone (ribs) and water-density soft tissue (i.e., solitary pulmonary masses). With this decreased contrast, the bone becomes less obvious and therefore less likely to obscure a small, solitary pulmonary mass. This is especially important in chest radiography, since up to 50% of the lung is obscured by bone and mediastinal structures. Increasing beam energy results in increased penetration of the mediastinum, allowing better visualization of small masses behind the heart and other mediastinal structures, and of those in the lower portions of the lungs that could be obscured by the upper abdomen. It is important to note that contrast between water-density structures, such as a solitary pulmonary mass, and air in the surrounding lung is also decreased with increasing kVp. This results in decreased contrast of the solitary pulmonary masses that are projected in the areas of the lung not covered by the ribs. This latter loss in contrast between water density and lung density, however, is much less than the decrease in contrast between bone and soft tissue. Proponents of higher-kVp techniques consider this compromise acceptable to obtain better visualization of the portions of the lung behind the ribs and mediastinal structures.

Appreciable controversy exists regarding the optimal beam energy for nodule detection. Christensen *et al.* (1977a), using a partial chest phantom, have shown an increase in nodule detection with increasing values up to 200 kVp. At energies higher than 200 kVp, nodule detection was not increased. Herman *et al.* (1980), using fixed lung specimens, also showed a decrease in visualization of small parenchymal lung abnormalities at 350 kVp when compared with 140- and 90-kVp images. Using paired radiographs, Haus *et al.* (1980) also showed a decrease in visualization of small pulmonary masses on 350-kVp images compared with 120-kVp images. A partial explanation for the decrased visibility of small structures at 350 kVp may be the relatively large focal spot (approximately 5 mm) used in the commercially available 350-kVp units.

Contrary observations regarding the image quality and visibility of small structures obtained with 350-kVp equipment are presented by Hallenbeck (1975) and Proto and Lane (1978). These authors report an improvement in visualization of small structures at 350 kVp.

The additional drawbacks of very high kVp include poor recognition of calcium in a pulmonary mass; the inability of this energy to study other areas of the body, e.g., the abdomen; and the paucity of X ray equipment manufacturers. These factors have contributed to a lack of general acceptance of 350-kVp equipment.

2. *Focal Spot Size*

Usually the smaller the effective focal spot size, the sharper the image. In the ordinary clinical range of focal spot sizes (0.3–2.0 mm), differences among them are not recognized visually, nor do they affect the detection of superimposed nodules in a chest phantom (Gray *et al.*, 1978). In Gray *et al.*'s (1978) study, there was in increase in false-positive rates at smaller focal spot sizes, possibly due to the visualization of small blood vessels not usually seen with standard radiographic techniques. The larger focal spots (2.0 mm or greater), however, may degrade the image and decrease the ability to see small pulmonary masses.

3. *Filtration*

The X ray beam, as it exits the tube, can contain a heterogeneous combination of energies. The lower-energy radiation adds to patient exposure but does not contribute to the final image. Attempts are therefore made to remove this radiation before it reaches the patient. A number of filters, including Ferlic, copper, and, more recently, yttrium, are being utilized to decrease radiation exposure while not significantly affecting the quality of higher (140–150 kVp) energy radiation.

4. *Antiscatter Measures*

Scattered radiation reduces image quality. At present, the majority of chest radiographs (especially at higher beam energies) are performed with the use of a grid. The grid is placed between the patient and the film–screen combination. It commonly consists of parallel strips of lead and aluminum. Grids are either stationary or are moved across the film during X ray exposure. The primary radiation has a straight course and readily passes through the aluminum portions of the grid, whereas scattered radiation exits at varying angles and is absorbed by the lead strips. Since some of the primary radiation is absorbed by the lead strips, more radiation is usually required with the use of grids. Another disadvantage of the grid technique is that, with fast exposure times, the moving grid may produce grid lines on the image, obscuring detail. In general practice, a 10-to-1 or 12-to-1 grid is commonly used with high-energy (130-150 kVp) radiographs.

A second method commonly used for scatter reduction is the air-gap technique. With this technique, the patient is moved 6–8 inches away from the film–screen combination. There is a consequent reduction in scatter because it exits at different angles and thus may not even hit the film or have enough energy to traverse the 6- to 8-inch gap. Radiation also decreases in intensity as it passes through air, so that the small amount of scattered radiation that may hit the film is usually of very low intensity.

Air-gap techniques are slightly less effective than grids in reducing scatter. When an air-gap technique is employed, the distance between the film and the X ray tube is about 9–12 feet. This increase in distance over the conventional chest radiograph taken at 6 feet introduces logistical problems in room design. For these reasons, the air-gap technique is not as popular as the grid technique.

Other techniques used to reduce scatter in chest radiography are the moving slit technique (Sotensen and Nelson, 1976), the multiple-slit scanning technique (Barnes *et al.*, 1977), and the raster technique (Plewes, 1983; Plewes and Vogelstein, 1983; Plewes and Wandtke, 1982; Wandtke and Plewes, 1983). With these techniques, a slot is placed at the X ray tube and a comparable slot is placed between the patient and the film, allowing only small portions of the film to be exposed. Although this slotted equipment is not commercially available at present, the concept may be used in future applications of chest radiography (Tesic *et al.*, 1984).

5. *Film–Screen Combinations*

The choice of film–screen combinations in the past was relatively simple; however, with the introduction of many rare earth film–screen combinations, the choice became more complex. In general, the film–screen combination is chosen on the basis of the radiologist's preference, taking into account resolution, cost, and radiation exposure. Rare earth film–screen combinations reduce radiation exposure (Rossi *et al.*, 1976; Thompson *et al.*, 1977) and can, because of the shorter exposure times, improve image quality. However, as radiation levels are decreased, the quantum mottle (film graininess) increases and can become objectionably high, to the point of obscuring solitary pulmonary masses. Gray *et al.* (1978), who measured quantum mottle with the root mean square (RMS) technique, showed a decreasing detection rate of small, solitary pulmonary masses with increasing RMS noise. This increase in noise was also associated with an increase in false-positive readings and intraobserver disagreements. Another possible drawback is that the very fast rare earth film–screen combinations may be too fast for accurate phototiming.

The characteristics of the film, whether paired with rare- earth or traditional calcium tungstate screens, also have to be considered. In general, the wide range of densities in the thorax described earlier present a special problem in film response. Again, a compromise is involved in choosing a film that will respond to low-density structures such as blood vessels behind the heart without becoming overpenetrated in the upper portions of the chest, i.e., burning out the pulmonary vascularity in the upper portions of the chest. As a rule, either standard or newer rare earth film–screen combinations with an adjusted speed of 200–400 appear to be optimal for current chest radiography. Anticrossover emulsion in the film base prevents the light of one screen from coming back through the film to expose its other side. These anticrossover emulsions are now available and may improve the resolution of chest radiographs in the future (Kelsey *et al.*, 1983).

6. *Number of Views*

In most instances, a standard radiographic examination of the chest includes a posteroanterior (PA) and a lateral view of the chest. In the past, the major value of the lateral view was to visualize areas of the lung not well seen with low-kVp PA chest radiographs—areas such as the posterior sulci, which can be obscured by the diaphragm in the frontal view, and the retrocardiac portions of the lung, which may be obscured by the heart. In modern practice, in which higher-kVp techniques are generally used, these benefits are not as important as they were formerly; however, the lateral view remains indispensable for confirming questionable abnormalities on the PA radiograph and for localizing obvious abnormalities in the frontal view.

We consider the lateral view a form of "double reading" and have noted that abnormalities may first be suspected on the lateral chest radiograph and then confirmed on review of the frontal film. The importance of the lateral view as a conscious or subconscious clue to pulmonary disease is often not appreciated later, since the PA radiograph is used to demonstrate the abnormality to clinicians, as well as in lectures and publications. Its value in screening for early lung cancer cannot be accurately judged, since there has been no prospective study analyzing the contribution of the lateral chest X ray alone to early lung cancer detection. Retrospective reviews of chest radiographs in patients with documented lung cancer have provided differing results, tabulated in Table I. Figure 1 illustrates an early lung cancer (seen in a Johns Hopkins Lung Project volunteer) that was identified only on the lateral view.

The second most common series of standard views is the stereo PA pair. Two PA views with minimal tube shift when viewed stereoscopically give the chest a three-dimensional appearance, thus allowing for better visualization of small masses behind the ribs and the mediastinal structures. Kelsey *et al.* (1982a) tested observers in detecting small pulmonary nodules when PA pairs were read as (1) one film only, (2) both films side by side, and (3) both films stereoscopically. The observer accuracy was 0.79, 0.87, and 0.89, respectively. It is clear that little is gained by stereoscopic viewing, but two PA views seen to-

TABLE I

Value of the Lateral View in Detecting Lung Cancer

Author	N	Better lat. view		Lat. view alone	
		(N)	(%)	(N)	(%)
Forrest and Sagel (1979)	99	4	4.0	0	0
Sagel *et al.* (1974)	4	0	0	0	0
Stitik and Tockman (1978)	74	2	2.7	1	1.4
Muhm *et al.* (1983)	80	—	—	2	2.5
F. P. Stitik, M. S. Tockman, and N. F. Khouri, unpublished data	203	14	6.9	4	2.0

gether—with a slight tube shift being the only difference between them—was enough to increase observer accuracy significantly over the reading of a single PA radiograph alone (0.79 to 0.87). The slight tube shift can be enough to displace a mass away from bone or confusing vascular shadows.

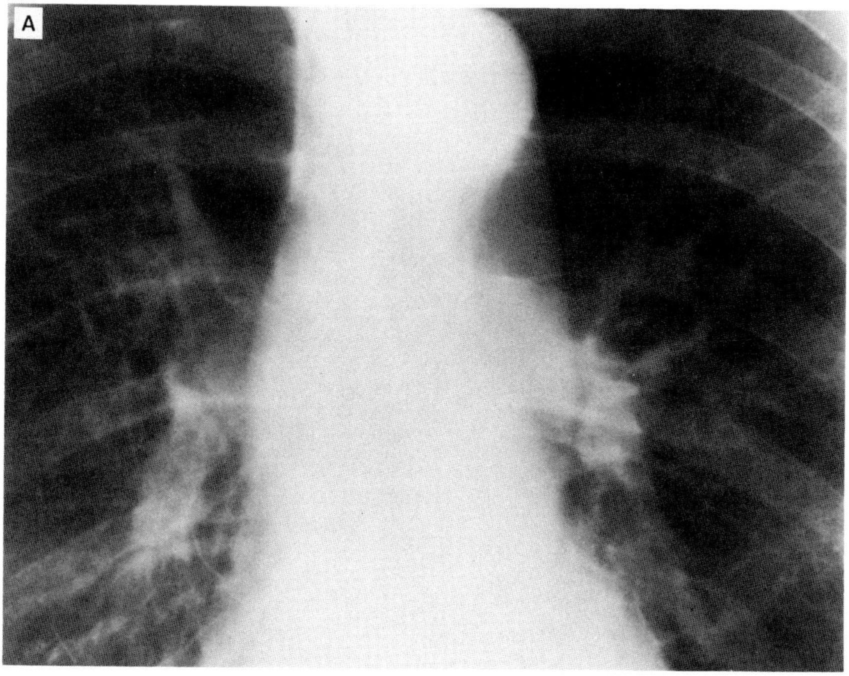

Fig. 1. Value of the lateral chest radiograph. This patient's squamous cell carcinoma is not seen on the closeup of the PA view (A) but is well seen anterior to the hilum on the closeup of the lateral view (B). The CT scan (C) confirms its location. *(continued)*

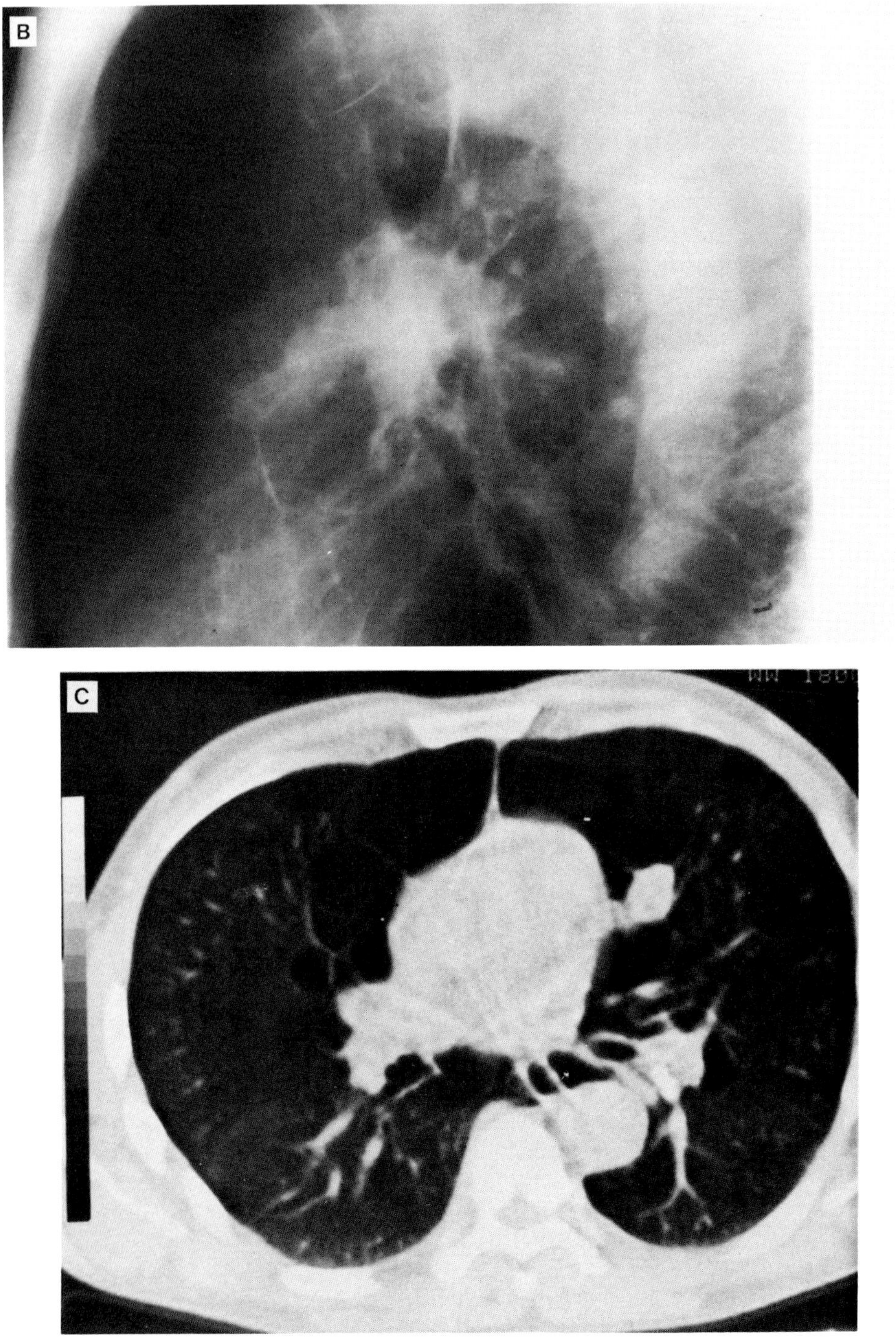

Fig. 1. (*Continued*)

Figure 2 shows close-ups of two PA chest radiographs, done minutes apart, of a patient with a small lung cancer. This patient's mass is barely seen on the close-up on the left but is readily detectable by a slight movement from underneath the rib, as shown in the close-up on the right. Kelsey *et al.* (1982a) postulate that a second PA chest radiograph could be added to the traditional PA and lateral and be cost effective in detecting small pulmonary masses in patients in whom the prevalence is high, e.g., in those with documented extrathoracic primary cancers known to metastisize to the lungs, but state that it would not be cost effective as a general screening procedure.

As a caution, however, it should be noted that the converse situation also exists. That is, a very small mass may be questionable on one PA radiograph, and the second follow-up radiograph may not show it clearly. For example, let us assume that only the first radiograph done in the patient shown in Fig. 2 was the one shown on the right. Once the abnormality was detected, the patient may have been asked to return for a follow-up chest radiograph. This conceivably could have been done with the technique and rotation shown on the left, and could have led to a false impression of a resolved pneumonia or disappearance of an artifact. Whenever a patient with a small, possible pulmonary mass is referred to us and the follow-up radiograph does not show any abnormality, we will fluoroscope

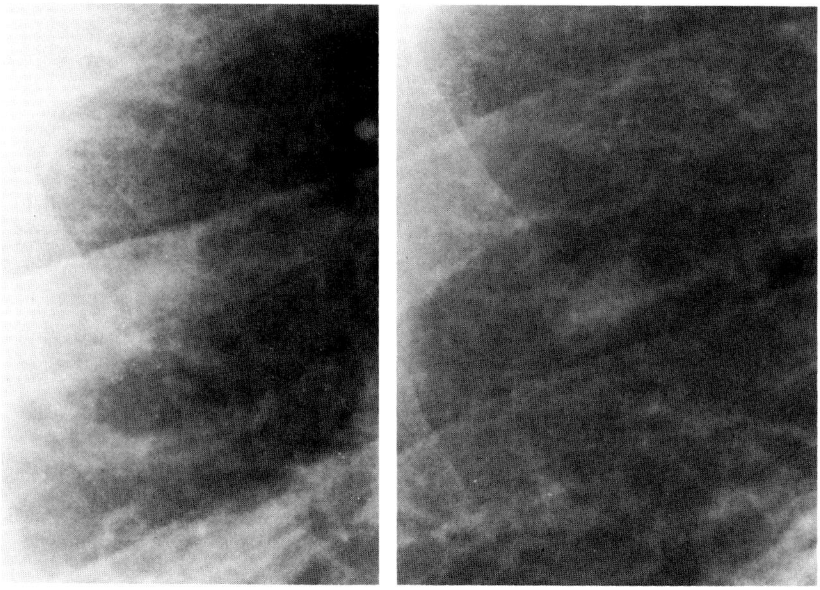

Fig. 2. Example of tube shift. The closeups of two PA radiographs that were obtained minutes apart show an early right lower lobe cancer. On the left, the small mass is barely seen because of the overlying ribs. On the right, the lesion is easily seen due to a slight tube shift and a slight difference in inspiration.

the chest, do thin section computed tomography (CT), or obtain a third follow-up radiograph in 3 months to ensure that we are not obscuring a small pulmonary parenchymal mass by slight differences in rotation and respiration.

C. Future Chest Radiographic Techniques

Using the localization device of modern CT scanners, i.e., the General Electric (GE) 8800 scout view, a computer-simulated chest radiograph can be obtained. This image is made by moving the patient through the gantry so that a narrow beam of radiation is passed through the body and accumulated by a series of detectors. Preliminary studies of computer chest radiography (Foley *et al.*, 1979, 1981; Huebener, 1983; Johnson and Ravin, 1983; Katragadda *et al.*, 1979) have prompted the development of devoted digital chest units. In one prototype (Fraser *et al.*, 1983; Tesic *et al.*, 1984) the chest is scanned by a narrow beam of radiation in 5 seconds or less. The digitalized image then appears on a cathode

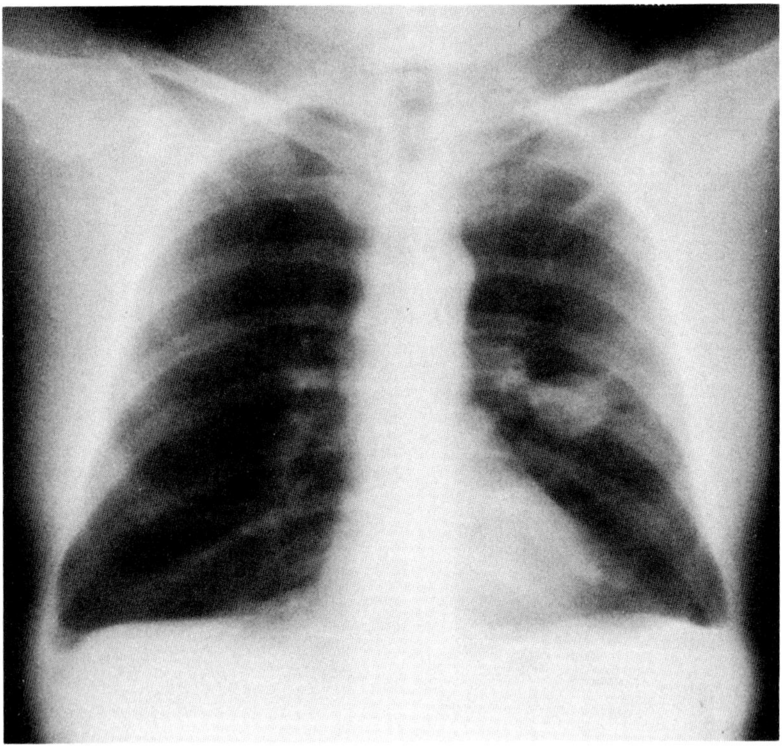

Fig. 3. Digital chest radiography. A left lower lobe lung cancer is readily demonstrated. (Case courtesy of Theresa C. McLoud, M.D.)

ray tube (CRT) 5 seconds later. Digital chest radiography remains experimental at this time, although its potential advantages of reduced scatter and therefore better contrast resolution, the wide latitude of densities displayed, the edge enhancement, the potential for reduced radiation exposure (especially since no repeat examinations should be necessary), the postprocessing image manipulation (as with CT), and storage and transfer in the digital mode may outweigh the disadvantages of increased physician interpretation time, equipment costs, and, at present, slightly poorer images (Fig. 3).

III. QUALITY CONTROL

All of the benefits of these carefully selected parameters just discussed can be negated unless a quality control program is established. Sudden drastic changes in radiographic quality are readily apparent, but the essence of a quality control program is to ensure against subtle, progressive degradation in image quality.

Radiographic film is stored in a cool, dry area, away from radiation and chemical sources. It is stored in such a manner that the oldest film is used first. A careful check is always made of expiration dates before the film is brought into the radiographic room.

The screens are cleaned on a monthly basis and replaced periodically.

Proper functioning of the radiographic equipment is checked annually by a physicist who measures the accuracy of parameters such as kVp, timer, mA, beam alignment, half-value layer, and repeatability. A reject/repeat study is performed periodically to provide a method for the analysis of the rejected radiographs.

Daily monitoring of film processors to measure developer temperature and film processing parameters such as speed (density), contrast, and base-plus-fog levels are integral to the quality control program. The developer temperature is checked daily with a digital thermometer, since the thermometers provided by the manufacturer are usually not accurate. The manufacturer's recommendations concerning chemistry, developer temperature, and replenishment rates should be followed exactly, and all tests should be carried out in the same manner each time. Every morning at an appointed time (at least one-half hour after startup), film set aside specifically for testing is exposed with a sensitometer on both sides of the emulsion. Ideally a 3- to 6-month supply of film with the same lot number is maintained for testing only. The appropriate density levels are then measured with a calibrated densitometer and plotted on a control chart for each processor. The upper and lower limits of acceptance are indicated on this chart, so that variances can be easily identified. The charts are then analyzed for trends or any points falling outside the control limits. If any point or points exceed the established limits, two additional exposed sensitometric films are run to verify the readings. This procedure often allows processing problems to be identified in the early stages before they become apparent to the practicing radiologist.

IV. THE VALUE OF SCREENING RADIOGRAPHY IN DETECTING LUNG CANCER

A. Introduction

To evaluate screening chest radiography, we analyzed the results of the Johns Hopkins Lung Project (JHLP). JHLP volunteers were recruited from the demographic groups at greatest risk of lung cancer, i.e., males aged 45 years or older (U.S. Department of Health, Education and Welfare, 1979). Direct mailings to those so identified were made from a list compiled by the Department of Motor Vehicles of the State of Maryland. Recruitment mailings were made from 1974 to 1978. These mailings included an invitation to join the JHLP program of screening for lung cancer if the participant smoked at least one pack of cigarettes per day at the current time or at some time during the previous year. Participants called the JHLP in response to this invitation. At the time of their call, participants were randomly placed in either of two groups, one to receive an annual radiographic screening, the other to be screened by annual radiography plus sputum cytology three times a year.

In a previous report, the results of the initial prevalence radiographic screening were presented (Stitik and Tockman, 1978). Here we will describe the features of the incidence screening radiographs taken by the JHLP following exclusion of the prevalence lung cancer cases. The radiographic screening techniques have remained constant over the duration of the study. In brief, all participants had PA and lateral chest radiographs taken at 140 kVp at 300 or 400 mA. Automatic exposure termination was routinely employed. The film–screen combination generally used was medium-speed film (DuPont Cronex 4) and medium-speed screens (DuPont Par Speed). A 10-to-1 stationary grid was employed. The focal spot film distance was 72 inches. The following day, the films were independently doubly read by two members of a pool of screeners, all of whom were board certified, diagnostic radiologists on the staff of The Johns Hopkins Hospital.

The radiographs were coded into the following categories:

Cancer (CAN)	Abnormality that probably represents cancer and needs immediate clinical evaluation.
Suspect (SUS)	Abnormality that probably is not cancer but needs additional examinations to exclude the possibility completely.—e.g., old films, repeat for artifact, repeat with nipple markers, oblique films, tomograms, etc., and follow-up films.
Negative (NEG)	No evidence of cancer.
Unsatisfactory (UNS)	Insufficient quality to enable detection of early lung cancer or exhibiting changes that could obscure early lung cancer.

Radiographs which probably showed lung cancer (CAN) were brought to the immediate attention of the clinical director of the JHLP (M.S.T.) for medical evaluation. Radiographs that possibly showed lung cancer (SUS) were sent to the referees (F.P.S. or N.F.K.) for final coding and disposition.

Secondary codes were assigned to the radiographs for conditions that may predispose to or be associated with lung cancer, including emphysema, bullae, pulmonary parenchymal scarring, probably the residua of previous tuberculosis, residua of other pulmonary parenchymal inflammatory disease, radiographic evidence of asbestosis, or diffuse interstitial fibrosis. The referee also resolved discrepancies in the recording of these secondary codes.

B. Results

The 10,307 participants free of lung cancer at the time of the initial JHLP screening were encouraged to continue their screening. For each individual, the worst JHLP incidence screening radiograph has been tabulated (Table II) by the presence or absence of confirmed lung cancer. A radiographic abnormality was detected during screening in 1792 (17.4%). A total of 352 (19.6%) of these participants had radiographs thought to show cancer (CAN), while 1440 (80.4%) were felt to be suspect (SUS), but probably not to have lung cancer. Of those

TABLE II

Interpretation of the Worst JHLP Screening Films (Entered Incidence Screening of 10,307 Persons)

	Abnormal 1792		Normal 8515	
	CAN (352)	SUS (1440)	NEG (8501)	UNS (14)
Confirmed cancer (354)	201		153	
True positives	171	30		
False positives (258)	181	77		
Probably benign				
Workup negative		1333		
< 2 years' stability				
False negatives[a]				
Interval since last screening				
≤ 14 months	6	17	75	
> 14 months	1	6	62	
Positive cytology	5	4	14	
Postscreening			2	

[a] False negatives are included above as confirmed cancer.

with positive radiographs, 171 (48.6%) were subsequently confirmed to have cancer. Conversely, 181 (51.4%) were falsely called positive. Similarly, 30 of the 1440 radiographs (2.1%) called SUS actually had detected a cancer, while 77 5.3%) falsely led to further medical management. The majority of the suspect films (1333/1440, 92.6%) merely required follow-up for 2 years to demonstrate radiographic stability and, thus, benignity.

Of the 8515 volunteers with negative results, 14 radiographs were unsatisfactory and 153 volunteers (1.8%) were subsequently found to have confirmed lung cancer. Of these false-negatives, 14 were detected by cytology only, and 2 were detected at other institutions shortly after screening concluded. The remaining 137 negative radiographs failed to show a cancer that presented clinically between screenings.

The association of the radiographic finding and the presence of lung cancer can be regrouped to calculate the sensitivity and specificity of radiographic screening for lung cancer (Table III). Of the 354 cases of lung cancer that occurred among the participants of the JHLP, 162 were detected by radiographic screening (sensitivity, 45.8%; 162/354). Conversely, of the 9953 J.H.L.P. participants who did not develop lung cancer, 9695 were correctly categorized by their screening radiograph (specificity, 97.4%; 9695/9953).

It is of more clinical relevance, however, to determine the predictive value of the radiograph. Among the 420 (159 CAN, true positives; 3 SUS, true positives; 181 CAN, false positives; 77 SUS, false positives undergoing medical evaluation) with a positive screening radiograph, 162 (38.6%) in fact had lung cancer. The low predictive value of a positive radiograph may be contrasted to the high predictive value of a negative one. Of the 9887 individuals with a negative chest radiograph, 9695 (98.1%) did not, in fact, have lung cancer.

It is reasonable to remove from consideration those 23 cancers detected by cytology only and the 2 cancers that occurred shortly after cessation of screening. Removal of these 25 cases leaves a total of 329 lung cancer cases in the JHLP. Screening radiography detected 162/329 of these, for a sensitivity of 49.2%. Removal of these cases, which might not have been eligible for radiographic detection, has the effect, therefore, of increasing the sensitivity from 45.8% to 49.2%. The specificity (97.4%) and the predictive value of a positive test (38.6%) would be unaffected by removal of these cases. The predictive value of a negative test would improve slightly. Of the remaining 9862 JHLP participants with negative chest radiographs, 9695 (98.3%) were correctly classified by their screening radiograph.

The American Joint Committee (AJC) (1983) stage distribution of the 354 cases of lung cancer is presented in Table IV by mode of detection. Cases detected during screening show the most advantageous stages. Of the 23 detected by cytology alone, 20 (87%) were detected either at an *in situ* (stage TIS) or a localized (stage 1) stage. Of the 162 cases detected by screening radiography, 86 (53.1%) were localized at the time of detection.

TABLE III

Determination of the Sensitivity and Specificity of Radiographic Screening for Lung Cancer

	Lung cancer present (chest X ray code)				Lung cancer absent (chest X ray code)		
	Abnormal		Normal				
	CAN	SUS	NEG	Total	Abnormal	Normal	Total
Mode of detection							
Radiograph	154	3		157	258	9695	9953
Cytology	5	4	14	23			
Both	5			5			
Interval[a]	7[a]	23[a]	137	167			
Postscreen			2	2			
	171	30	153	354	258	9659	9953
True positive				162			
Lung cancer present							
X ray–abnormal		157					
X ray, cytology abnormal		5					
False positive				258			
Lung cancer absent							
X ray CAN		181					
X ray SUS		77					
False negative				192			
Lung cancer present							
Cytology abnormal		23					
Interval		167					
Postscreen		2					
True negative				9695			
X ray SUS, probably benign		1333					
X ray NEG		8362					

[a] Abnormalities called CAN or SUS were not the site of eventual lung cancer.

TABLE IV

Stage Distribution of Confirmed Lung Cancer by Mode of Detection

			X ray–negative cases									
	X ray–positive cases		≤ 14 months since last screen		> 14 months since last screen		Cytology-detected cases		Postscreening cases		Total	
Stage	(*N*)	(%)	(*N*)	(%)	(*N*)	(%)	(*N*)	(%)	(*N*)	(%)	(*N*)	(%)
TIS	0	—	3	3.1	0	—	10	43.5	0	—	13	3.7
1	86	53.1	13	13.3	13	18.8	10	43.5	1	50.0	123	34.7
2	18	11.1	6	6.1	7	10.1	1	4.3	0	—	32	9.0
3	58	35.8	76	77.6	49	71.0	2	8.7	1	50.0	186	52.5
Total	162	100.0	98	100.0[a]	69	100.0[a]	23	100.0[a]	2	100.0	354	100.0

[a] Distribution significantly different from that of X ray–detected cases; $p < 0.005$.

The cases that could not be detected by screening showed the least advantageous distribution of stage at the time of their presentation. These interval cases, which arose between regularly attended screenings (less than or equal to 14 months since the last screen), were found in stage 1 only (16.4%, 16/98). Among these interval cases, it did not matter whether screenings were regularly attended (less than or equal to 14 months since the last screen) or not (greater than 14 months since the last screen). Only 18.8% (13 cases) of the latter group presented in stage 1. With the exception of the postscreening cases, whose number is small, each of the stage distributions by mode of detection noted above is significantly different from the stage distribution in the X ray–detected cases. The cases detected by cytology have a significantly better stage distribution. That of the interval cases is significantly worse.

The lung cancer cell type seems to influence the likelihood of radiographic detection (Table V). Significant differences are seen between the cell type distributions of lung cancers detected by radiography, those detected by cytology, and those X ray–negative cases that arose between regular screenings. Adenocarcinoma was the most frequent cell type detected by radiography (36.4%), squamous cell cancer was the most frequent cell type detected by sputum cytology (95.6%) and small-cell undifferentiated cancer was the most frequent cell type that arose between regular screenings (30.6%). Clinically detected (X ray-negative) cancers that arose outside of regular screening (beyond 14 months and after screening) showed no significant difference in cell type distribution from those detected by radiography.

There is an association between the radiographic appearance and the stage of confirmed lung cancer in the JHLP, although the association is somewhat counterintuitive (Table VI). Those individuals whose radiographs showed no evidence of cancer, but who subsequently developed cancer, were found to have lung neoplasms at an advanced stage. Interestingly, there was no difference in the clinical severity distribution among those with completely negative chest radiographs, and those with SUS radiographs that were being followed over time because they were thought probably to indicate a benign condition (SUP). The clinical severity of the radiographs called CAN was significantly better. There was no difference in the stage distribution between individuals whose radiograph was called CAN and those whose film was felt to be suspicious for cancer (SUS).

The annual radiograph prior to the one that resulted in a positive screen (led to detection of a lung cancer) was evaluated. All of these prior radiographs had been called normal. However, on several, a retrospective review showed the presence of a lesion. Factors that may have led to a prior miss of these lesions are listed in Table VII in the column headed "X Ray–positive Cases." Similarly, the annual screening radiographs that preceded the nonradiographic detection of lung cancer cases (those detected by clinical presentation, i.e., interval cases or those detected by cytology alone) were evaluated. On retrospective review,

TABLE V

Cell Type Distribution of Confirmed Lung Cancer by Mode of Detection

Cell type	X ray–positive cases		X ray–negative cases: ≤ 14 months since last screen		X ray–negative cases: > 14 months since last screen		X ray–negative cases: Cytology-detected cases		Postscreening cases		Total	
	(*N*)	(%)	(*N*)	(%)	(*N*)	(%)	(*N*)	(%)	(*N*)	(%)	(*N*)	(%)
Squamous	35	21.6	25	25.5	15	21.7	22	95.6	0	—	97	27.4
Adeno	59	36.4	23	23.5	16	23.2	1	4.3	2	100.0	101	28.5
Large cell	41	25.3	17	17.3	20	29.0	0	—	0	—	78	22.0
Small cell	21	13.0	30	30.6	16	23.2	0	—	0	—	67	18.9
Other	6	3.7	3	3.1	2	2.9	0	—	0	—	11	3.1
Total	162	100.0	98	100.0[a]	69	100.0	23	100.0[a]	2	100.0	354	100.0

[a] Distribution significantly different from that of X ray–detected cases; $p < 0.01$.

TABLE VI

Clinical Severity of Confirmed Cancers (AJC Stage) by Radiographic Appearance

	SUS		CAN		SUP		NEG		Total	
Stage	(*N*)	(%)	(*N*)	(%)	(*N*)	(%)	(*N*)	(%)	(*N*)	(%)
TIS	0	—	1	0.9	3	10.7	9	5.8	13	3.7
1	41	66.1	48	44.0	5	17.8	29	18.7	123	34.7
2	6	9.7	13	11.9	—	—	13	8.4	32	9.0
3	15	24.2	49	44.1	20	71.4	102	66.7	186	52.5
Total	62	100.0[a]	111	100.0[a]	28	100.0	153	100.0	354	100.0

[a] Distribution significantly different from that of X ray–negative cases; $p < 0.005$.

several of these radiographs also showed the presence of a lesion. Factors that may have led to the miss of these interval or cytologically positive cases are listed in Table VII in the column headed "X Ray–Negative Cases."

Films that, in retrospect, showed a radiographically detectable lesion are thus compared in Table VII by whether the presence of lung cancer was determined by subsequent radiologic screening or by clinical presentation or positive sputum cytology.

Overall, the radiographs of patients in whom a lung cancer was later detected by radiographic screening were more often abnormal than those radiographs that

TABLE VII

Retrospective Review of Missed Lesions

	X ray–negative cases[a]	X ray–positive cases[b]
Observer error	21	35[a]
Ill-defined	14	33[a]
Overlying mediastinum	15	11
Overlying bone	13	30[a]
Small (< 1 cm)	6	17[a]
Suboptimal film	2	5
Complex films	18	10
Total reviewed	137	97
Total lung cancers[c]	190	162
[a]Interval, cytologic detection		

[a] Factor is found significantly more often in X ray–positive than in X ray–negative cases; $p < 0.005$.

[b] Distribution is significantly different from that of X ray–negative cases; $p < 0.05$.

[c] Excludes two postscreening cases.

preceded detection by clinical presentation or by positive sputum cytology alone. Specific factors that contribute significantly to this difference include observer error, ill-defined lesions, overlying bone, and small (less than 1 cm) lesions. All of these features are found more often on radiographs that later led to a radiographic screening detection than those that did not, suggesting that the negative screening radiographs that preceded the clinical and/or cytologic detection were truly negative.

Of the 329 cases of lung cancer detected by radiologic screening or clinical presentation during this project, 203 had both PA and lateral chest radiographs available for retrospective review (frequently, outside hospitals would send only a PA view for our records). The lateral film was compared to the frontal film for visibility of lung cancer and coded as (1) cancer seen worse on the lateral view, (2) cancer seen equally well in both views, (3) cancer seen better in the lateral view, or (4) cancer seen only on the lateral view (Table 1).

In approximately two-thirds of these cases, 138/203 (68%), the cancer was better seen on the frontal view. In 47/203 (23%) it was seen equally well in both views. In 14/203 (7%) and 4/203 (2%), the cancer was better seen on the lateral view or seen only on the lateral view, respectively.

V. CONCLUSIONS

The wide variety of radiographic densities on a chest radiograph precludes a single optimal technique. The truly optimal technique must visualize both very dense structures, such as the thoracic spine behind the mediastinum, and much less dense structures, such as small upper lobe pulmonary masses. However, where the primary task is to detect a solitary pulmonary mass, the current techniques afford excellent means of visualization.

Usually, a modern generator should be employed in a devoted chest room equipped with automatic exposure control. To visualize all portions of the lung, a high-energy technique in the range of 135–150 kVp is our preference. The effective focal spot should be between 0.3 and 2.0 mm. Usually a focal spot of about 0.6 mm effective size is optimal. Appropriate filtration is a matter of individual choice. We use a grid as an antiscatter device. In facilities where air-gap techniques have been developed, these may be an adequate substitute. The film–screen combinations can be varied according to individual preference, although generally they should be in the adjusted speed of 200–400, have an anticrossover base, and allow a PA and lateral chest radiograph to be performed, with the total radiation exposure for both views being under 30 mR.

Although retrospective reviews (Table 1) have shown that a few bronchogenic carcinomas are seen only on the lateral view, we consider this view indispensable as a prospective form of double reading. Frequently, the abnormality on the chest radiograph is brought to one's attention initially on the lateral view, although, with the search now being focused in a definite area, it will eventually be better seen or documented on the frontal view. The use of a second PA radiograph performed with a slight tube shift may be considered an adjunct to a standard PA and lateral chest examination. Studies of cost effectiveness indicate, however, that this would not be feasible in a standard population, although it could possibly be justified in very-high-risk groups (Kelsey *et al.*, 1982a).

Further radiographic screening efforts will undoubtedly employ digital screening radiography, with its ability to increase contrast resolution and postprocessing capabilities. Future studies should consider this modality.

Quality control of chest radiography is as critical as any other radiographic quality control measure. It mandates careful monitoring of film dates, radiation actually delivered by the machine, and developing techniques. Standardized, regular quality control evaluation is an important part of any facility performing radiographic examinations.

The sensitivity of modern-day chest radiography, despite the improvements mentioned in this chapter, remains remarkably similar to that of photofluorograms obtained during screening for tuberculosis or bronchogenic carcinoma (Boucot *et al.*, 1961; Brett, 1968; Groth-Petersen *et al.*, 1952; Guiss and Kuenstler, 1960; Yerushalmy *et al.*, 1950). Our study shows that approximately

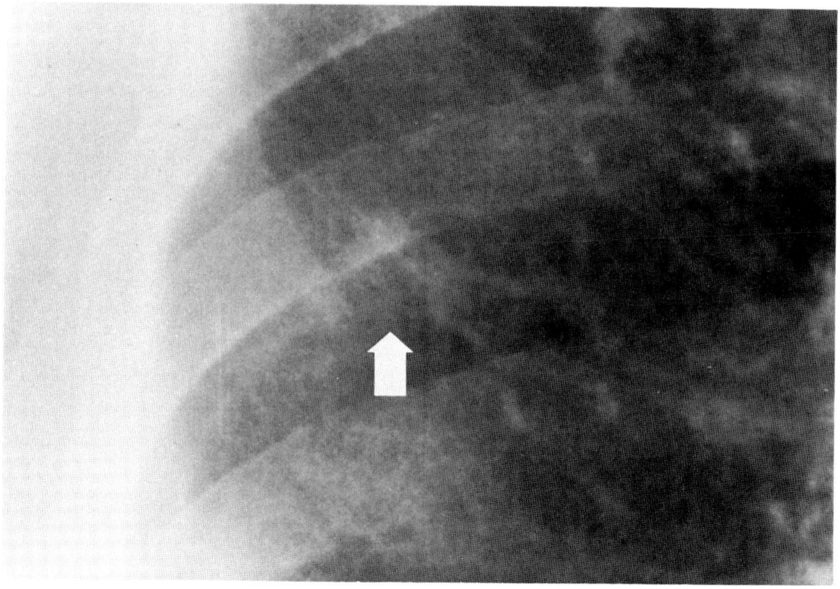

Fig. 4. Subtle bronchogenic carcinoma. This small, irregular right upper lobe lesion (arrow) was missed by one of our screeners and labeled SUS by the second. This very small early lung cancer could easily be confused with a pleural plaque and therefore ignored.

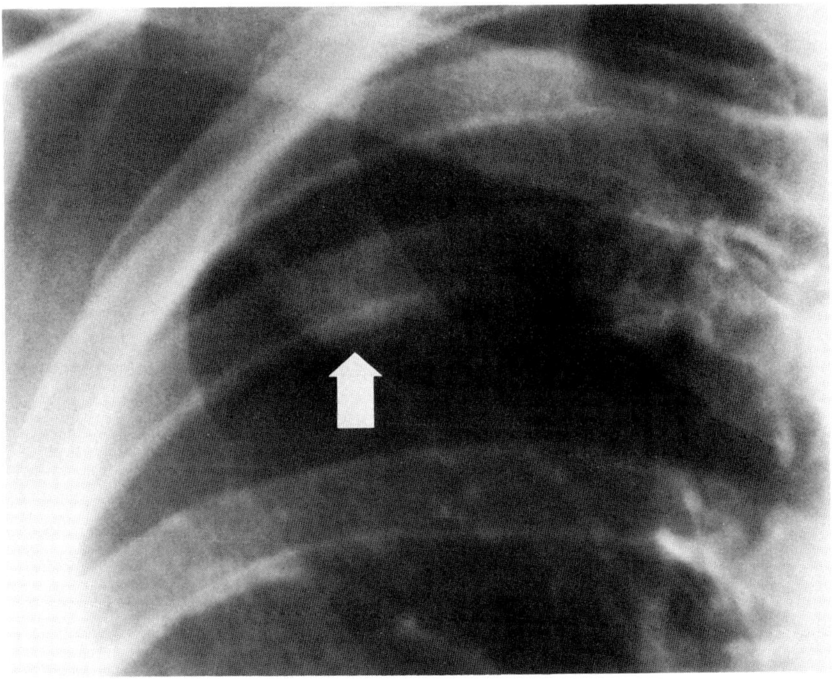

Fig. 5. Lung cancer hidden by bone. The right upper lobe adenocarcinoma (arrow) was almost completely obscured by the anterior second rib. This lesion was detected by only one of our screeners.

50% of bronchogenic carcinomas will be missed by screening radiography. The reason for this high rate is two-fold.

First, the lung cancers are not apparent on the radiograph even in retrospective review. These interval cases are generally rapidly growing small-cell carcinoma of the lung. The second reason is failure to detect small abnormalities on the chest radiographs that subsequently are shown to represent lung cancer. These small masses can be easily overlooked as nonsignificant abnormalities (Fig. 4) or can be partially obscured by the overlying mediastinum or osseous structures (Fig. 5). In patients with multiple abnormalities on their chest radiographs, the radiologist may focus on more striking findings on the chest radiograph while ignoring a small lung cancer in another region of the lung (Fig. 6). Our observa-

Fig. 6. Complex films. This PA chest film shows extensive left pleural fibrosis, linear fibrosis in the left lower lobe, scattered calcified granuloma, and scoliosis of the thoracic spine. These findings prevented one of the screeners from seeing a small, newly appearing cancer (arrow) in the right upper lobe (closeup).

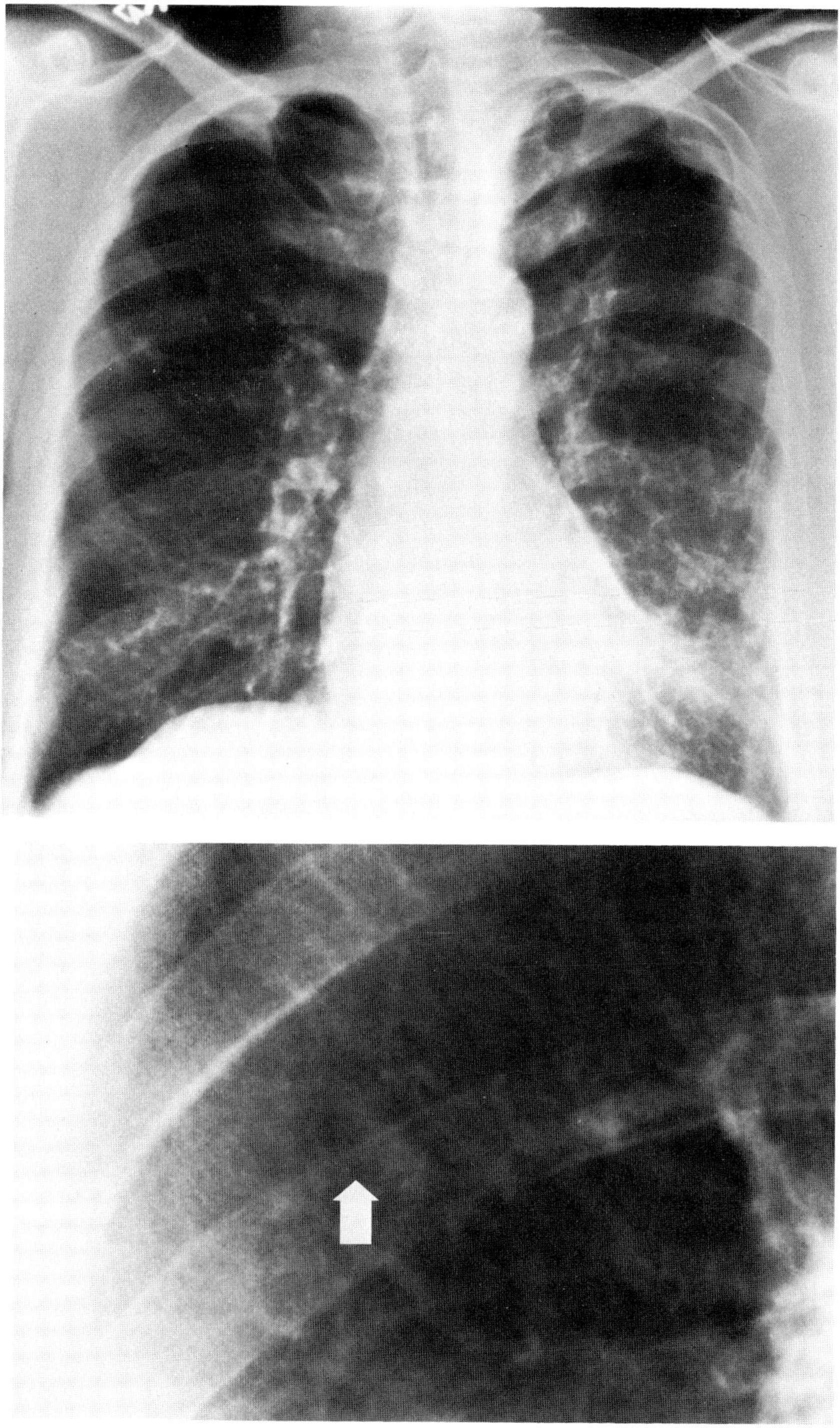

tions agree with those of Muhm *et al.* (1983) in that both small peripheral lesions (Fig. 7) and central lesions (Fig. 8) can be missed.

Observer error is an important problem in diagnostic radiology. The addition of a second reader decreases the miss rate by approximately 13% (Stitik and Tockman, 1978). A second reader introduces, however, an increase in the false-positive rate. This false-positive rate can be kept to an acceptable level by the addition of a referee. The referee strategy that we adopted and recommend is the one of true arbitration (the referee is asked to address only a specific difference) rather than pseudo-arbitration (a third blind reading, after which the discrepancy is resolved by majority opinion (Hessel *et al.*, 1978).

If future screening programs for lung cancer are undertaken, independent double reading and a referee system should be employed. Studies from Memorial Hospital (Flehinger *et al.*, 1978) have indicated that specially trained technologists may detect early lung cancer with appreciable skill.

Our data suggest a bimodal distribution of lung cancer growth rates (patterns of natural history). The rapid pattern may represent very-fast-growing cancers that arise in the interval between a truly negative chest radiograph and a clinically apparent, widespread bronchogenic carcinoma. The slow pattern may represent small peripheral lesions, which, although missed on a number of successive screens, are still in a localized, resectable stage when finally detected (Fig. 7). This concept is strengthened by a retrospective review of the missed lesions

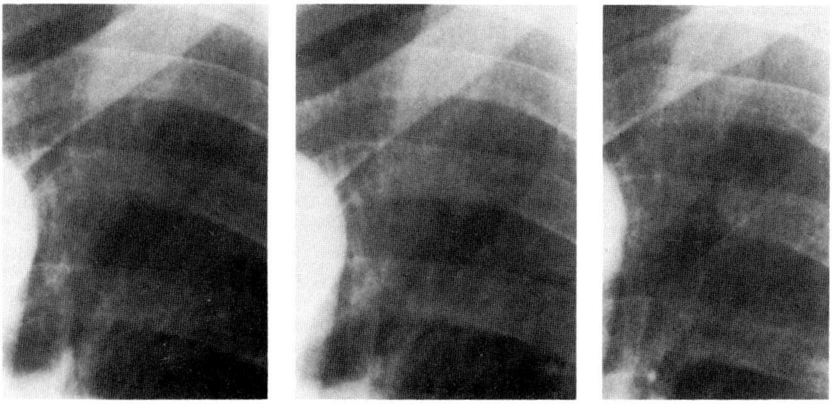

Fig. 7. Slowly growing peripheral cancer. Three closeups of PA chest radiographs in a patient who had a slowly growing left upper lobe adenocarcinoma are presented. The closeup on the left is of the first film, where the lesion was visible in retrospect. The mass was not seen by either screener at that time. The middle closeup was obtained 11 months later. Again, the cancer was missed by both of our screeners. The closeup on the right was obtained another 8 months later. The lesion was detected by both of our screeners at that time.

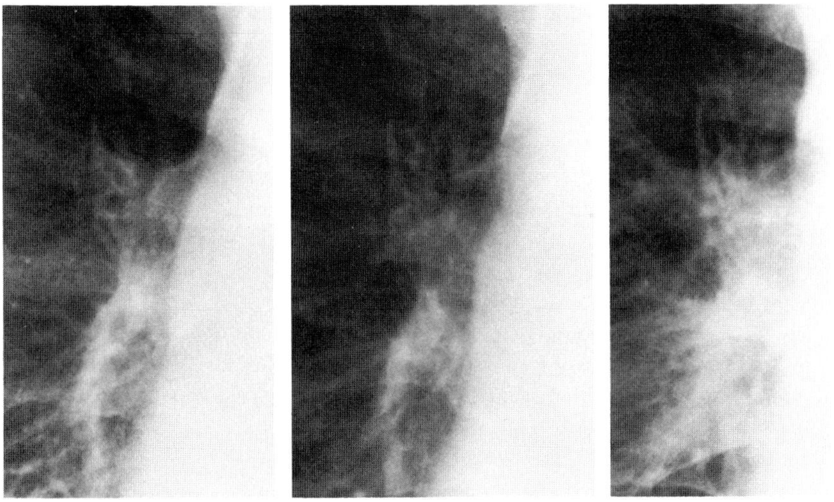

Fig. 8. Example of a missed central cancer. Three closeups of PA chest radiographs centering on the right hilum are compiled. The closeup on the left, even in retrospect, is normal. The middle closeup, obtained 11 months later, shows a subtle increase in density in the upper portion of the right hilum. This change was not appreciated by either screener. The closeup on the right was obtained 12 months later and shows a moderate increase in the hilum. This change was detected by only one of the two screeners. It is especially apparent when compared to the close-up shown on the far left.

demonstrating a statistically significant difference between the previous radiographs of cancers that were subsequently radiographically detected at the next screen and those that became clinically apparent between screens (Table VII). Those coded as cancer were often more sharply defined, rounded lesions that in retrospect were noted to have been growing over several screening intervals. The similarity of stage distribution between patients with a SUS code who eventually had cancer and those with a CAN code (true positives) is not immediately explainable. These true-positive SUS cancers may represent an intermediate form of cancer or a very rapidly growing cancer caught in an early stage. Our findings here are consistent with those radiographic observations made by the National Lung Program (NLP) (Heelan and Flehinger, 1984) and the Mayo Lung Project (MLP) (Muhm *et al.*, 1983).*

The specificity (even in the range of 97–98%) is somewhat low for screening large populations. At the incidence rate experienced in the JHLP, for every 1000 high-risk male smokers screened each year, 5 would have been found to have

*The JHLP, NLP, and MLP are the three clinical arms of the National Institutes of Health-National Cancer Institute Early Lung Cancer Cooperative Group.

lung cancer. Radiographic screening sensitivity was somewhat less than 50%, indicating, therefore, that two or three of these new cases would have been detected by radiographic screening. In addition, radiographic screening would produce another 26 who would be either falsely positive or suspicious for lung cancer (1 − specificity equals 2.6%). Thus, for every 2 or 3 persons with truly positive lung cancers, an additional 26 would undergo medical evaluation or frequent radiographic follow-up to determine that the lesion was benign. This 10-fold false-positive/true-positive ratio would result in additional expense and patient annoyance, which should be considered in advance of any future screening programs.

Board-certified radiologists using varied criteria cannot reliably separate benign from malignant, noncalcified solitary masses. At present, the only radiographic criteria to ensure that the lesion is benign are (1) absolutely no growth on serial radiographs for 24 or more months and (2) the presence of diffuse, laminated or central calcification on CT or plain film tomography. The inability of the chest radiograph to separate accurately benign from malignant disease is generally not of direct clinical concern, since modern diagnostic techniques such as exfoliative sputum cytology, bronchoscopy with transbronchial biopsy, and transthoracic needle biopsy are very accurate methods of diagnosing solitary pulmonary lesions. At The Johns Hopkins Hospital, it is extremely rare for a patient to go to thoracotomy without a definite previous histologic diagnosis of malignant disease.

The authors wish to emphasize that the results presented here represent our experience with annual screening radiography. Direct extrapolations cannot be made to other current or future projects in which radiographic screening is performed at shorter intervals.

In addition, our conclusions about radiographic screening in this population cannot be directly applied to the clinical practice of radiology. Since small, asymptomatic lung cancers tend to be still localized and, therefore, resectable, early lung cancer detection should be an ongoing project of every diagnostic radiologist. The practicing radiologist should consider early lung cancer detection as a major objective when interpreting a chest radiograph in any male or female smoker over the age of 35.

ACKNOWLEDGMENTS

The authors wish to acknowledge the roles of Drs. John K. Frost, Wilmot C. Ball, Jr., and Morton L. Levin in the design and direction of the JHLP.

This study was supported in part by "Lung Cancer Control-Detection and Therapy, Phase II," NCI No. NO1–CN–45037; the Inpatient General Clinical Research Center (Osler 5), NIH No. MO1–RR–00035–23; and the Outpatient General Clinical Research Center, NIH No. RR–00722–12.

REFERENCES

American Joint Committee (1983). "Manual for Staging of Cancer" 2nd ed. Lippincott, Philadelphia, Pennsylvania.

Barnes, G. T., Brezovich, I. A., and Witten, D. M. (1977). Scanning multiple slit assembly: A practical and efficient device to reduce scatter. *AJR, Am. J. Roentgenol.*, **129,** 497–501.

Boucot, K. R., Cooper, D. A., and Weiss, W. (1961). The Philadelphia pulmonary neoplasm research project: An interim report. *Ann. Intern. Med.*, **54,** 363–378.

Breckenridge, J. W., and Bird, G. C. (1977). Errors of omission in pulmonary nodule detection. *Appl. Radiol.* **6,** 51–54.

Brett, G. Z. (1968). The value of lung cancer detection by six-month chest radiographs. *Thorax* **23,** 414–420.

Brett, G. Z. (1969). Earlier diagnosis and survival in lung cancer. *Br. Med. J.*, **4,** 260–262.

Brogdon, B. G., Moseley, R. D., Kelsey, C. A., and Hallberg, J. R. (1978). Perception of simulated lung lesions. *Invest. Radiol.*, **13,** 12–15.

Christensen, E. E., Dietz, G. W., Murry, R. C., Moore, J. G., and Stokely, E. M. (1977a). Effect of kilovoltage on detectability of pulmonary nudules in a chest phantom. *AJR, Am. J. Roentgenol.*, **128,** 789–793.

Christensen, E. E., Dietz, G. W., Murry, R. C., Stokely, E. M., and Moore J. G. (1977b). Grid versus non-grid techniques for the detection of pulmonary nodules in a chest phantom. *Invest. Radiol.*, **12,** 462–463.

Flehinger, B. J., Melamed, M. R., Heelan, R. T., McGinnis, C. M., Zaman, M. B., and Martini, N. (1978). Accuracy of chest film screening by technologists in the New York early lung cancer detection program. *AJR, Am. J. Roentgenol.*, **131,** 593–597.

Foley, W. D., Lawson, T. L., Scanlon, G. T., Heeschen, R. C., and DiBianca, F. (1979). Digital radiography of the chest using a computed tomography instrument. *Radiology* **133,** 231–234.

Foley, W. D., Wilson, C. R., Keyes, G. S., DiBianca, F. A., Scanlon, G. T., Schleuter, D., and Lawson, T. L. (1981). The effect of varying spatial resolution on the detectability of diffuse pulmonary nodules. *Radiology* **141,** 25–31.

Forrest, J. V., and Sagel, S. S. (1979). The lateral radiograph for early diagnosis of lung cancer. *Radiology* **131,** 309–310.

Fraser, R. G., Breatnach, E., and Barnes, G. T. (1983). Digital radiography of the chest: Clinical experience with a prototype. *Radiology* **148,** 1–5.

Gray, J. E., Taylor, K. W., and Hobbs, B. B. (1978). Detection accuracy in chest radiography. *AJR. Am. J. Roentgenol.*, **131,** 247–253.

Groth-Petersen, E., Løvgreen, A., and Thillemann, J. (1952). On the reliability of the reading of photofluorograms and the value of dual reading. *Acta Tuberc. Scand.*, **26,** 13–37.

Guiss, L. W., and Kuenstler, P. (1960). A retrospective view of survey photofluorgrams of persons with lung cancer. *Cancer* **13,** 91–95.

Hallenbeck, G. S. (1975). Clinical evaluation of the 350-kV chest radiography system. *Radiology* **117,** 1–4.

Haus, A. G., Meyer, J., and North, L. B. (1980). Effects of geometric and screen-film unsharpness in conventional and 350-kVp chest radiography. *Radiology* **137,** 197–202.

Heelan, R., Flehinger, B. J., Melamed, M. R., Zaman, M. B., Perchick, W. B., Caravelli, J. F., and Martini, N. (1984). Non-small-cell lung cancer: Results of the New York screening program. *Radiology* **151,** 289–293.

Herman, P. G., Goldstein, J., Balikian, J., Sandor, T., Hessel, S. J., and Drummey, J. (1980). Visibility and sharpness of lung structure at 90, 140, and 350 kV. *Radiology* **134,** 591–597.

Hessel, S. J., Herman, P. G., and Swensson, R. G. (1978). Improving performance by multiple interpretations of chest radiographs: Effectiveness and cost. *Radiology* **127,** 589–594.

Huebener, K. H. (1983). Scanned projection radiography of the chest versus film radiography: A comparison of 250 cases. *Radiology* **148,** 363–368.

Johnson, G. A., and Ravin, C. E. (1983). A survey of digital chest radiography. *Radiol. Clin. North Am.,* **21,** 655–665.

Katragadda, C. S., Fogel, S. R., Cohen, G., Wagner, K. L., Morgan, C., III, Handel, S. F., Amtey, S. R., and Lester, R. G. (1979). Digital radiography using a computed tomographic instrument. *Radiology* **133,** 83–87.

Kelsey, C. A., Moseley, R. D., Brogdon, B. G., Bhave, D. G., and Hallberg, J. (1977). Effect of size and position on chest lesion detection. *AJR, Am. J. Roentgenol.,* **129,** 205–208.

Kelsey, C. A., Moseley, R. D., Jr., Mettler, F. A., Jr., and Briscoe, D. E. (1982a). Cost-effectiveness of stereoscopic radiographs in detection of lung nodules. *Radiology* **142,** 611–613.

Kelsey, C. A., Moseley, R. D., Mettler, F. A., Garcia, J. F., Parker, T. W., and Briscoe, D. E. (1982b). Comparison of nodule detection with 70-kVp and 120-kVp chest radiographs. *Radiology* **143,** 609–611.

Kelsey, C. A., Moseley, R. D., Mettler, F. A., Garcia, J. F., Parker, T. W., Juhl, J. H., and Briscoe, D. E. (1983). Anticrossover emulsions evaluated by observer performance tests. *Radiology* **146,** 209–211.

Kundel, H. L. (1981). Predictive value and threshold detectability of lung tumors. *Radiology* **139,** 25–29.

Kundel, H. L., and Revesz, G. (1976). Lesion conspicuity, structured noise, and film reader error. *AJR, Am. J. Roentgenol.,* **126,** 1233–1238.

Kundel, H. L., Nodine, C. F., and Carmody, D. (1978). Visual scanning, pattern recognition and decision-making in pulmonary nodule detection. *Invest. Radiol.,* **13,** 175–181.

Lindheim, R. (1971). "Uncoupling the Radiology System." Hospital Research and Educational Trust, Chicago, Illinois.

Muhm, J. R., Miller, W. E., Fontana, R. S., Sanderson, D. R., and Uhlenhopp, M. A. (1983). Lung cancer detected during a screening program using four month chest radiographs. *Radiology* **148,** 609–615.

Nash, F. A., Morgan, J. M., and Tomkins, J. G. (1968). South London lung cancer study. *Br. Med. J.,* **2,** 715–721.

Plewes, D. B. (1983). A scanning system for chest radiography with regional exposure control: Theoretical considerations. *Med. Phys.,* **10,** 646–654.

Plewes, D. B., and Vogelstein, E. (1983). A scanning system for chest radiography with regional exposure control: Practical implementation. *Med. Phys.,* **10,** 655–663.

Plewes, D. B., and Wandtke, J. C. (1982). A scanning equalization system for improved chest radiography. *Radiology* **142,** 765–768.

Proto, A. V., and Lane, E. J. (1978). 350 kVp chest radiography: Review and comparison with 120 kVp. *AJR, Am. J. Roentgenol.,* **130,** 859–866.

Revesz, G., and Kundel, H. L. (1977). Psychophysical studies of detection errors in chest radiology. *Radiology* **123,** 559–562.

Rossi, R. P., Hendee, W. R., and Ahrens, R. T. (1976). An evaluation of rare earth screen/film combinations. *Radiology* **121,** 465–471.

Sagel, S. S., Evens, R. G., Forrest, J. V., and Bramson, R. T. (1974). Efficacy of routine screening and lateral chest radiographs in a hospital-based population. *N. Engl. J. Med.,* **291,** 1001–1004.

Sorensen, J. A., and Nelson, J. A. (1976). Investigations of moving-slit radiography. *Radiology* **120,** 705–711.

Stitik, F. P., and Tockman, M. S. (1978). Radiographic screening in the early detection of lung cancer. *Radiol. Clin. North Am.,* **16,** 347–366.

Tesic, M. M., Sones, R. A., and Morgan, D. R. (1984). Single-slit digital radiography: Some practical considerations. *AJR, Am. J. Roentgenol.*, **142,** 697–702.

Theros, E. G. (1977). Varying manifestations of peripheral pulmonary neoplasms: A radiologic-pathologic correlative study. *AJR, Am. J. Roentgenol.*, **128,** 893–914.

Thompson, T. T., Radford, E. L., and Kirby, C. C. (1977). A look at rare-earth and high-speed intensifying screens. *Appl. Radiol.*, **6,** 71–72.

U.S. Department of Health, Education and Welfare (1978). "The Chest X-ray as a Screening Procedure for Cardiopulmonary Disease," Publ. No. (FDA) 78–8036. U.S. Gov. Printing Office, Washington, D.C.

U.S. Department of Health, Education and Welfare. (1979). "Smoking and Health: A report of the Surgeon General," Publ. No. (PHS) 79–5006. U.S. Govt. Printing Office, Washington, D.C.

U.S. Department of Health and Human Services (1980). "Optimization of Chest Radiography," HHS Publ. (FDA) 80–8124. U.S. Govt. Printing Office, Washington, D.C.

Wandtke, J. C., and Plewes, D. B. (1983). Improved chest radiography with equalization. *Radio-Graphics* **3,** 141–154.

Yerushalmy, J., Harkness, J. T., Cope, J. H., and Kennedy, B. R. (1950). The role of dual reading in mass radiography. *Am. Rev. Tuberc.* **61,** 443–464.

11

Double Contrast Radiography of the Stomach

HEIZABURO ICHIKAWA AND TATSUYA YAMADA

I. Introduction 193
II. Method 194
III. Presentation of Films Taken with the Double Contrast Method 196
IV. Results 207
V. Discussion 208
VI. Summary 213
References 213

I. INTRODUCTION

Double contrast radiography of the stomach was developed by a group of doctors, who were organized mainly by Drs. Shirakabe, Ichikawa, Kumakura, and their colleagues in the early 1950s. It was improved by further investigations and has now reached a level of almost complete perfection.

Since very tiny lesions of the gastric mucosa can be clearly and accurately revealed by the double contrast method, we are now able to diagnose even carcinoma of the so-called superficial spreading type, whose preoperative diagnosis has so far been considered impractical. As a result, not only are the many cases of tiny peptic ulcers, multiple ulcers, and even small ulcer scars well diagnosed with this technique, but also the number of cases of cancer of the stomach detected early enough for an absolute cure to be expected has rapidly increased. In fact, the number of patients whose cancer was detected at an early stage (carcinoma limited to the gastric mucosa and/or to the gastric mucosa and submucosa) exceeded 1000 as of 1978 at the National Cancer Center Hospital, Tokyo, which was established in 1962. Thus, this technique is now widely

ISBN 0-12-496720-5

employed, and is considered an essential roentgenologic examination in screening for stomach cancer in Japan. Furthermore, this technique has been widely disseminated in Japan through several thousand lectures and demonstrations by the pioneer group over the past 20 years. At present, not only in leading big hospitals but also in small private practices interested in gastrointestinal radiology, this technique is well used in almost 100% of patients, and statistics now show that more than 4000 cases of early gastric cancer are detected every year in Japan.

The authors have been pleased to learn that during the past few years, many radiologists and physicians in East Asia, South America, and Australia, as well as in Europe and North America, have become interested in this technique and have visited Japan to study it (Laufer, 1979). These doctors have been enthusiastic in studying and applying it in their practice. Indeed, in January 1980, the Department of Radiology of the University of Pennsylvania planned and sponsored a course entitled "Double Contrast Radiography." The development of a course with this title in a country other than Japan is an epochal event. It is one proof that the importance and usefulness of this technique are now being recognized on a global scale.

II. METHOD

Double contrast radiography is a method of obtaining high-radiopacity barium coated thinly over the mucus membrane of the gastrointestinal tract by allowing positive contrast medium (barium meal) and negative contrast medium (air) to exist concurrently in the gastrointestinal tract. With this method, very slight unevenness of the mucosa can be clearly demonstrated.

It is common knowledge that when a barium meal is swallowed, a small amount of air is also taken into the stomach, even in normal cases, and remains in the fornix of the stomach; the quantity varies with the case. If the patient shifts from upright to supine and then to the right anterior oblique position, the air in the fornix flows into the prepyloric antrum and inflates this area, and sometimes the duodenal bulb as well. Double contrast radiography occurs if these areas are X-rayed at this time. Many radiologists have been calling this method *double contrast radiography*. However, the area that can be covered in this way is no more than one-fifth of the entire stomach. X-ray examination of the stomach has to cover every area of the stomach, and for that purpose, air has to be purposely injected, since the amount of air swallowed spontaneously is usually not sufficient.

Fischer (1923) showed that injected air was effective for X ray examination of the large intestine, although the method was not then popular on a global scale. Attempts to use this method for X ray examination of the stomach were made by

Hilpert (1929), Vallenbona (1931), Poppel (1937), and other authors, but they were not successful, particularly in coating the gastric mucosa with barium—an important part of the technique. It may indeed be more appropriate to call this method *air contrast radiography,* since the images these authors obtained showed only the outline or size of large tumors in the stomach, not the delicate lesions of the mucosal surface. Therefore, not much attention was subsequently paid to double contrast radiography, because it had not been fully evaluated.

Since the end of the 1940s, Shirakabe and Ichikawa and their colleagues (Ichikawa *et al.*, 1964; Ichikawa, 1976, 1978; Matsue *et al.*, 1970; Shirakabe *et al.*, 1966, 1982; Shirakabe, 1971; Shirakabe and Ichikawa, 1973) have investigated the extent of X ray diagnosis of intestinal tuberculosis utilizing Fischer's method for imaging tuberculous ulcers in the large intestine. In such cases, surgery was indicated where successful diagnosis of the accurate number and site of such ulcers had been achieved. Radiograms of a resected stomach specimen were prepared, and the advantages and disadvantages of double contrast radiography as well as those of the filling method, compression method, mucosal relief method, and others were investigated in detail.

As a result, it was found that well-demonstrated double contrast radiograms could show, naturally and accurately, the detailed morphological pattern of the lesions. Far better than expected X ray films were also taken in similar experiments on the resected specimen of the stomach.

In attempts to take double contrast radiograms in clinical trials on patients in 1955, a narrow tube was inserted into the stomach to inject the necessary amount of air. The size of the stomach varies with the patient, and it was found necessary to regulate the amount of barium for each patient. Since some gastric juice remains in the stomach even after fasting, it was found that a fairly large amount of barium is necessary in order to ignore this remaining gastric juice. It was also found that when almost no gastric juice existed in the stomach, considerable viscous mucus covered the mucosal surface of the stomach, preventing sufficient adhesion of the barium meal. We believe that double contrast examination of the stomach did not succeed for a long time, while double contrast examination of the colon succeeded fairly easy, mainly for this reason: the viscous mucus that exists in the stomach but not in the colon.

Many years of investigation were required before these difficulties were overcome and the amount of barium meal and air needed to produce a sufficient coating could be determined.

Since it is inconvenient to insert a tube into the stomach of every patient, an effervescent powder or fine-quality granules was introduced by the authors in 1962, when the National Cancer Center Hospital opened. This powder or granules are now used for almost all examinations, greatly reducing the inconvenience to patients of double contrast X ray examinations.

III. PRESENTATION OF FILMS TAKEN WITH THE DOUBLE CONTRAST METHOD

The quality of the diagnosis obtained with the double contrast examination is greatly dependent upon the quality of the film. The quality of the film is evaluated in terms of how much detail of the surface unevenness of the gastric mucosa

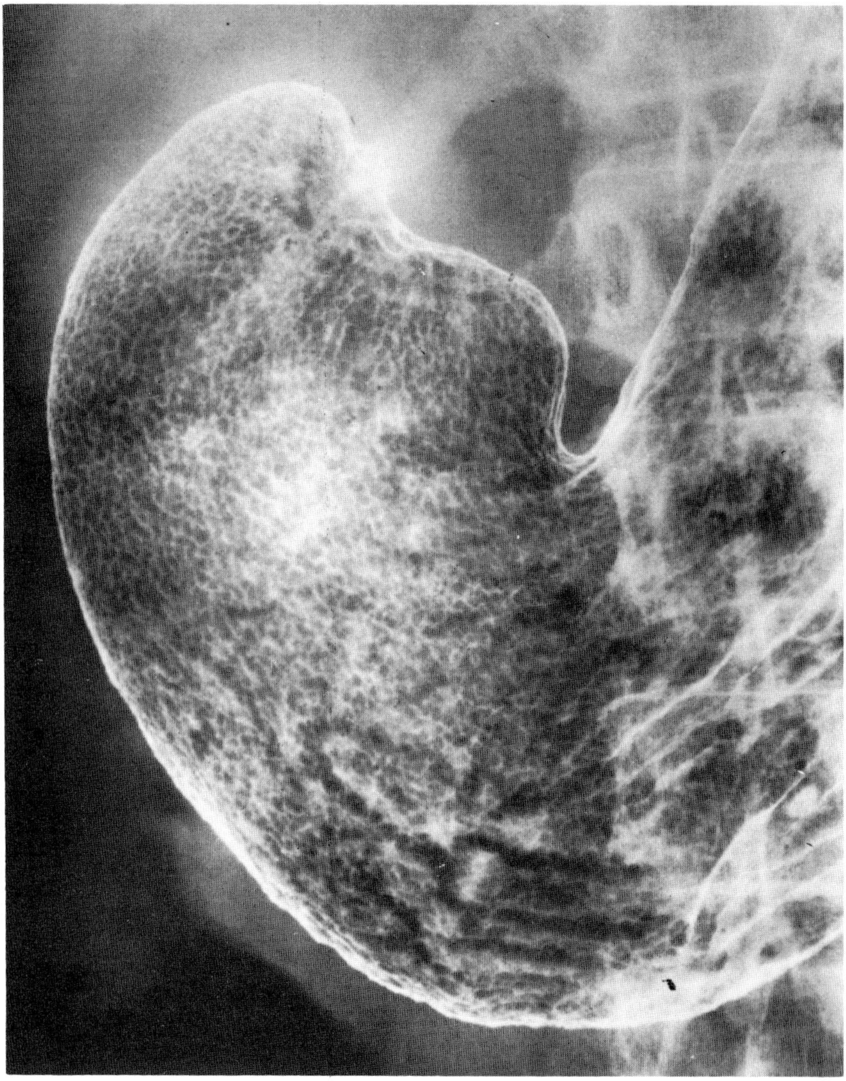

Fig. 1. Radiograph showing area gastricae of the antrum.

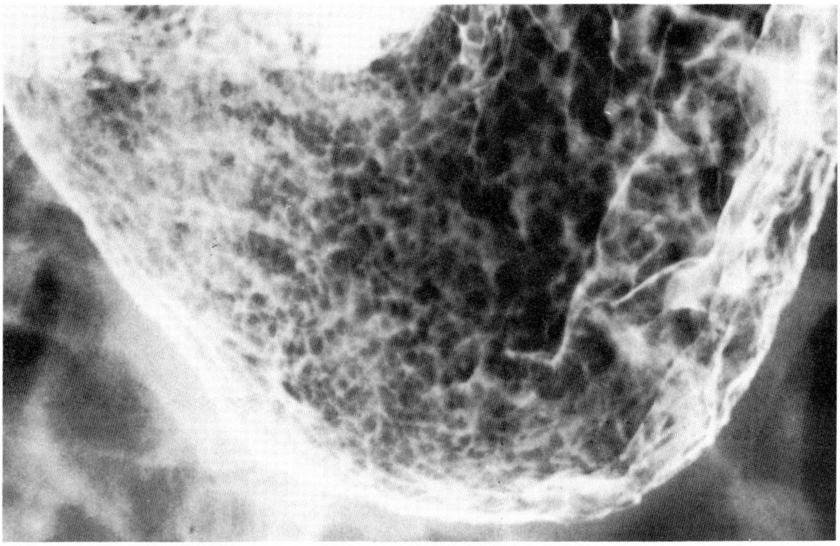

Fig. 2. Granulous changes of the gastric mucosa.

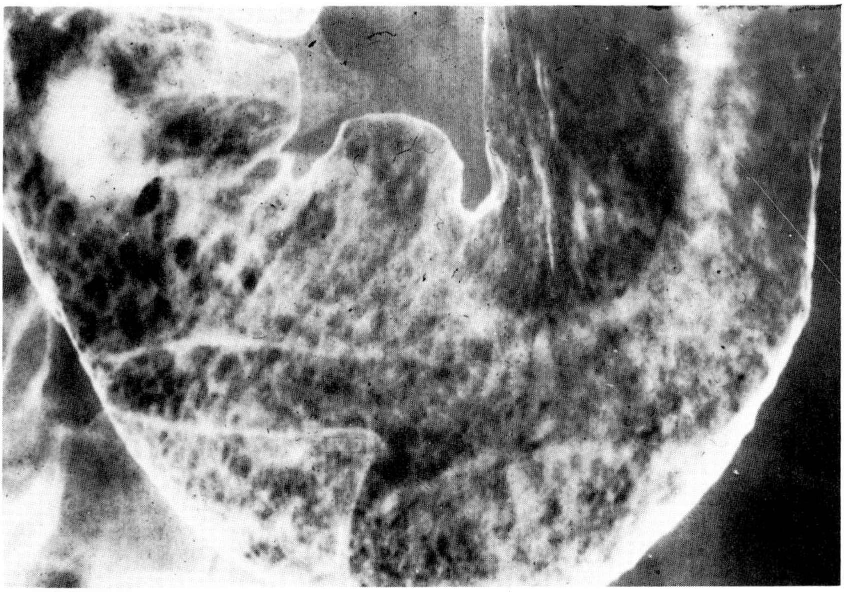

Fig. 3. Intestinal metaplasia of the gastric mucosa.

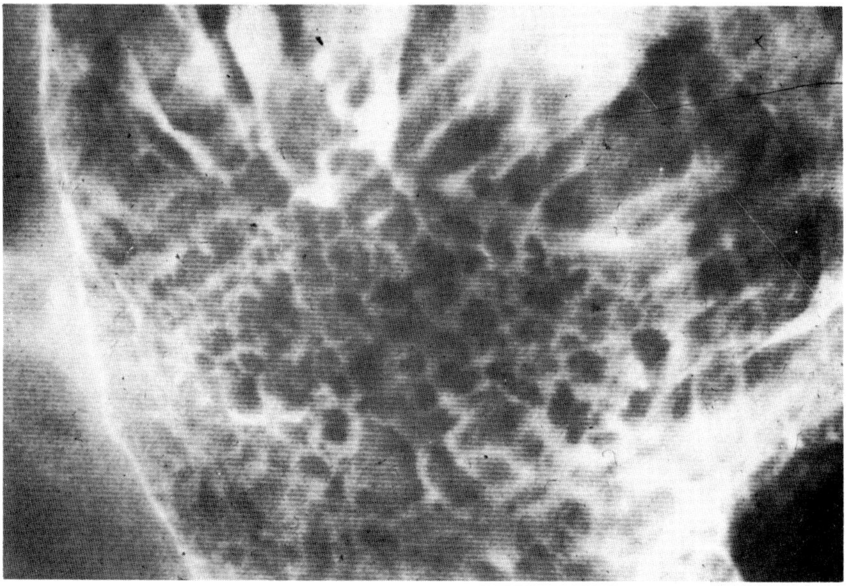

Fig. 4. Early gastric cancer of the superficial flat type.

is demonstrated. From this standpoint, the demonstration of area gastricae—the smallest macroscopic unit of the gastric surface—is considered one of the most important markers. Figure 1 is an example of a well-coated mucosal surface demonstrating the fine pattern of area gastricae of the antrum.

In the early stage of experience with double contrast radiography, radiologists can often see the very characteristic finding shown in Fig. 2, which demonstrates a large number of fairly big granulous changes of the gastric mucosa. This is a typical appearance of hyperplastic change of the gastric mucosa.

In cases of intestinal metaplasia of the gastric mucosa, nodules are not regular, as seen in hyperplastic changes, but are generally irregular in size and shape, as shown in Fig. 3. There are some small spaces, shown by thin pooling of barium between the nodules, which are not usually seen with hyperplastic changes.

Around the central part of Fig. 4, a large number of nodules are gathered, the sizes of which are quite irregular; the shape of each nodule is also irregularly outlined. These are typical findings of early gastric cancer of the superficial flat type. Such cancerous changes are usually quite hard to recognize by macroscopic inspection of the mucosal surface after opening of the resected specimen. Carcinoma was limited to the mucosa in this case.

In Fig. 5, large and small nodules are gathered near the cardiac orifice, indicating an early gastric cancer lesion of the superficial elevated type. Irregularity of nodule size and irregularity of the outline of each nodule are much

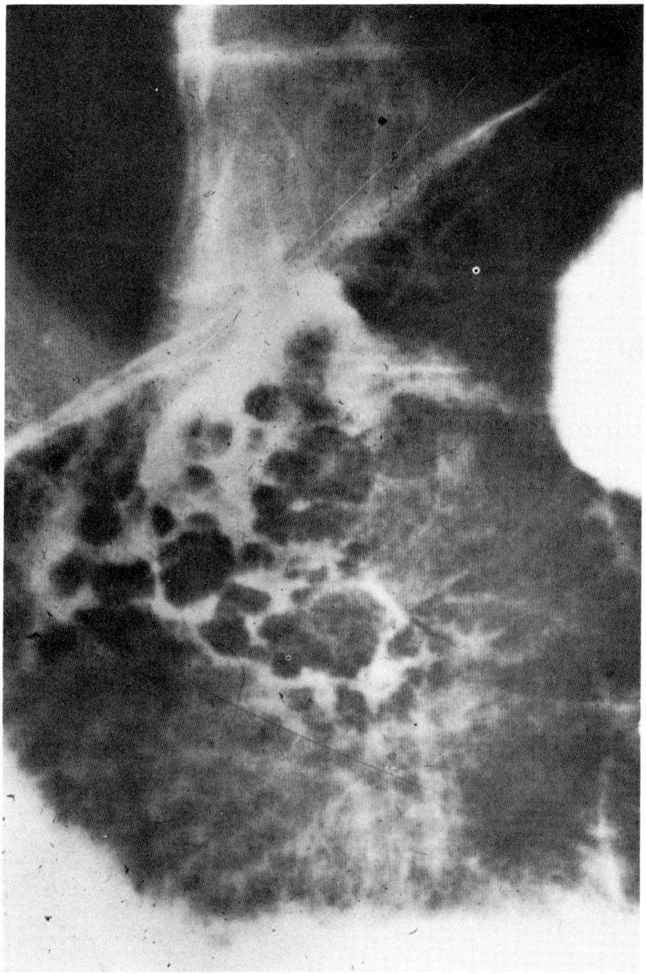

Fig. 5. Early gastric cancer of the superficial elevated type near the cardiac orifice.

more remarkable than those seen in Fig. 4, but most of the carcinomatous invasion was still limited to the mucosa and only a very small part of the lesion had invaded the submucosa.

In Fig. 6, there is a fairly big polypoid lesion at the posterior wall of the gastric body, with an irregular outline and surface suggesting a malignant polypoid cancer. But if the area surrounding the polypoid lesion is inspected very carefully, a sharply demarcated, radiolucent area with an irregular outline is well demonstrated, suggesting that there is an irregularly shaped, flat, elevated lesion extending from the polypoid lesion. In other words, this lesion consists of two

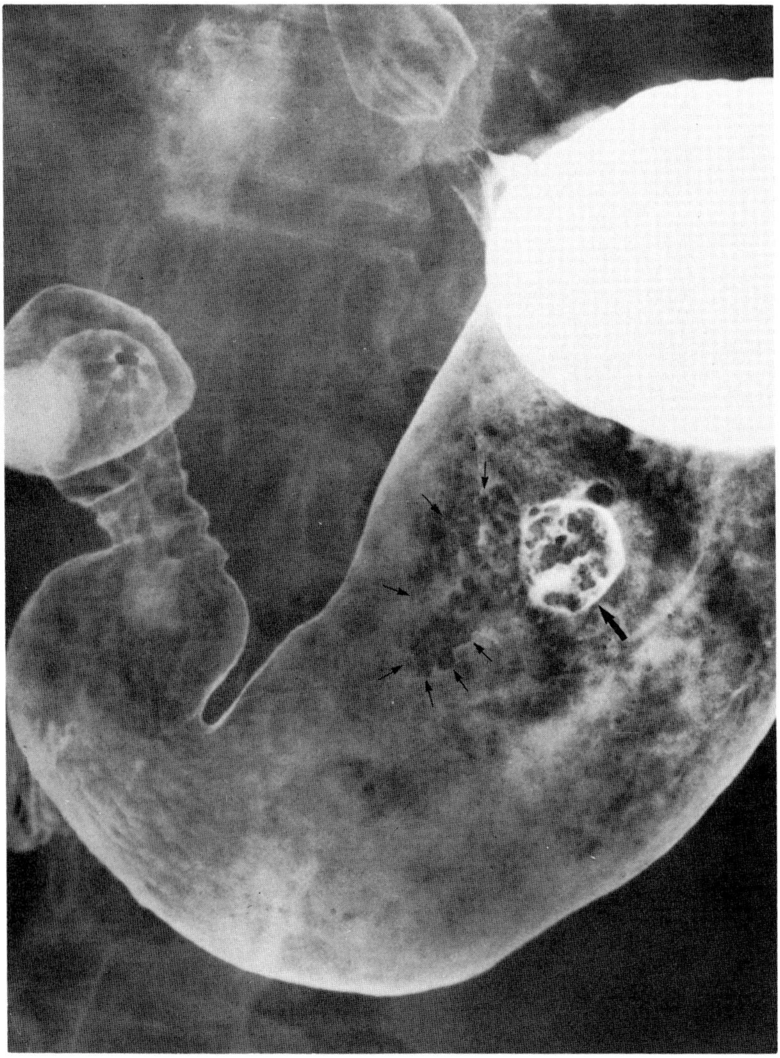

Fig. 6. Two different types of early gastric cancer (see text).

different types of early gastric cancer. Carcinoma was limited to the mucosa in both types.

In the right upper quarter of Fig. 7, there is a very thin but fairly wide pool of barium with an irregular outline. Multiple irregular nodules are scattered within this pool. These findings indicate one of the typical superficial, depressed types of early gastric cancer. Carcinoma in this case was limited to the mucosa in

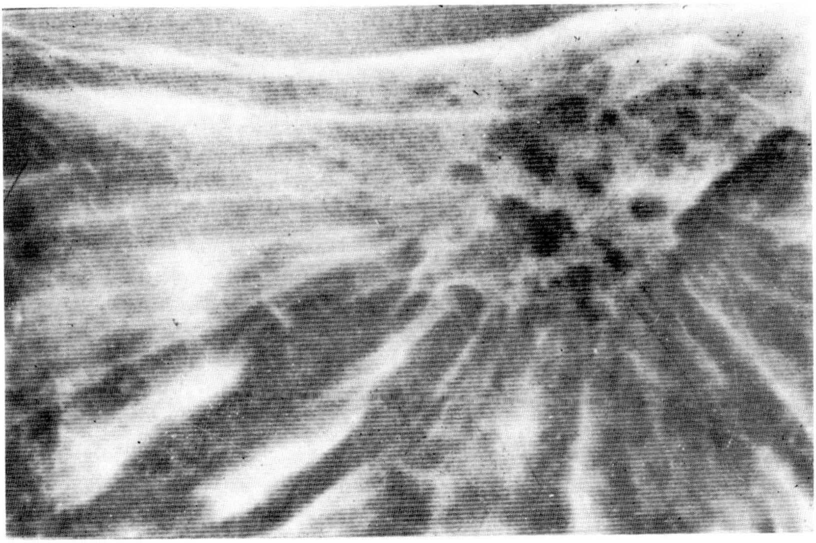

Fig. 7. Superficial depressed type of gastric cancer.

almost all of the lesion except for a very small part near the largest nodule, where it had invaded the submucosa.

In Fig. 8, there is a small, star-shaped barium pool at the posterior wall and the proximal part of the antrum near the greater curvature. Some folds are converging toward the lesion. A radiolucent area at the center of the pool indicates that there is a slight elevation of the base of the depressed lesion. This is a case of early gastric cancer of the superficial depressed type. Carcinoma was limited to the mucosa.

Figure 9 shows the macroscopic findings of a resected specimen with an early gastric cancer. When this case was presented at the sixth World Congress of Gastroenterology in 1978 in Madrid, no person from the floor could show where the lesion was located. In fact, when this case was sent to a surgical pathologist of the National Cancer Center just after surgical removal, he could not find the lesion. He therefore asked the surgeon, and the surgeon asked the radiologist where it was, since the surgeon could not feel any pathology, including even a slight thickness of the stomach wall, by palpation during the surgical operation. According to the radiologist, the pathologist then found the lesion. But the lesion was clearly demonstrated with the double contrast method, as seen in Fig. 10. It was 1.3 × 0.9 cm in diameter, carcinoma was limited to the mucosa, and no metastasis was found in 29 lymph nodes removed and examined histologically.

A radiograph of a stomach full of barium in the upright position is shown in Fig. 11. The lesion is in the middle of the gastric body, but no evidence of a

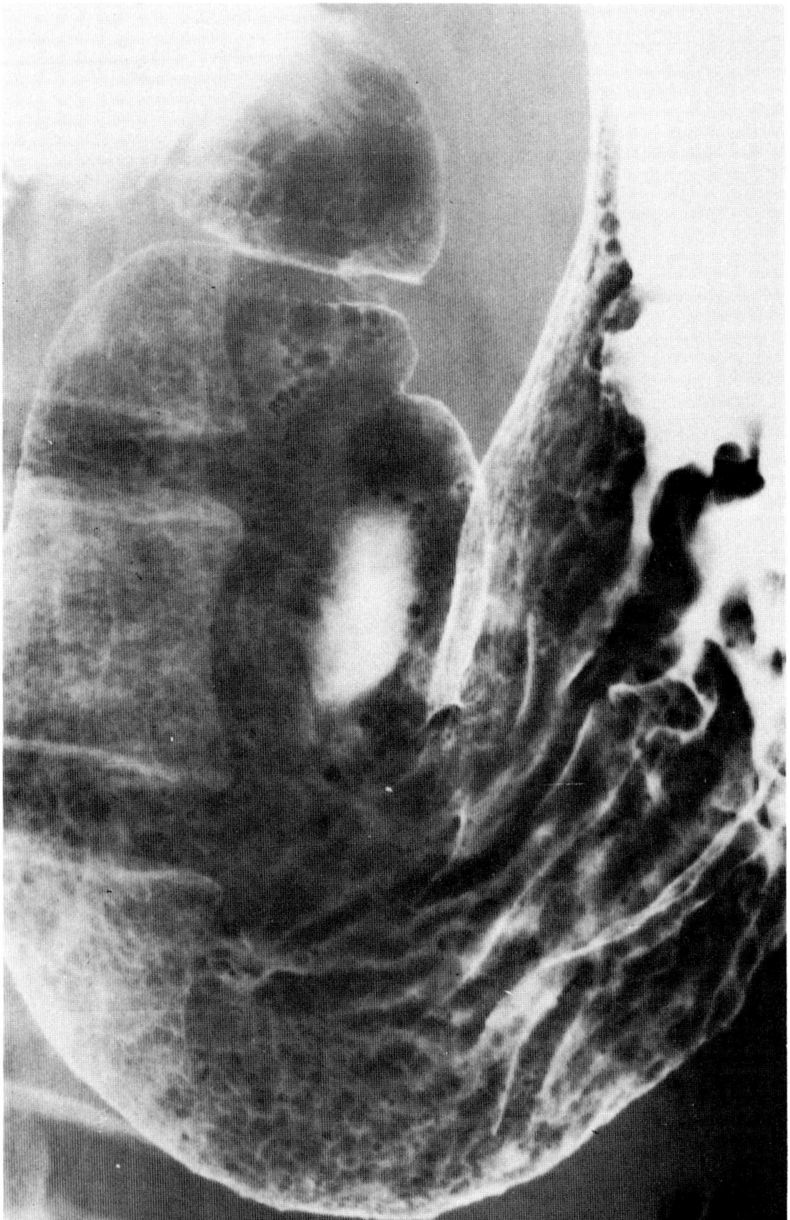

Fig. 8. Early gastric cancer of the superficial depressed type.

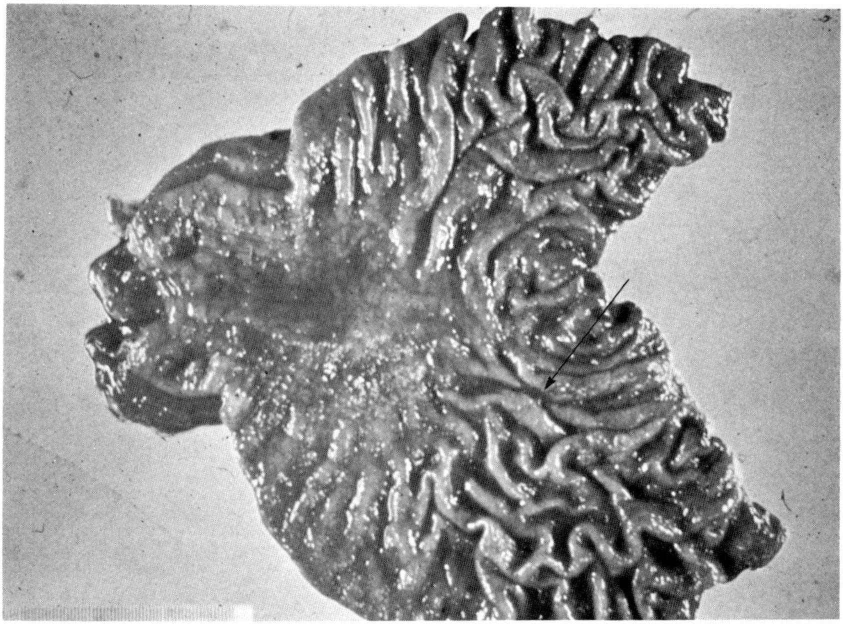

Fig. 9. Resected specimen of early gastric cancer.

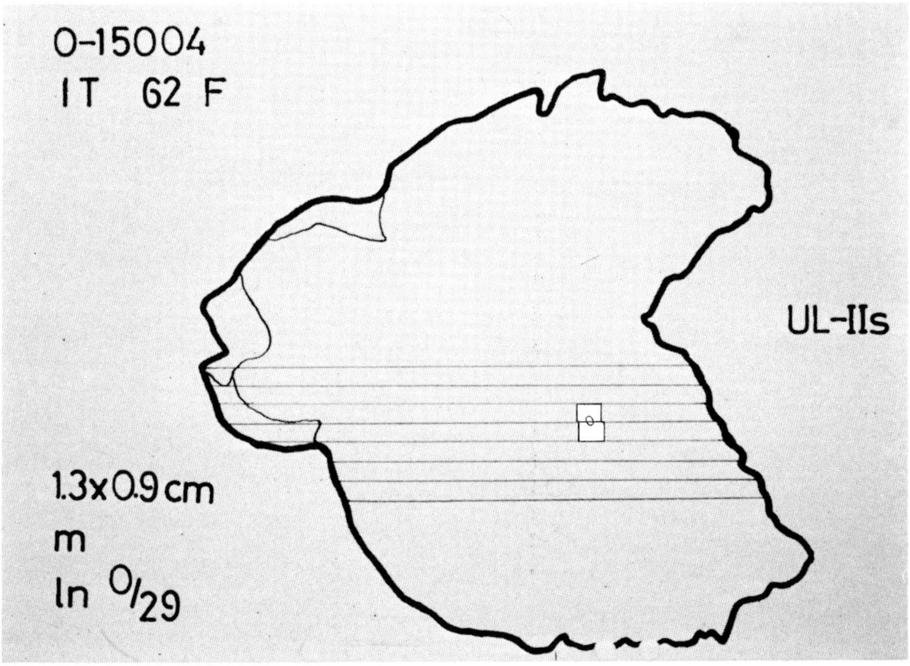

Fig. 10. Position of the lesion in Fig. 9.

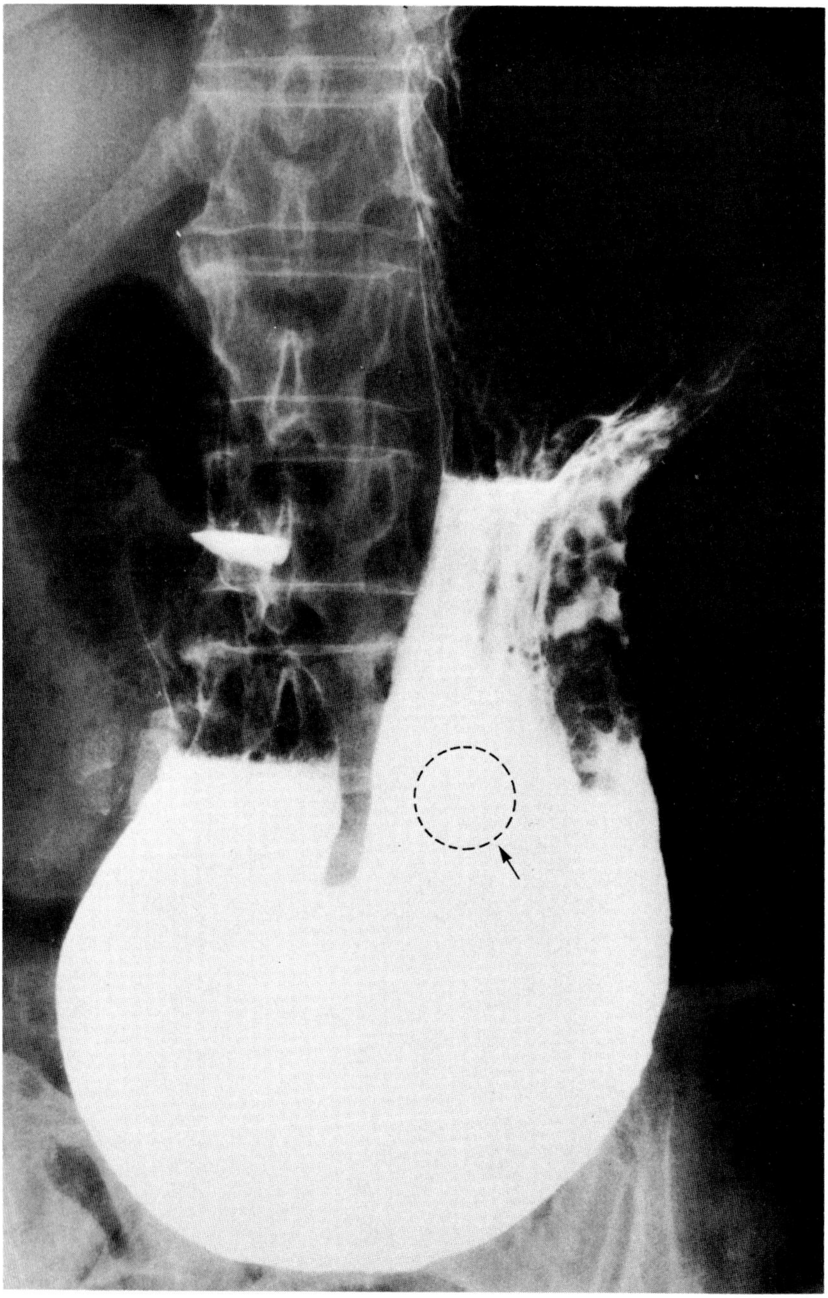

Fig. 11. Radiograph with no lesion visible (upright position).

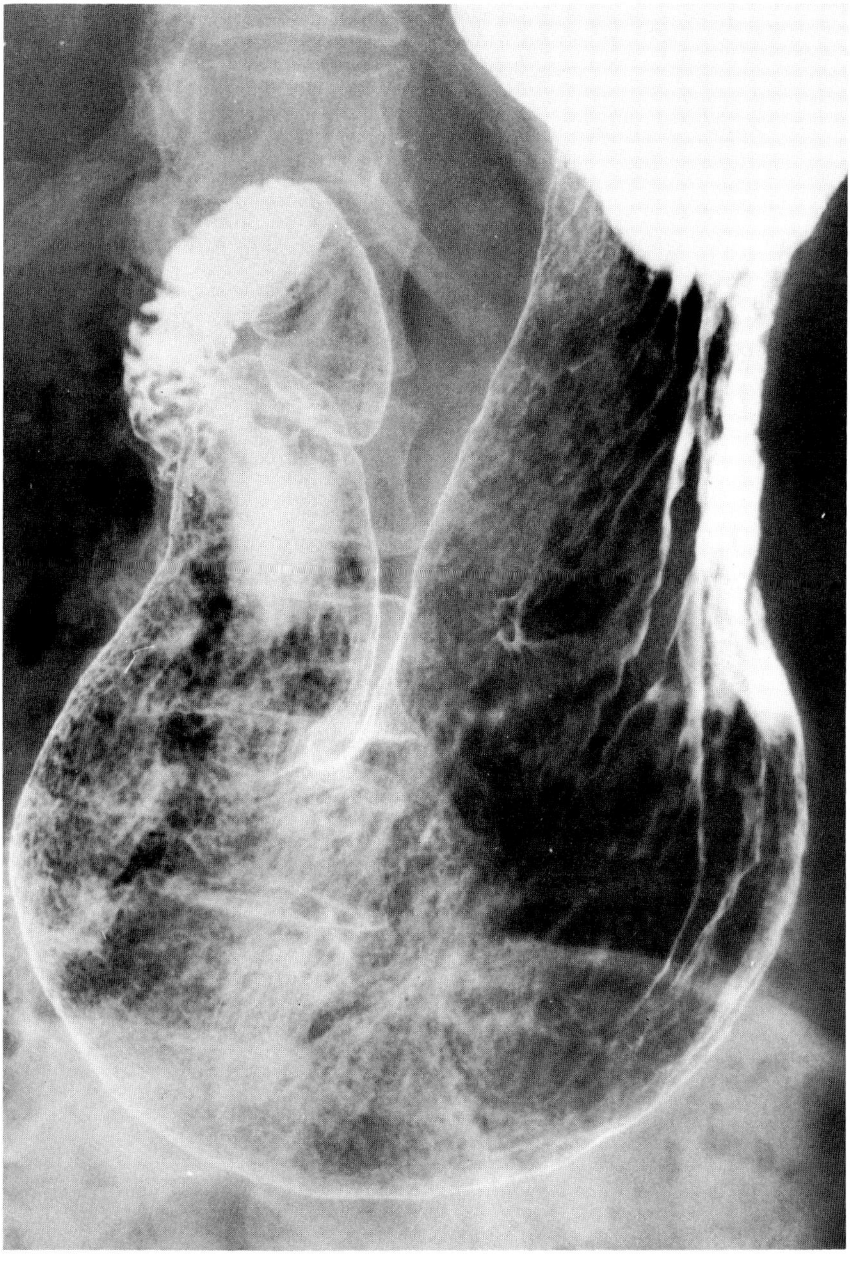

Fig. 12. Lesion seen with the patient in a supine position (same patient as in Fig. 11).

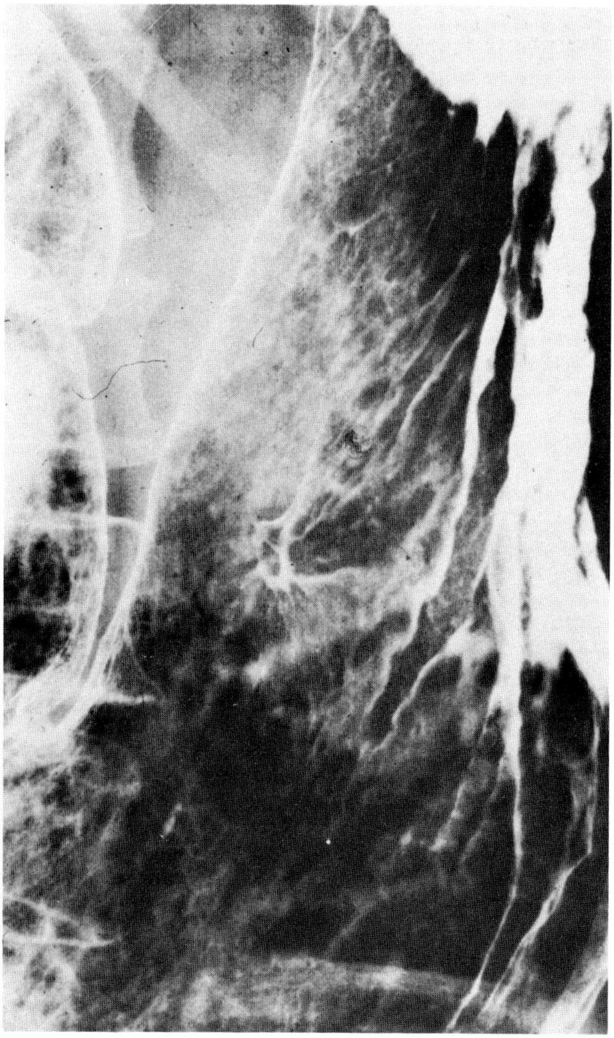

Fig. 13. Enlarged view of the lesion in Fig. 12.

pathological finding was seen in this film. With the patient in the supine position, a beautiful double contrast radiograph was produced, as seen in Fig. 12. A small but clearly demonstrated shadow with characteristic findings of cancer was revealed. An enlarged picture (Fig. 13) shows the findings, including a very thin pool of barium, with two central elevations combining several mucosal folds converging toward the pool, making the outline of the pool a delicate irregularity. These findings suggest a small, superficial cancerous erosion.

IV. RESULTS

The value of double contrast radiography has been illustrated by the above cases. Some of the data that will help us to understand the diagnostic results will now be presented.

Figure 14 summarizes 1300 cases of gastric cancer operated on at the National Cancer Center Hospital. Black and white dots represent each case, with and without lymph node metastases, respectively, plotted according to the size (in millimeters) and the depth of invasion. The larger and deeper the lesion, the more cases with lymph node metastases are observed. A particularly important point in this figure is that in about 25% of the cases with submucosal invasion, lymph node metastases were revealed. However, these metastases were minute, and were found only with very detailed histological examination, so that no pathological finding was observed macroscopically during the surgical operation. Furthermore, these lymph nodes are usually located close to the lesion and are easily removed during the regular surgical operation for gastric cancer. Therefore, as seen in Fig. 15, the 20-year survival rate of submucosal cancer patients is quite high: 90%. Since the survival rate of mucosal cancer patients is almost 100%, the survival rate of those with early gastric cancer, which is defined in Japan as carcinoma limited to the mucosa or mucosa and submucosa, is approximately 95%. The number of patients with early gastric cancer detected and operated on in the National Cancer Center Hospital since its opening in 1962

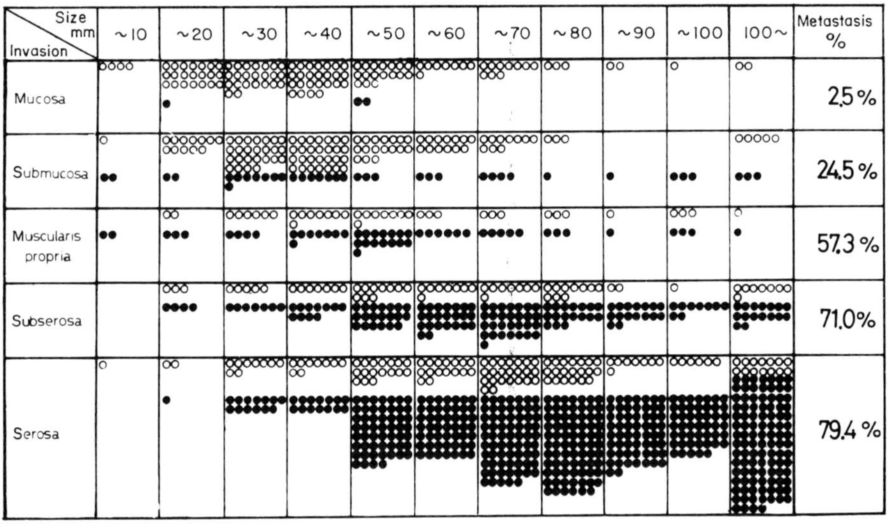

Fig. 14. Summary of size and invasion of 1300 cases of gastric cancer operated on at the National Cancer Center Hospital. ○, Metastasis (−); •, Metastasis (+).

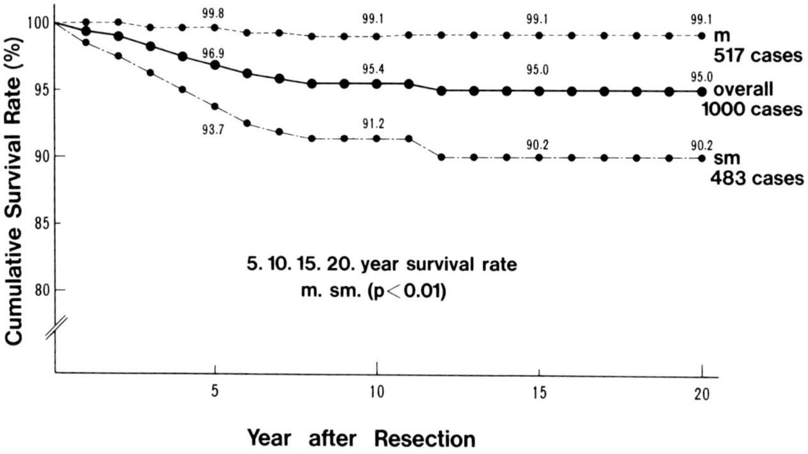

Fig. 15. Survival rate after surgery for early gastric cancer, National Cancer Center Hospital (1962–1980).

exceeded 1300 at the end of 1983. This high detection rate for early gastric cancer has been made possible by the application of the double contrast method and by the cooperative work with gastric endoscopy.

However, the role of the double contrast method in screening cannot be overestimated. Recent statistics reveal that the detection rate of early gastric cancer as a percentage of all detected gastric cancers has increased rapidly year after year in the mass screening field after application of the double contrast method. (see Chapter 19). In some pioneer groups, it was 16% when they started in 1960 and reached 62% in 1974. This technique has now been disseminated widely throughout Japan, and a total of 4,365,238 people received mass screening for cancer of the stomach in 1982. The double contrast method was used in 100% of these examination, although there is still a range in its quality. However, the average rate of detection of early gastric cancer throughout Japan using mass screening was 52.9%.

V. DISCUSSION

We must mention a common misunderstanding concerning double contrast radiography. When it was reported that early cancer could be diagnosed by this method, some workers assumed that it was effective only for detecting early cancers. It has also been assumed that double contrast radiography is ineffective in the diagnosis of progressive cancer, gastric ulcer, polyps, and so on, and that it is not required in countries where gastric cancer occurs less frequently.

However, as already mentioned, the investigations carried out by Shirakabe's group primarily concerned the clear demonstration of intestinal tuberculous ulcers. They resulted in the successful demonstration of accurate numbers of multiple tuberculous ulcers of the colon and small intestine with double contrast radiography. When this method was applied to the examination of the stomach, the number and images of peptic ulcers and polyps, and even the linear ulcer, which was not well known to clinicians in those days, was well demonstrated and properly diagnosed (Shirakabe, 1971). Later, this method even made it possible to diagnose superficial spreading carcinomas that had been very difficult to detect. Thus, early-stage cancer can now be diagnosed. The authors believe that the above-mentioned misunderstandings were caused by Japanese researchers who overemphasized that double contrast radiography is so effective that even the superficial spreading early gastric cancer can be demonstrated, because they believed that this type of lesion is one of the most difficult to demonstrate and also *most crucial* for the patient. They were so delighted to have discovered the technique by which such a difficult lesion can be detected, and to know that they had succeeded in revealing a completely curable cancer, that they overemphasized early gastric cancer and did not adequately discuss other minute lesions.

In short, delicate lesions can be diagnosed effectively with double contrast radiography alone, and furthermore, all large lesions can be described more accurately than with other conventional methods. Not only can almost all lesions recognizable by macroscopic inspection be clearly demonstrated with this method, but in some cases, minute changes hardly detectable macroscopically can also be clearly shown.

However, it took at least 10 years in Japan for almost all leaders of institutes to evaluate double contrast radiography of the stomach. And there are still many radiodiagnosticians in other countries who criticize the usefulness of this technique, although a large and increasing number of radiologists are very interested in using it routinely. The reason evaluation of this method by different specialists varies so much is, we believe, that the quality of the films obtained with double contrast radiography differs greatly from one specialist to another, and all of them evaluate it on the basis of their own experience.

There are many factors that radiologists must always keep in mind when taking pictures with the double contrast method. If they miss or forget even one of them, the quality of each picture will be inferior. Of these factors, the most important one is the coating of barium on the mucosal surface of the stomach. On the films taken with the double contrast method in departments of radiology where the leader is not interested in this method, the coating of barium is usually not satisfactory. The Japanese technique is the result of research work focusing on how to obtain a good coating of barium on the mucosal surface of the stomach.

In the history of double contrast radiography of the colon, a successful technique was developed about 60 years ago. However, after 1970, the so-called direct method of double contrast radiography of the colon was generally adopted. This has made it possible to take clear pictures of polypoid lesions with a diameter of less than 5 mm and to demonstrate the delicate features of ulcerative colitis or Crohn's disease. In fact, the number of cases of early cancer of the colon detected by this method has been rapidly increasing. Around 1976, double contrast radiography of the small intestine was developed and is now becoming widely popular.

However, we must recognize that a coating of barium is easier to apply in the colon and small intestine than it is in the stomach. This is because the mucosal surfaces of the colon and small intestine are usually clean after proper preparation, even dry in the colon, and because these organs are the sites where the liquid parts of the contents are usually absorbed. In contrast, in the stomach, a large amount of liquid as well as very sticky mucus is secreted. This, we believe, is why it was very difficult to get a good coating of barium in the stomach. Our group solved this problem using the experience of radiography of hundreds of resected specimens of the colon, the small intestine, and the stomach. We noticed from these experiences that even in the stomach, the mucosal surface can be well demonstrated with double contrast radiography when it is well prepared. Therefore, during the initial stage of our research, we tried to wash the inner surface of the stomach with water instilled through a tube. This did not succeed because some of the water usually remained and interfered with coating of barium. Finally, we found that a fairly large amount, 200–300 ml, of barium meal with a high concentration of barium sulfate and low viscosity is effective in washing the surface of the mucosa merely by changing the patient's position.

Another important factor is distension of the gastric wall. Small lesions easily hidden among the mucosal folds are well demonstrated after distension of the wall with enough air.

Transparency is another condition that can be produced merely by introducing air. The more air introduced, the wider the area of the stomach that becomes transparent. However, the amount of air that can be introduced is limited, and the patient must be allowed to change position in order to get the transparent area needed.

Pooling is also a very important factor, because delicate unevenness of the surface can be demonstrated by regulating the size of the barium pool covering the lesion. For that reason, when a suspicious lesion is noticed during fluoroscopy, the radiologist has to change the patient's position very delicately in order to get good double contrast films that are easy to be read.

Although the double contrast examination can cover every part of the stomach, some parts are less easy to examine than others. Furthermore, it is not wise to deny some advantages of the conventional techniques in reconstructing the series of positions in routine examinations of the stomach. From this point of view, the authors have divided the inner surface of the stomach into 77 sections, as shown in Figs. 16 and 17 (Matsue *et al.*, 1970). This map has been used widely by specialists in this field in Japan, who have nicknamed it as "Stomap." In November 1983, the Committee on Standardization of Indirect X Ray Examination (chairman, H. Ichikawa) of the Japanese Society of Gastrointestinal Mass

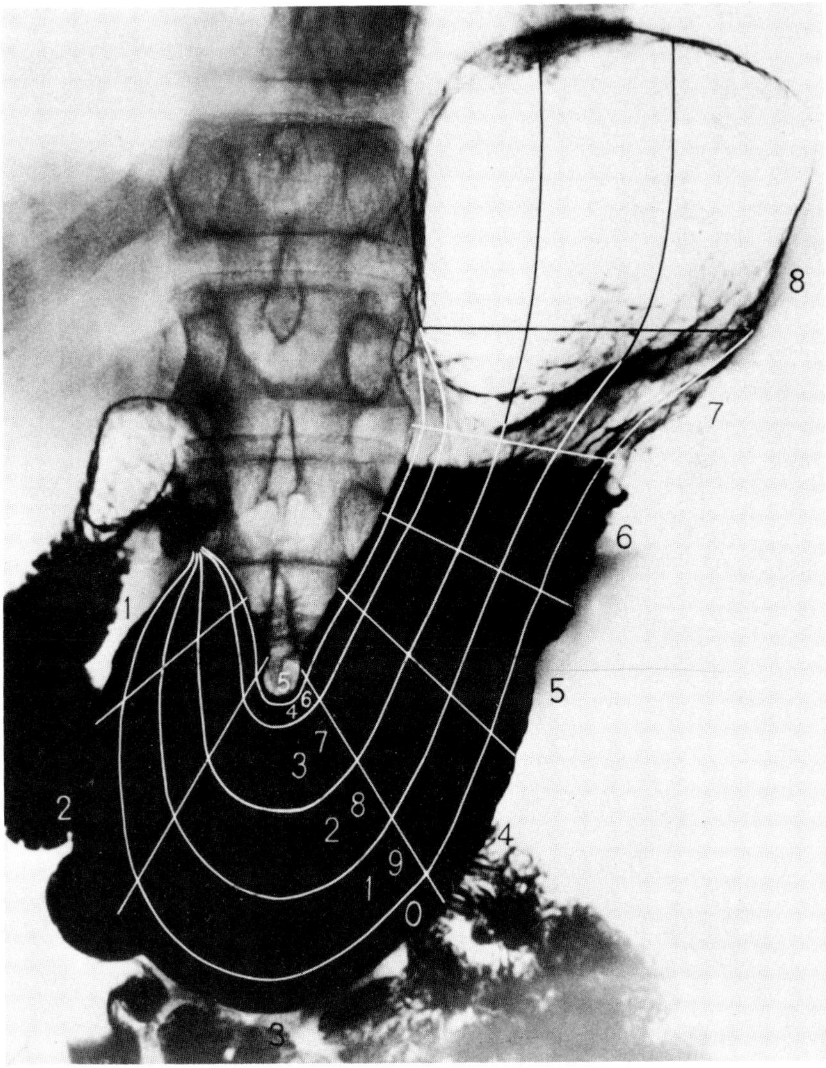

Fig. 16. Seventy-seven sections of stomach.

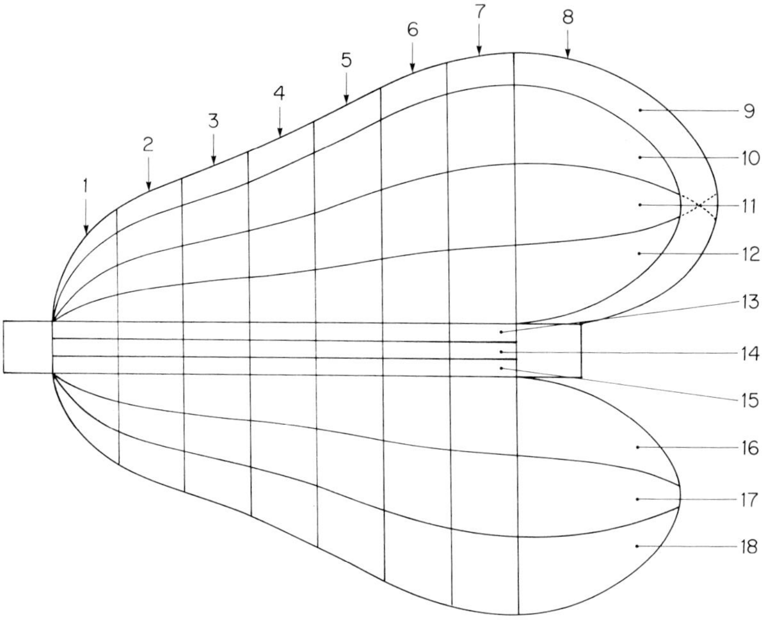

Fig. 17. Sections of stomach comprising the stomap.

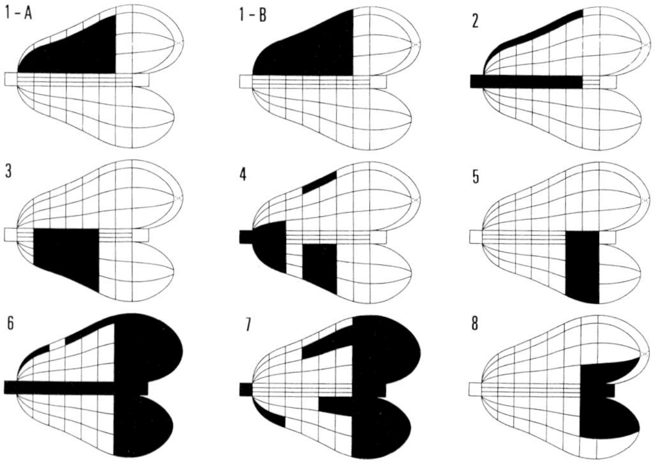

Fig. 18. Combinations of positions to cover the stomach in double contrast radiography (see text).

Survey reported, after 2 years of discussion, combinations of required positioning, as shown in Fig. 18.

In this figure, each number and stomap represent the required positioning:

1A Mucosal relief study in the prone position
1B Double contrast radiography in the prone position
2 Full of barium in the prone position
3 Double contrast radiography in the supine position
4 Double contrast radiography in the supine and right anterior oblique positions
5 Double contrast radiography in the supine and left anterior oblique positions
6 Double contrast radiography in the supine, semirecumbent, and left anterior oblique positions
7 Upright and right anterior oblique positions
8 Upright and sagittal positions

The black-stained area in each stomap represents the sections of the stomach usually covered by each position. It is clear that the combination of these eight positions can cover all of the sections.

We believe that this concept is also applicable in the routine examination of the stomach.

VI. SUMMARY

After giving a short history of double contrast radiography of the stomach, the authors presented some cases diagnosed with this method. Fine and delicate features of the lesions are well demonstrated using the technique, and some characteristic findings are explained.

Using this method, a large number of minute lesions representing early gastric cancer have been diagnosed and treated, with extremely high 5- and 20-year survival rates.

Some technical points in regard to this method and the combination of positions in routine X ray examination of the stomach are discussed.

REFERENCES

Fischer, A. W. (1923). Uber eine neue roentgenologische Untersuchungs-methode des dickdarms: Kombination von Kontrasteinlauf und Luftaufblahung. *Klin. Wochenscher.* **2,** 1595–1598.

Hilpert, F. (1929). Das Pneumo-Relief des Magens. *Fortschr. Roentgenstr.* **38,** 80–87.

Ichikawa, H. (1976). Differential diagnosis between benign and malignant ulcers of the stomach. *Clin. Gastroenterol.* **2,** 239.

Ichikawa, H. (1978). Mass screening for stomach cancer in Japan. *In* "Screening in Cancer" (A. B. Miller, ed.), UICC Tech. Rep. Ser., Vol. 40, pp. 279–305. Int. Union Against Cancer, Geneva.

Ichikawa, H., Yamada, T., and Doi, H. (1964). "Practice of X ray Diagnosis of the Stomach, for the Diagnosis of Early Gastric Cancer." Bunkodo Ltd., Tokyo.

Laufer, I. (1979). "Double Contrast Gastrointestinal Radiology with Endoscopic Correlation." Saunders, Philadelphia, Pennsylvania.

Matsue, H., Tobayashi, K., Yamada, T., Horikoshi, H., Doi, H., Suko, H., and Ichikawa, H. (1970). X-ray diagnosis of lesions in the upper portions of the stomach. *"I to Cho"* *(Stomach & Intestine)* **5,** 1071–1083.

Poppel, M. H. (1937). Double contrast method in Roentgenograph of the gastrointestinal tract. *Am. J. Roentgenol. Radium, Ther.* **37,** 379–381.

Shirakabe, H. (1971). "Double Contrast Studies of the Stomach." Bunkodo Ltd., Tokyo.

Shirakabe, H., and Ichikawa, H. (1973). Early gastric cancer. *In* "The Esophagus and Stomach," An Atlas of Tumor Radiology. (P. J. Hodes, ed.), pp. 277–357. Am. Coll. Radiol., Year Book Med. Publ., Chicago, Illinois.

Shirakabe, H., Ichikawa, H., Kumakura, K., Nishizawa, M., Higurashi, K., Hayakawa, H., and Murakami, T. (1966). "Atlas of X-ray Diagnosis of Early Gastric Cancer." Lippincott, Philadelphia, Pennsylvania.

Shirakabe, H., Nishizawa, M., Maruyama, M., and Kobayashi, S. (1982). "Atlas of X-ray Diagnosis of Early Gastric Cancer," 2nd ed. Igaku Shoin, Ltd., Tokyo.

Vallebona, A. (1931). A new combined method of iconography. *Rep. Commun. Int. Congr. Radiol., 3rd, 1930,* p. 309.

12

Ultrasound: Screening for Early Breast Cancer by Echography

TOSHIJI KOBAYASHI

I.	Introduction	215
II.	History of Breast Echography	216
III.	Equipment for Gray-Scale Echography	218
IV.	Technique Used for the Water-Bag Examination	220
V.	Echographic Characteristics of the Normal Female Breast	220
VI.	Diagnostic Criteria	223
VII.	Demonstration of Typical Echograms in Various Abnormalities	226
VIII.	Malignant Disease (Breast Cancer)	226
	A. Diagnostic Accuracy	228
	B. Expanded Echography	228
	C. Ultrasonic Tissue Characterization for Breast Cancer	229
IX.	Application of Ultrasound to Screening for Breast Cancer	231
	A. Methods of Screening	232
	B. Results of Screening	232
X.	Conclusion	234
	References	235

I. INTRODUCTION

Early detection and correct diagnosis of breast cancer is mandatory and is an important determinant of the prognosis because of its high incidence, affecting 1 out of 13 women in Western countries. Gray-scale ultrasonography offers considerable potential as a diagnostic technique for the visualization of soft tissue structures and pathologies. It is noninvasive, presents no physical hazard of ionizing radiation, and is simple and easy to apply clinically. Breast ultrasonography, in particular, has high diagnostic accuracy because of the recently developed gray-scale image display.

ISBN 0-12-496720-5

This chapter deals with the historical development of breast echography; techniques of water coupling approaches, especially the water-bag technique; diagnostic criteria; diagnostic accuracy; the demonstration of typical gray-scale echograms from various breast diseases; and a brief review of its current status and use in screening. Throughout, we should bear in mind the definition of screening tests. *Screening tests* are designed to differentiate apparently well persons who have a disease from those who probably do not. A screening test is not intended to be diagnostic. Persons with positive or suspicious findings must be referred for diagnosis or treatment.

II. HISTORY OF BREAST ECHOGRAPHY

As early as 1951, Wild and co-workers (Wild and Neal, 1951; Wild and Reid, 1952a,b) demonstrated the potential usefulness of ultrasonic visualization in detecting benign and malignant breast tumors by the A-mode display, designated the *echoscope* (Table I). They further developed this technique for two-dimensional imaging and devised a new method of display using a linear scanner that

TABLE I

History of Breast Echography

Investigator	Year reported	Type of examination or equipment used	Clinical comments
Wild and Neal	1951	A-mode	Qualitative differences in records of cancerous and benign lesions of breast noted
Wild and Reid	1952a	Echoscope A-mode 15 MHz used	Diagnostic criteria Echographic ratio (tumor/control) Malignant and benign accuracy rate Malignant 12/12 (100%) Benign 7/9 (78%)
Wild and Reid	1952b	Echograph linear scanner B-mode 15 MHz used	First report for echographic visualization of the breast
Wild and Reid	1954	Echoscope Echograph A-mode B-mode 15 MHz used	Echographic diagnosis by A-scope Diagnostic accuracy rate Malignant 19/20 (95%) Benign 19/21 (90%)

(*continued*)

TABLE I *(Continued)*

Investigator	Year reported	Type of examination or equipment used	Clinical comments
Howry *et al.*	1954	Somascope B-mode Radial scanner 2 MHz used	Echographic visualization of breast cancer (scirrhous carcinoma)
Kikuchi *et al.*	1957	Ultrasonotomography B-mode 5–10 MHz used	Echographic visualization of breast tumor
Kikuchi	1968	Sensitivity-graded tomogram pairs of ultrasonotomography devised	Method of sensitivity-graded tomogram pairs of ultrasonotomography introduced in clinical application
Kossoff	1972	Octoson Gray scale	Diagnostic accuracy rate Overall 90% Malignant 85%
Kobayashi *et al.*	1972	Sensitivity-graded method of ultrasonotomography Sonolayergraph	Diagnostic accuracy rate Medullary carcinoma 81% Papillary carcinoma 88% Scirrhous carcinoma 100% TNM classification T1 82% T2 94% T3 100%
Kobayashi	1977	Gray-scale echography Sonlayergraph Correlation of echographic findings (acoustic middle shadow sign): attenuation and content of connective tissue in breast cancer	Connective tissue Rich: Scirrhous carcinoma Moderate: Papillary carcinoma Poor: Medullary carcinoma Attenuation Strong: Scirrhous carcinoma Moderate: Papillary carcinoma Weak: Medullary carcinoma
Wagai *et al.*	1982	Serial echography Hitachi EUB	Application of echography to the screening of early breast cancer; 20,323 women screened during the last 6 years 14 cases of breast cancer detected Detection rate 0.06%
Kobayashi	1983	Hitachi EUB	Screening was carried out at the Kouchi Screening Center 6031 women screened during the last 3 years 4 case of breast cancer detected Detection rate 0.06%

they designated an *echograph*. This echographic visualization of the normal and the diseased breast was a milestone in the field of clinical ultrasound.

During the same period, Howry *et al.* (1954) devised an ultrasound compound scanning technique called *somascope,* consisting of a B-mode display with a radial scanner. They reported the first echographic demonstration of scirrhous carcinoma. After this epoch-making introduction by these American investigators, there were no further clinical reports in the literature of this field, except for the important basic research contributions made by the outstanding investigator Fry (1977) in the ultrasonic detection of breast tumors.

In addition to the American research, extensive ultrasound investigations and clinical applications were carried out in Japan by Kikuchi *et al.* (1957), an outstanding microwave engineer and physicist, who devised a technique called *ultrasonotomography* and an apparatus named the *ultrasonotomograph.* This instrument used a scanner, mainly for the visualization of neoplastic lesions of various tissues and organs in the human body, but especially for brain, abdominal, and breast tumors.

Kossoff (1972), an outstanding Australian investigator and pioneer in ultrasound, used a unique technique of display called *gray-scale echography* in an instrument called an *Octoson.* This instrument was an important development in the history of echography. It can visualize fine structural features and the pathologic status of the breast.

At the same time, Kobayashi *et al.* (1972; 1974), using the sensitivity-graded method of ultrasonotomography, reported diagnostic criteria, mainly three differential points: the boundary echo and shape, internal echoes, and the retrotumorous shadowing, including the tadpole-tail sign and the lateral shadow sign for benign tumors and the acoustic middle shadow sign for malignant tumors. Kobayashi (1977) described the correlation between echographic signs, especially the acoustic middle shadow sign, and collagen fiber or connective tissue. He suggested that connective tissue may play an important role in producing the acoustic middle shadow sign or posterior shadowing, which is the parameter of ultrasonic attenuation and absorption by cancerous tissue (Table I).

In 1978, Wagai and co-workers first introduced this technique into the field of screening to detect early breast cancer in Japan (Wagai *et al.,* 1976). Later on, Kobayashi (1983) used the same technique at a local screening center.

III. EQUIPMENT FOR GRAY-SCALE ECHOGRAPHY

Since the breast is a superficial soft tissue organ, water coupling techniques such as a water-bath or water-bag approach can be routinely used. Equipment for these approaches is commercially available (Table II). These instruments can all be used in screening for breast cancer.

TABLE II

Present Status of Echographic Approaches to Breast Cancer Using the Water-Coupling Technique

	Scanning in water-bath	Scanning in water-bag
Equipment available:	UI Octoson (Australia) Life instrument (United States) Ausonic System I (Australia) Technicare System (United States) breast scanner	Toshiba Sonolaryergraph (Japan) Hitachi EUB (Japan) Aloka SSD (Japan)
Clinical applicability	Good for large dense breast	Small and fibrous atrophic breast
Position in examination	Prone	Supine
Applicability to screening	(+)	(+)
Display quality	Gray-scale image	Gray-scale image
Diagnostic accuracy rate	Good (over 85%)	Good (over 85%)
Diagnostic points	Boundary echo—internal echo—posterior echo	Boundary echo—internal echo—posterior echo
Diagnostic superiority	Scirrhous carcinoma > Papillary carcinoma > Medullary carcinoma >	Scirrhous carcinoma > Papillary carcinoma > Medullary carcinoma >

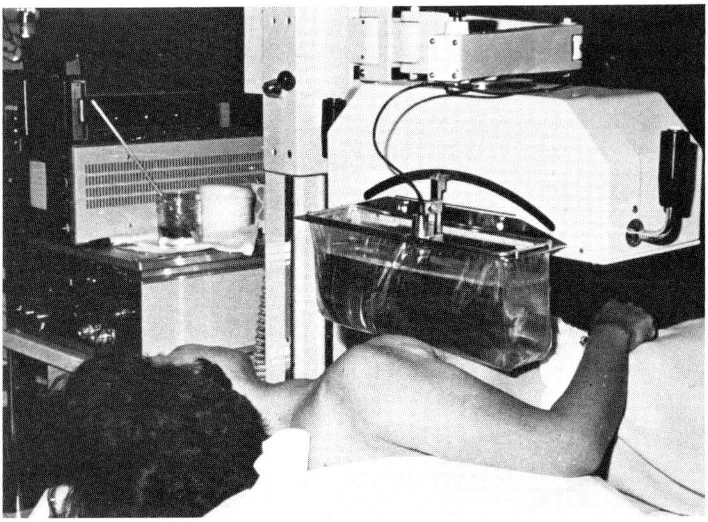

Fig. 1. Water-bag technique used arc fashion. A palpable breast mass is positioned by placing a pillow or soft pad under the shoulder for an optimal scanning level while patient is in a supine position. A degased water bag at a temperature of approximately 37°C is lowered to a position just above the breast mass; olive oil is applied to the overlying skin to provide acoustic coupling between the water-bag and the skin. The water depth is kept a constant 5 cm from the transducer surface to the overlying skin, and the ultrasonic transducer of 5 MHz is mechanically oscillated in a 60-degree arc within the water bag. The time gain compensation is kept constant at 5 dB/cm, and various other instrumentation settings in the receiving amplifier are also kept constant.

IV. TECHNIQUE USED FOR THE WATER-BAG EXAMINATION

For the water-bag examination, the patient is in the supine position and a polyvinyl water bag containing degased water is placed on the skin overlying the breast after the contact medium is applied. The transducer–skin distance is kept constant, and scanning is performed in an arc fashion (Fig. 1).

V. ECHOGRAPHIC CHARACTERISTICS OF THE NORMAL FEMALE BREAST

With the gray-scale echograph utilizing the water-bag technique, the breast tissue, Cooper's ligament, fat layers, muscle layers, and chest wall are clearly

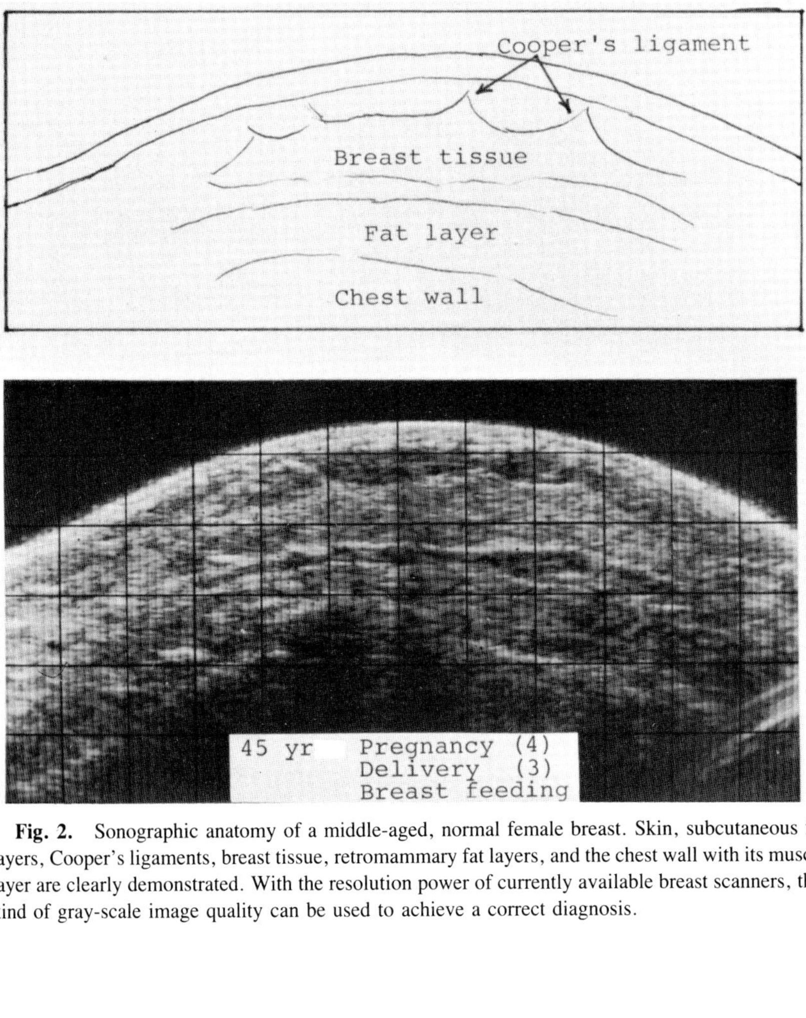

Fig. 2. Sonographic anatomy of a middle-aged, normal female breast. Skin, subcutaneous fat layers, Cooper's ligaments, breast tissue, retromammary fat layers, and the chest wall with its muscle layer are clearly demonstrated. With the resolution power of currently available breast scanners, this kind of gray-scale image quality can be used to achieve a correct diagnosis.

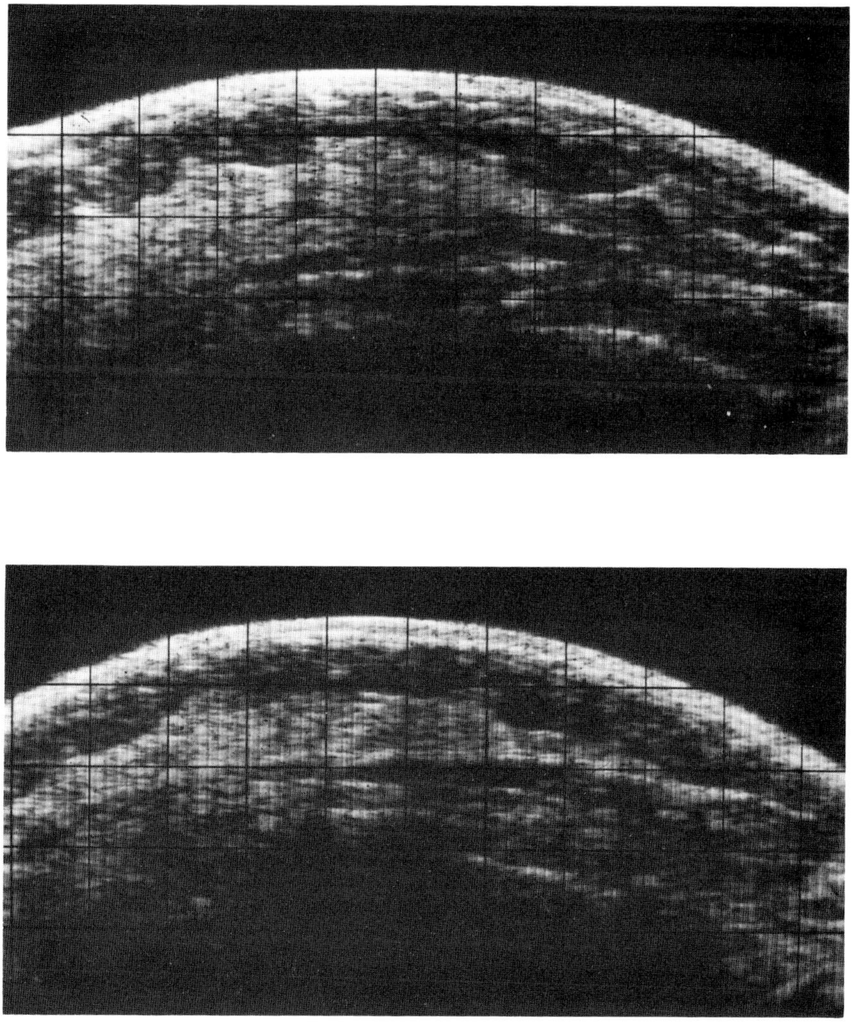

Fig. 3. Similarity in the sonographic characteristics of bilateral breasts. Both echograms were recorded 1 cm below the nipple in a normal 48-year-old female with a gestational history of five pregnancies, three deliveries, and breast feeding. In order to detect early breast cancer, comparison of the parenchymal pattern in both breasts may be very helpful in reaching a correct diagnosis.

visualized (Fig. 2). This echogram was recorded by a linear scanner from a 45-year-old female with a history of four pregnancies and three deliveries; all infants were breast-fed.

Echograms recorded from the breasts of a 48-year-old normal female are shown in Fig. 3 for comparison. There is no difference in visualization of the fine

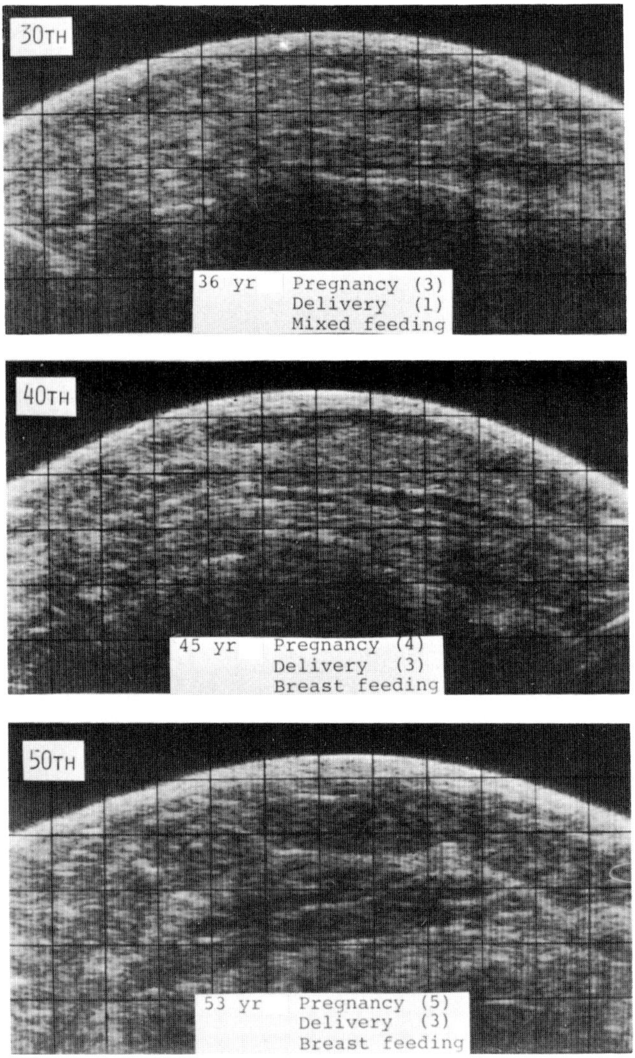

Fig. 4. Changes in glandular tissue and connective tissue contents due to aging. Breast glandular tissue may regress in amount with aging, and the echogenic level may increase in sonographic intensity because the amount of connective tissue within the fat layers increases.

structures of the breast. Bilateral comparison easily enables one to recognize fine pathology in early carcinoma.

The aging process involved in breast tissue is shown in Fig. 4. In general, breast tissue is rich and dense in the third decade and poor and atrophied in the fifth decade.

VI. DIAGNOSTIC CRITERIA

The characteristics that differentiate breast cancer from benign breast tumors are shown in Fig. 5. Differential points can be divided into three categories:

1. *Boundary echo and shape.* These are regular, smooth, and round, oval, or hemioval in benign disease, whereas they are irregular, jagged, and crablike or polymorphous in malignant disease.
2. *Internal echo.* In benign disease it is homogeneous, uniformly sized, or echo free (anechoic), whereas it is nonhomogeneous in breast cancer.
3. *Posterior shadowing or retromammary shadowing.* The tadpole-tail sign, the lateral shadow sign, or accentuation of the posterior echo may appear in benign disease, whereas the acoustic middle shadow sign or attenuation of the posterior echo may appear in breast cancer as the result of sonic attenuation and absorption by cancerous tissue (Kobayashi, 1975).

These criteria are very useful in the evaluation of a routine clinical echogram. Very similar criteria were reported by several investigators (Baum, 1977; Cole-Beuglet and Beique, 1975; Fry, 1977; Gros *et al.*, 1975; Huber, 1981; Jellins *et al.*, 1975; Kossoff *et al.*, 1978; Pluygers *et al.*, 1977a; Rombaut *et al.*, 1981; Rubin *et al.*, 1979).

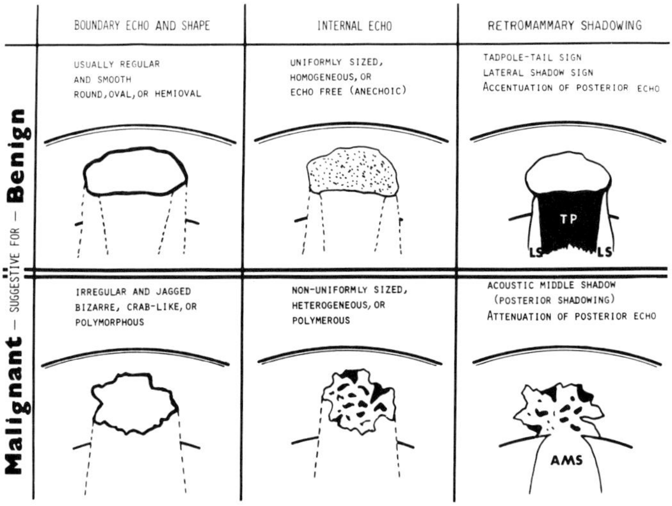

Fig. 5. Diagnostic criteria. Points in differentiation: The upper and lower schemas are findings suggestive of benign and malignant tumors, respectively. It is important to check points such as the boundary echo and shape, the internal echoes, and the retromammary or retrotumorous shadowing.

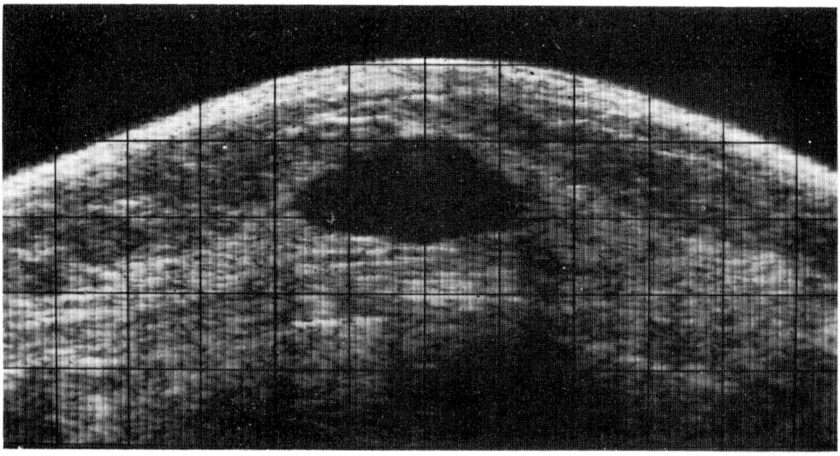

Fig. 6. This large benign cyst measures 3.0 × 1.4 cm and shows a regular, smooth boundary echo with an anechoic area within the breast tissue (47-year-old female, gravida 4, para 2; artificial feeding).

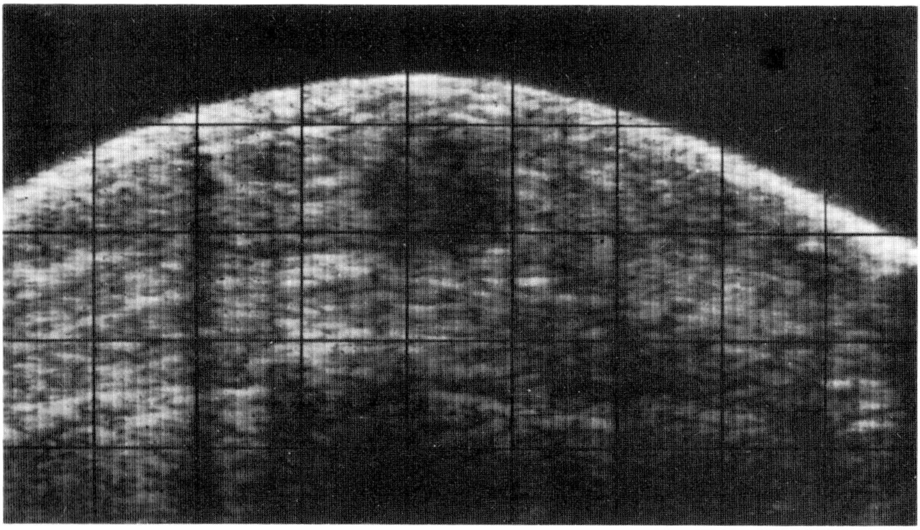

Fig. 7. Typical echo pattern of fibroadenoma, characterized by a regular, smooth boundary echo and shape, homogeneous internal echoes, and tumor mass echoes with rather low-level intensity compared with those of the normal surrounding breast tissue. The tumor measured 1.4 × 1.2 cm (39-year-old female, gravida 5, para 3; mixed feeding).

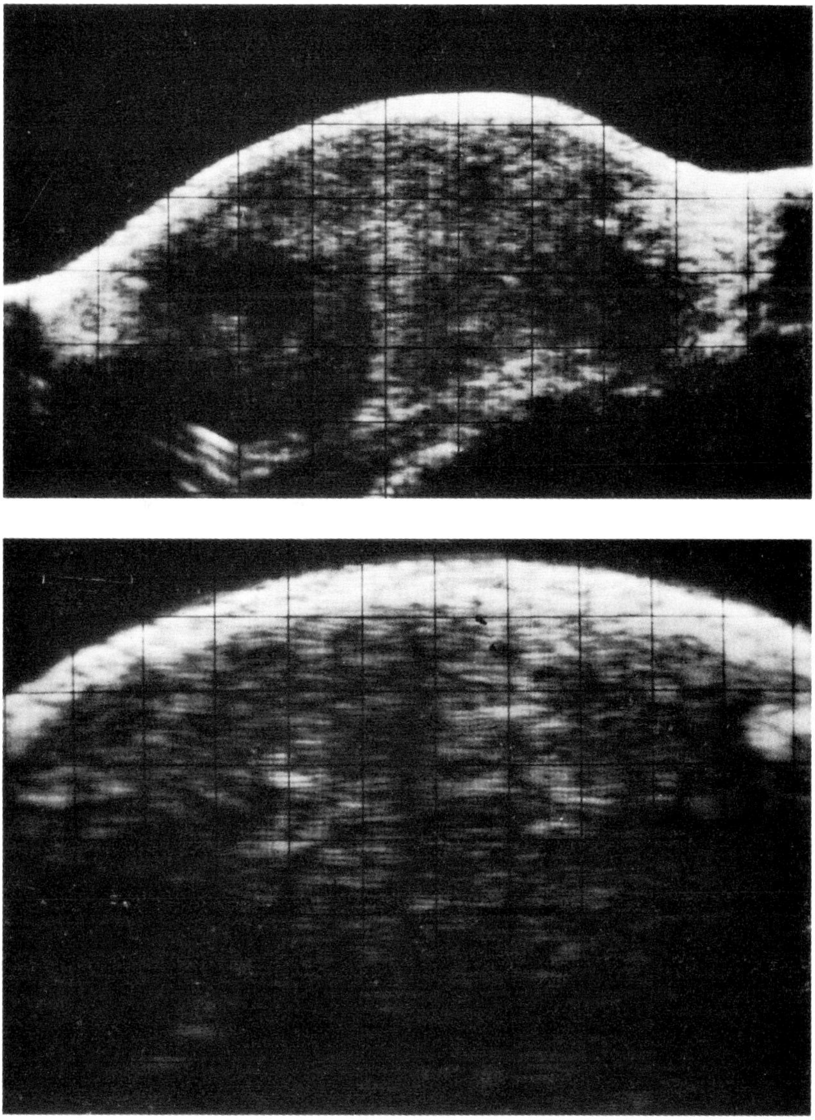

Fig. 8. Typical echogram of cystosarcoma phylloides, the central portion of which became cystic as a degenerative change. The echographic characteristics are homogeneous, fine dotted internal echoes compared with those of a malignant tumor. Attenuation of the posterior shadowing is less notable than that of a malignant tumor. On the left side of the tumor mass, an anechoic area is seen as the cyst. A low echo-level area surrounds it, and an area of cystosarcoma is distributed throughout under the skin. The tumor measured 8 × 4 cm; the cyst was 1.5 × 1.5 cm. The patient was a 21-year-old female.

VII. DEMONSTRATION OF TYPICAL ECHOGRAMS IN VARIOUS ABNORMALITIES

1. *Benign cyst.* A typical echogram of a large benign cyst is shown in Fig. 6, illustrating a rather smooth boundary echo with no echo rising from the inside of the cyst, i.e., sonolucent or anechoic. The surrounding breast tissue and the fat layer are clearly visualized.

2. *Fibroadenoma.* This common breast tumor is shown in Fig. 7, illustrating a regular, smooth boundary echo and a homogeneous internal echo with less ultrasonic attenuation behind it.

3. *Cytosarcoma phylloides.* This common benign tumor frequently seen in the young female is shown in Fig. 8, demonstrating homogeneous internal echoes with partial cystic degeneration at the left corner as a sonolucent area.

VIII. MALIGNANT DISEASE (BREAST CANCER)

Typical echograms seen in scirrhous carcinoma are shown in Fig. 9. There is rather strong ultrasonic attenuation behind the tumor mass echo, forming the acoustic middle shadow sign or posterior shadowing; also, the bottom echo of the

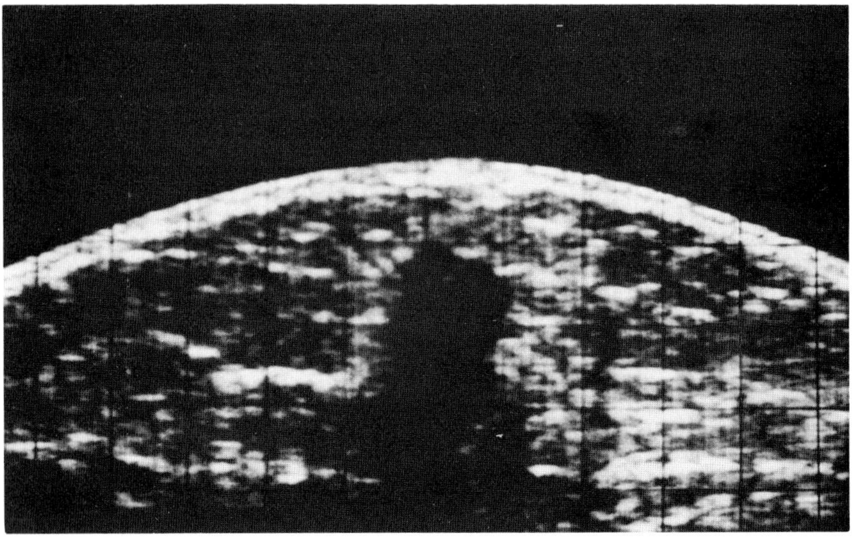

Fig. 9. Early breast cancer (Scirrhous carcinoma). Echogram shows strong ultrasonic attenuation behind tumor mass, thus forming complete absence of bottom echo of tumor mass. Boundary echo is irregular and uneven, suggesting malignant tumor echographically. Tumor measured 1.5 × 1.5 cm.

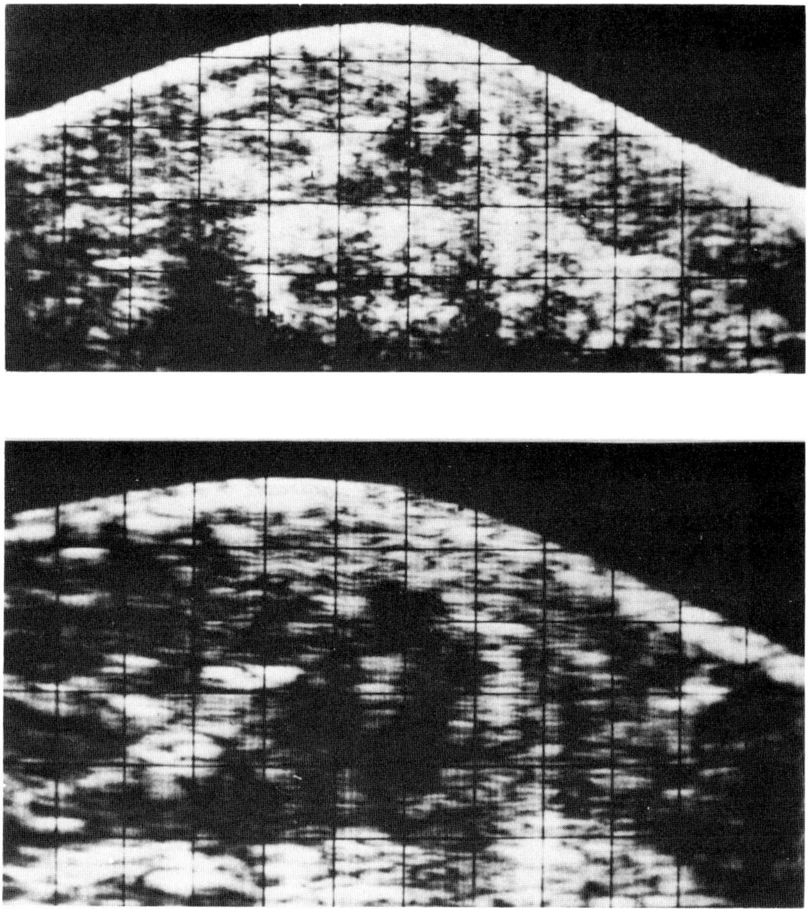

Fig. 10. Typical echograms of medullary carcinoma. A completely irregular, uneven boundary echo, nonhomogeneous internal echoes, and less attenuation of retrotumorous shadowing are clearly demonstrated within the breast tissue. This type of echogram may often be seen in medullary carcinoma and papillary carcinoma. The tumor measured 2.0 × 1.8 cm (T1). The patient was a 49-year-old female. Upper: ordinary echogram. Lower: expanded echogram.

tumor mass has completely disappeared. The boundary echo of the tumor mass is completely irregular and uneven, and its internal echoes are nonhomogeneous in size.

The echograms in Figs. 10 and 11 were recorded from cases of medullary carcinoma and show rather weak ultrasonic attenuation, i.e., unchanged or accentuated ultrasonic energy throughout the tumor mass. Its boundary echo is completely irregular and polymorphous, and its internal echoes are nonhomogen-

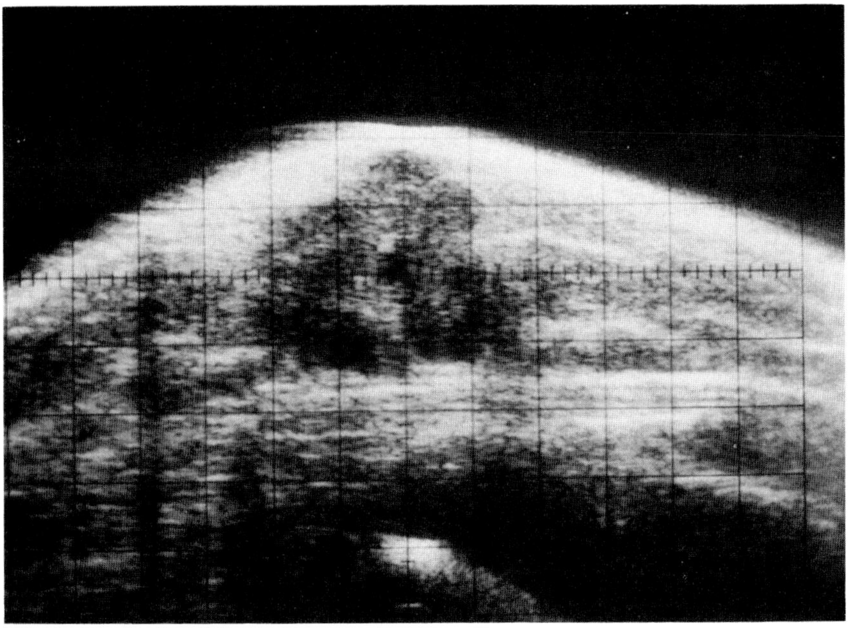

Fig. 11. Medullary carcinoma (T2) of the breast, showing a rather unchanged bottom echo behind the tumor mass or ultrasonically accentuated in the retrotumorous area, in contrast to the echo pattern of scirrhous carcinoma. This pattern often makes differentiation from a benign tumor, i.e., fibroadenoma, difficult. The only points that differentiate it from a fibroadenoma are an irregular, nonsmooth, uneven boundary echo and nonhomogeneous internal echoes.

eous in size. These echographic characteristics are often seen in cases of medullary carcinoma.

A. Diagnostic Accuracy

Diagnostic accuracy rates are shown in Table III according to the TNM classification, comparing echography and mammography. Accuracy rates are also shown according to histologic type. The rates are highest in scirrhous carcinoma, followed in order by papillary carcinoma and medullary carcinoma. The overall accuracy is approximately 85% (Kobayashi, 1978a; Kobayashi and Hayashi, 1980).

B. Expanded Echography

Expanded echography is another approach used to improve the diagnostic accuracy rate in early breast cancer, especially for T1 tumors less than 2 cm in

TABLE III

Diagnostic Accuracy of Ultrasound Compared with Mammography

A. According to Tumor Size				
TNM	Ultrasound	Percentage	Mammography	Percentage
T1	31/40	78	28/37	76
T2	52/58	90	49/56	88
T3	13/14	93	12/14	86
Total	112 cases		107 cases	

B. According to Histologic Type				
Histologic type	Ultrasound	Percentage	Mammography	Percentage
Scirrhous carcinoma	32/35	91	30/33	91
Medullary carcinoma	33/42	79	26/40	65
Papillary carcinoma	26/31	84	25/32	78
Total	108 cases		105 cases	

size. The target lesion is magnified 16 times on a cathode ray tube (CRT) display, so that all diagnostic information can be easily recognized by this technique. A typical example of early breast cancer is presented in Fig. 12. The ordinary echogram at the upper left did not show the acoustic middle shadow sign, whereas it was clearly shown in the expanded echogram at the lower right. Expanded echography is indicated in cases of suspected tumors less than 1 cm in size (Kobayashi *et al.*, 1977; Kobayashi, 1981).

C. Ultrasonic Tissue Characterization for Breast Cancer

The tissue characterization or tissue signature for breast cancer has been evaluated recently from the clinical echographic point of view. Retromammary or posterior shadowing is important diagnostic information in breast cancer, i.e., the acoustic middle shadow sign as seen in Fig. 5, lower right. This sign may be considered to be closely related to the acoustic mechanism of ultrasonic attenuation. Therefore, consecutive histologic specimens from the cases that showed strong posterior shadowing or retromammary shadowing were examined microscopically, especially to determine the collagen fiber content or connective tissue content in breast cancer tissue. It was found that the cases in which the collagen fiber content was greater than 75% in 12 consecutive sliced specimens in a given tumor mass demonstrated strong posterior shadowing or ultrasonic attenuation echographically. In contrast, little attenuation occurred in cases with a collagen fiber content of less than 25%. Thus, scirrhous carcinomas with a collagen fiber

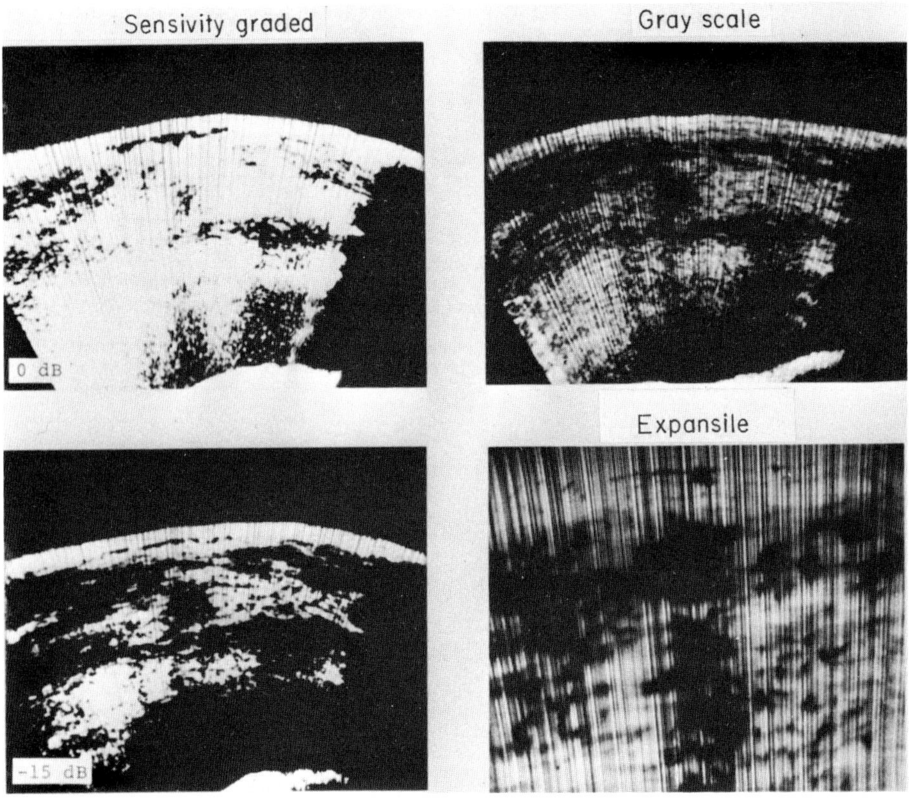

Fig. 12. Expanded echogram of early breast cancer. The acoustic middle shadow sign indicative of malignancy is poorly visualized in all but the expansile echogram (lower right). This sign is important in diagnosing malignancy.

content of over 75% cast strong acoustic middle shadow signs (Fig. 9) Medullary carcinomas, on the other hand, which often have a collagen fiber content of less than 25%, show a rather unchanged bottom echo of the tumor mass or ultrasonic attenuation behind the mass (Fig. 11).

Figure 13 gives a better understanding and visualization of echo patterns and various amounts of collagen fiber content; the echogram in the top left shows strong attenuation, with a collagen fiber content of over 75%; the middle echogram demonstrates the intermediate shadow from a cancer with 50% collagen; and the lower one represents less than 25% collagen, showing less attenuation.

The correlation between the echographic findings, especially the appearance of an acoustic middle shadow sign, and the collagen fiber content may give some clinical insight into the histologic type in a given case. This is schematically shown in Fig. 14 (Kobayashi, 1979a; Kobayashi, 1979b).

IX. APPLICATION OF ULTRASOUND TO SCREENING FOR BREAST CANCER

Breast echography was first used in screening for early breast cancer by Wagai and co-workers in 1976 in Japan, but there has been no report about its screening use in the literature up to now. Later on, this technique was applied to detect early breast cancer in another screening center; the results have been reported by Kobayashi (1983).

Kobayashi and his co-worker carried out screening using ultrasound to detect

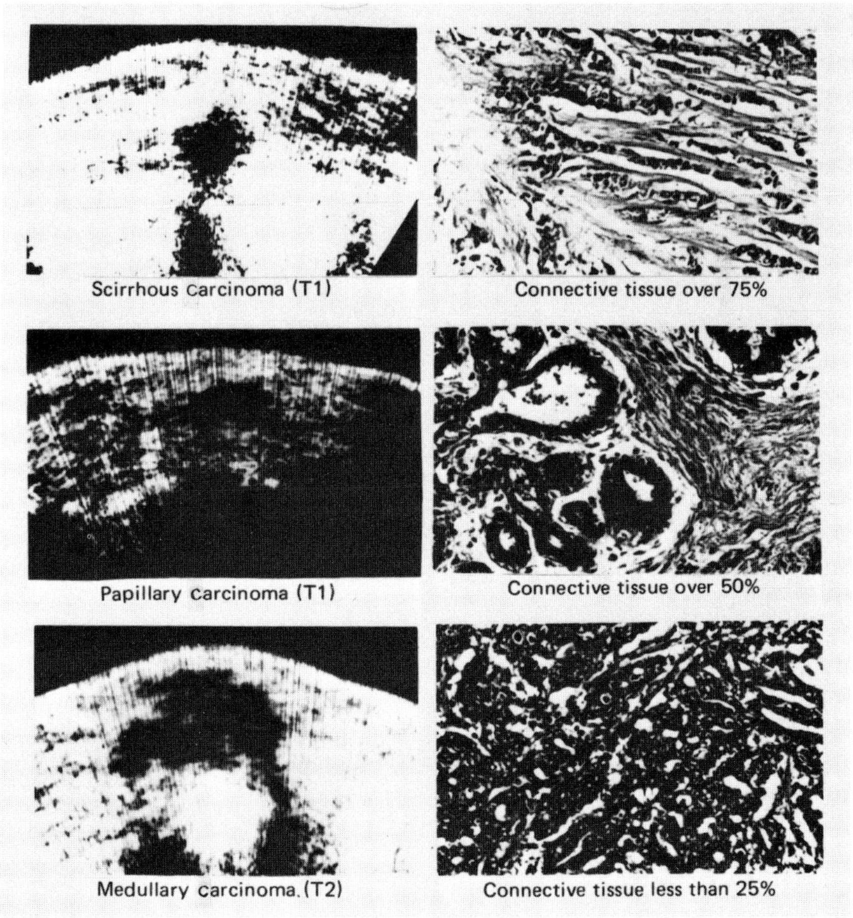

Fig. 13. Comparison of different breast cancers by analysis of echo patterns and amounts of connective tissue within tumors.

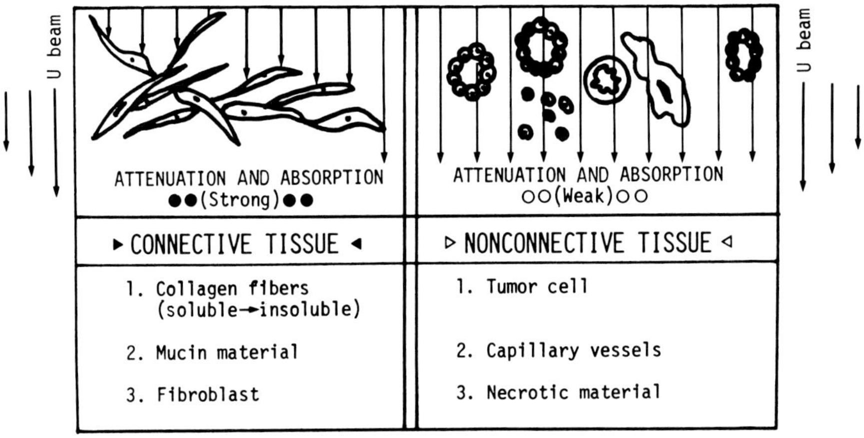

Fig. 14. Schematic illustration of the correlation between collagen fibers or connective tissue and ultrasonic attenuation, especially the formation of the acoustic middle shadow sign.

early breast cancer in the Kouchi Screening Clinic, the screening center for adult diseases in Kouchi City, Shikoku Island, Japan.

In outline, the program was as follows:

1. Screening subjects: self-applicants from the general screening population
2. Institution: Kouchi Screening Clinic
3. Age for screening: not restricted to any age group
4. Term of observation: April 6, 1979, to August 6, 1982

A. Methods of Screening

Breast history taking was performed by a public health nurse, and then breast palpation was performed by a surgeon who selected the location of the breast to be examined by echography. Palpation was performed first because the surgeon's experience in detecting small nodules was considered to be superior to self-examination by the applicant.

A water-bag linear scanner with a pitch of 5 mm and a scanning length of 150 mm, and the breast area covered by scanning of 4 cm, was used; nine consecutive echograms were obtained from each applicant, as shown in Fig. 15. The flow chart for screening is shown in Fig. 16.

B. Results of Screening

The yearly number of screening examinations performed, the age distribution of those examined, and the diagnosed disease entities are listed in Table IV. Four carcinomas, three fibroadenomas, and four cysts were diagnosed during this

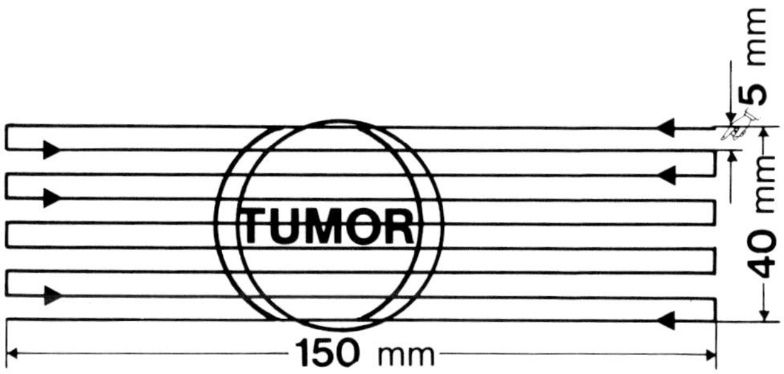

Fig. 15. Scanning or screening equipment is illustrated. Nine consecutive echograms can be obtained by this scanning technique. Length, 150 mm; pitch, 5 mm; area covered, 5 mm.

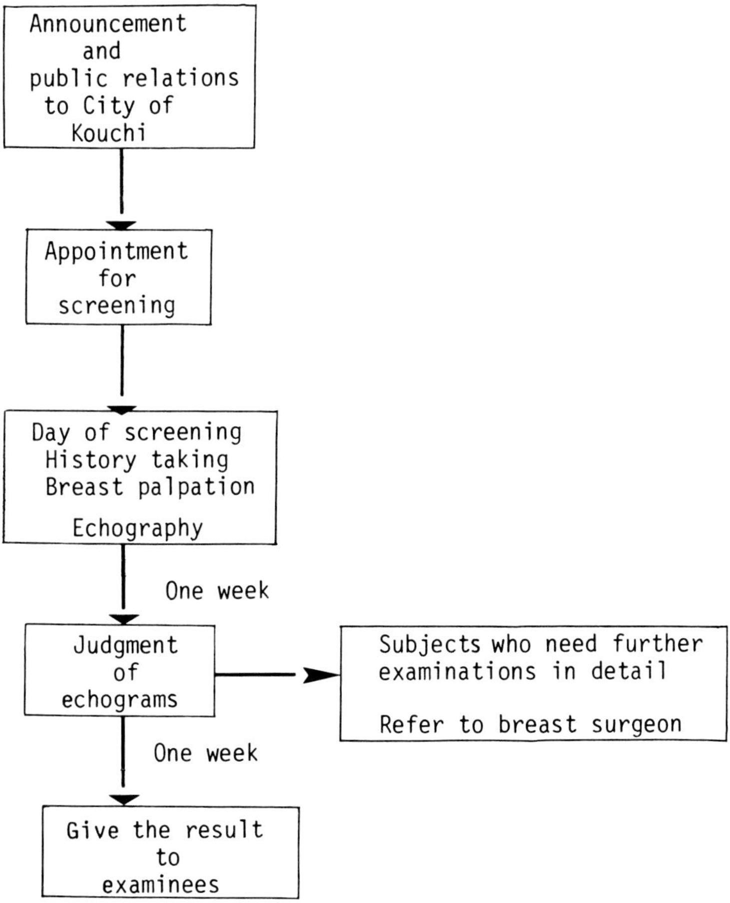

Fig. 16. Flow chart for screening.

TABLE IV

Yearly Number of Screening Examinations and Results

Age Distribution	Year 1979	1980	1981	1982	Total
20–29	21	23	25	25	94
30–39	331	364	451	237	1383
40–49	552	745	888	490	2675
50–59	318	438	582	374	1712
60–69	29	35	57	41	162
70 +	1	2	1	1	5
Total	1252	1607	2004	1168	6031
Diagnosed					
Carcinoma	0	1	1	2	4
Fibroadenoma	3	1	2	1	7
Cyst	0	1	1	2	4

TABLE V

Detection Rate of Breast Cancer

Investigator period covered	Wagai and Tsutsumi (1982) (6 years)	Kobayashi (1983) (3 Years, 4 months)
Number of screened examinees	20,323	6031
Cancer detected	14	4
Detection rate	0.06%	0.06%

observation period. The cancer detection rate was therefore 0.6 per 1000, which was the same as the rate previously reported by Wagai and Tsutsumi (1982) (Table V).

X. CONCLUSION

I sincerely hope that this chapter has provided guidelines for the use of echography in diagnosing breast cancer in screening, as well as evidence of its efficacy, so that this technique can become more widespread and can help to rescue many women from breast cancer.

REFERENCES

Baum, G. (1977). Ultrasound mammography. *Radiology* **122,** 199–205.

Cole-Beuglet, C., and Beique, R. A. (1975). Continuous ultrasound B-scanning of palpable breast masses. *Radiology* **117,** 123–128.

Fry, K. E. (1977). The use of ultrasound methods to detect changes in breast tissue which precede the formation of a malignant tumor. *In* "Acoustical Holography" (L. W. Kessler, ed.), Vol. 7, pp. 1–20. Plenum, New York.

Gros, C. H., Dale, G., Gautherie, M., Gairard, B., and Haehnel, P. (1975). Echography-radiography-histology correlation in breast cancer. *In* "Ultrasonics in Medicine" (E. Kazner, ed.), pp. 253–261. Excerpta Medica, Amsterdam.

Howry, D. H., Stott, D. A., and Bliss, W. R. (1954). The ultrasonic visualization of carcinoma of the breast and other soft-tissue structures. *Cancer* **7,** 354–358.

Huber, C. (1981). "Echographie en pathologie mammaire." Vigot, Paris.

Jellins, J., Kossoff, G., Reeve, T. S., and Barraclough, B. H. (1975). Ultrasonic gray scale visualization of breast disease. *Ultrasound Med. Biol.* **1,** 393–404.

Kikuchi, Y. (1968). Way to quantitative examination in ultrasonic diagnosis. *Med. Ultrason.* **5,** 1.

Kikuchi, Y., Uchida, R., Tanaka, T., and Wagai, T. (1957). Early cancer diagnosis through ultrasonics. *J. Acoust. Soc. Am.* **29,** 824–833.

Kobayashi, T. (1975). Review: Ultrasonic diagnosis of breast cancer. *Ultrasound Med. Biol.* **1,** 383–391.

Kobayashi, T. (1977). Gray scale echography for breast cancer. *Radiology* **122,** 207–214.

Kobayashi, T. (1978a). "Clinical Ultrasound of the Breast." Plenum, New York.

Kobayashi, T. (1978b). Ultrasonic tissue characterization of breast cancer: Correlation of attenuation and echo-pattern. *In* "Recent Advances in Ultrasound Diagnosis" (A. Kurjak, ed.), pp. 281–291. Excerpta Medica, Amsterdam.

Kobayashi, T. (1979a). Correlation of ultrasonic attenuation with connective tissue content in breast cancers. *In* "Ultrasonic Tissue Characterization II" (M. Linzer, ed.), pp. 93–99. U.S. Govt. Printing Office, Washington, D.C.

Kobayashi, T. (1979b). Diagnostic ultrasound in breast cancer: Analysis of retrotumorous echo patterns correlated with sonic attenuation by cancerous connective tissue. *J. Clin. Ultrasound* **7,** 471–479.

Kobayashi, T. (1981). Current status of breast echography. *In* "Progress in Medical Ultrasound" (A. Kurjak, ed.), pp. 123–125. Excerpta Medica, Amsterdam.

Kobayashi, T. (1983). Screening of breast cancer by ultrasound. *Proc. Jpn. Soc. Ultrason. Med.* **42,** 645–646.

Kobayashi, T., and Hayashi, M. (1980). Manual contact scanning in gray-scale echography. *J. Univ. Occup. Environ. Health* **2,** 469–479.

Kobayashi, T., Takatani, O., Kimura, K., Watanabe, H., and Abe, O. (1972). Clinical investigation for the differential diagnosis of breast tumor by means of the graded sensitivity method of ultrasonotomography (2nd report). Proposal of new differential diagnostic criteria: Tadpole-tail sign with bilateral shadow (Benign) and acoustic middle shadow sign (Malignant) and its clinical significance and evaluation. *Med. Ultrason.* **10,** 81–86.

Kobayashi, T., Takatani, O., Hattori, N., and Kimura, K. (1974). Differential diagnosis of breast tumors: The sensitivity graded method of ultrasonotomography and clinical evaluation of its diagnostic accuracy. *Cancer* **33,** 940–951.

Kobayashi, T., Nagata, F., Shinoda, A., Nakamura, S., Tanabe, S., and Takatani, O. (1977). Ultrasonic diagnosis of early breast cancer: Clinical significance of gray scale expanded echography. *Jpn. J. Clin. Oncol.* **7,** 55–66.

Kossoff, G. (1972). Improved techniques in ultrasonic cross sectional echography. *Ultrasonics* **10,** 221–227.

Kossoff, G., Jellins, J., and Reeve, T. S. (1978). Ultrasound in the detection of early breast cancer. *In* "Early Diagnosis of Breast Cancer" (E. Grundmann, ed.), pp. 149–158. Fischer, Stuttgart.

Pluygers, E., Beauduin, M., Devergnies, F., Pieron, A., and Rombaut, M. (1977a). Seméiologie echographique du sein normal et du sein dysplasique. *Senologia* **1,** 3–9.

Pluygers, E., Rombaut, M., Beauduin, M., Hendricks, B., Devergnies, F., Pieron, A., and Tamignaux, G. (1977b). Possibilities, results and indications of breast echography. *J. Belge Radiol.* **60,** 181–196.

Rombaut, M., and Pluygers, E. (1981). "Guide pratique d'ultrasonographie mammaire." Masson, Paris.

Rubin, C. S., Kurtz, A. B., Goldberg, B. B., Feig, S., and Cole-Beuglet, C. (1979). Ultrasonic mammographic parenchymal patterns: A preliminary report. *Radiology* **130,** 515–517.

Wagai, T. and Tsutsumi, M. (1982). Screening of breast cancer by echography. *In* "Ultrasound and Cancer" (S. Levi, ed.), pp. 315–322. Excerpta Medica, Amsterdam.

Wagai, T., Tsutsumi, M., and Takeuchi, H. (1976). Diagnostic ultrasound in breast diseases. *In* "Present and Future of Diagnostic Ultrasound" (I. Donald, ed.), pp. 148–161.

Wild, J. J., and Neal, D. (1951). Use of high-frequency ultrasonic waves for detecting changes of texture in living tissues. *Lancet* **1,** 655–662.

Wild, J. J., and Reid, J. M. (1952a). Application of echo-ranging techniques to the determination of structure of biological tissues. *Science* **115,** 226–230.

Wild, J. J., and Reid, J. M. (1952b). Further pilot echographic studies of the histologic structure of tumors of the living intact human breast. *Am. J. Pathol.* **28,** 839–861.

Wild, J. J., and Reid, J. M. (1954). Echographic visualization of lesions of the living intact human breast. *Cancer Res.* **14,** 277–283.

13

Fecal Occult Blood Testing

MARTIN FLEISHER, MORTON K. SCHWARTZ, AND SIDNEY J. WINAWER

I.	Introduction	237
II.	Test Characteristics	238
III.	Diet	240
IV.	Sensitivity	241
V.	Storage and Rehydration	242
VI.	Quality Control of Fecal Occult Blood Tests	242
VII.	Available Tests	244
	References	246

I. INTRODUCTION

The possible value of the fecal occult blood test was proposed in 1901 by Boas (1901), who used the gum guaiac method developed by Van Deen (1864). Adler and Adler (1904) reported that benzidine produced a better color reaction than that obtained with guaiac. The production of color was shown to be related to the pseudoperoxidase activity of hemoglobin by Wu (1922). A modified benzidine test developed by Gregersen (1919) was found to be exquisitely sensitive, an 8% solution of which detected fecal blood in a dilution of 1:20,000. Numerous other tests that depend on the ability of hemoglobin or its derivatives to oxidize chromogenic substances were subsequently developed. These reactant substances included ferrocyanide, 3-aminophthalic acid, hydrazide, paraphenylenediamine, chlorohydrate, pyramidon, aloin, phenolpthalein, and orthotolidine. The last compound, marketed as Occultest and Hematest tablets, received the greatest attention but proved to be clinically unreliable and consequently disenchanted the medical community. The major difficulty with qualitative fecal occult blood tests is their lack of standardization *vis-á-vis* different test products

ISBN 0-12-496720-5

and screening program testing conditions (Fleisher *et al.*, 1980). Some of these factors, such as diet, test sensitivity, test conditions, and quality controls, are considered below.

II. TEST CHARACTERISTICS

An ideal fecal occult blood (FOB) test should have the following characteristics: (1) sufficient sensitivity to detect clinically significant amounts of blood beyond physiologic blood loss; (2) unaffected by an ordinary diet or by commonly used medications; (3) simplicity and ease of performance, requiring minimum equipment; and (4) reasonably inoffensive and hygienic.

Most FOB tests are based on the pseudoperoxidase activity of hemoglobin, which reacts with exogenous peroxide in the presence of a leucodye. The production of color suggests the presence of blood (hemoglobin). Because of its carcinogenicity, the benzidine test is no longer performed. Orthotolidine is still used to detect FOB, but it lacks specificity and reliability. Guaiac is the most widely used chromogen; its interaction with hemoglobin and peroxide is shown in Fig. 1. Although there are physical and chemical (sensitivity) differences between the various FOB tests products (Winawer and Fleisher, 1982), the basic test characteristics are similar (Table I).

Several factors may influence the accuracy of the FOB test (Table II). The amount of enzymatically active hemoglobin in the stool sample tested does not necessarily reflect the total amount of blood in the stool. Shedding of blood from neoplasms may not be constant or continuous. Even large cancers do not all bleed persistently. Isotope studies have confirmed the fluctuation of occult bleeding from colorectal tumors (Macrae and St. John, 1982). Furthermore, the distribution of blood in the stool may depend on the site of origin, i.e., the right or

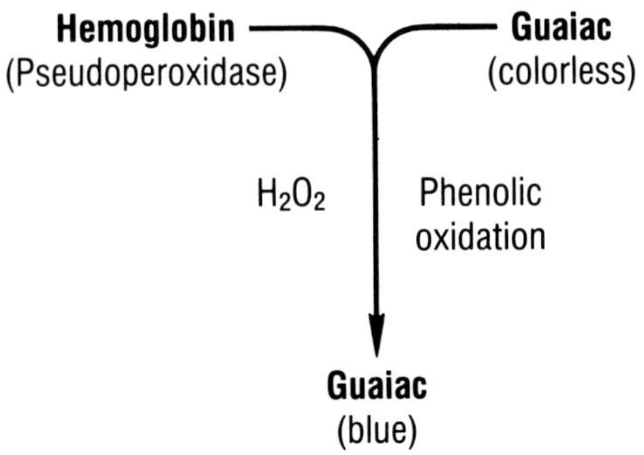

Fig. 1 Principle of phenolic oxidation of guaiac in the presence of hemoglobin (a pseudoperoxidase) and H_2O_2.

TABLE I

Test Characteristics of the Fecal Occult Blood Test[a]

Test reagents	Filter paper–impregnated guaiac; hydrogen peroxide and denatured alcohol
Analyte	Hemoglobin
Test rationale	Phenolic oxidation of guaiac in the presence of hemoglobin
Known chemical interference	Compounds with peroxidase activity
Minimum sensitivity	Varies with the manufacturer of the test. For standardization of the test the recommended sensitivity should be approximately 1 μg crystalline human hemoglobin in aqueous solution; 0.2 g hemoglobin/100 g stool under simulated conditions[b]
Stability following specimen application	30 days if the test is strongly positive (+4) on day 1; 4–5 days if the test is weakly positive (+1) on day 1
Stability related to hemoglobin concentration	Yes
Effect of rehydration on sensitivity	Increased sensitivity with increased rate of false-positive reactions
Effect of diet on sensitivity	Foods containing peroxidase activity

[a] Modified from Fleisher *et al.*, 1980.
[b] Blood added to stool *in vitro*.

left colon. Herzog and associates (1982) reported that left-sided colonic polyps gave a positive FOB test in 54% of tests from 22 patients. Stools from five patients with right-sided lesions gave only 19% positive tests. Further data are needed to corroborate this observation. The number and density of stool samples may produce variable results. Macrae and St. John (1982) demonstrated that increasing the number of test days improved the screening sensitivity for cancers. The current test protocol requires duplicate stool sampling over 3 consecutive days.

TABLE II

Fecal Occult Blood Testing: Possible Sources of Error

Fluctuation of bleeding from colorectal neoplasm
Site of bleeding in colon
Site and number of stool samples taken for analysis
Amount of enzymatically active hemoglobin in the stool sample taken
Hemoglobin present in rare meat
Vegetable peroxidases

III. DIET

By virtue of its pseudoperoxidase activity, hemoglobin reacts with hydrogen peroxide to induce a phenolic oxidation of guaiac, thus producing a blue coloration. Unfortunately, this peroxidase activity is not limited to human hemoglobin, but is also found in high concentration in fresh fruits and vegetables and bacteria, as well as in animal hemoglobin and myoglobin. Thus, dietary factors may potentially cause false-positive reactions. Ostrow and associates (1973) have found that meat restriction has no bearing on Hemoccult positivity. Conversely, Glober and Peskoe (1974), in their study of Japanese-Americans in Hawaii, noted a significant decline in positive Hemoccult reactions after adding bulk to and eliminating red meat from the diet. Complete elimination of all meat from the diet has been shown to reduce the false positivity of FOB tests. In addition to foodstuffs, certain minerals and vitamins may influence FOB test reactivity. It has been demonstrated, *in vitro* and *in vivo,* that dietary ferrous compounds can produce a false-positive reaction (Lifton and Kreiser, 1982). Reducing agents, particularly ascorbic acids, may interfere with the oxidation of guaiac, resulting in a false-negative reaction. Bassett and Goulston (1980) have shown that the restriction of high peroxidase-containing foods, vitamin C, salicylates, and nonsteroidal anti-inflammatory agents significantly reduced the false positivity of Hemoccult on single fecal samples but not that of Hemoccult II.

Dietary peroxidase activity in stool can be virtually eliminated if a low-peroxidase diet is adopted or if a specific inhibitor of nonhemoglobin peroxidase activity is used. Table III lists the vegetables that contain high concentrations of peroxidase activity and that should be avoided if dietary restrictions call for low peroxidase intake. The use of a vegetable peroxidase inhibitor referred to as VPI (Helena Laboratories, Beaumont, TX) involves the addition of a few drops of this reagent to the test slide prior to color development, thus obviating the imposition of dietary restrictions. Although additional confirmatory data are needed, early indications suggest that VPI can be helpful in eliminating false-positive FOB tests resulting from dietary food peroxidase interference. Treat-

TABLE III

Vegetables Containing Peroxidase Activity

High activity	Moderate activity
Turnip	Cabbage
Horseradish	Potato
Broccoli	Cucumber
Cauliflower	Mushroom
Radish	Artichoke

ment with VPI selectivity denatures vegetable peroxidase present in stool, while the pseudoperoxidase activity exhibited by hemoglobin remains unaffected. This suggests that rehydration (see below) combined with VPI treatment may improve the specificity of the FOB test.

At present, it seems reasonable to place patients on a low-peroxidase diet or to incorporate the use of VPI in protocols for FOB testing, particularly if slides are to be rehydrated. Bulk is included in the diet, presumably for tumor absorption and the stimulation of bleeding. This last point remains to be documented.

IV. SENSITIVITY

The sensitivity of the impregnated guaiac slide test for FOB has been a controversial topic (Winawer and Fleisher, 1982). *In vitro,* the Hemoccult slide is sensitive to less than 1 ug of human hemoglobin in aqueous solution (Fleisher *et al.*, 1980). Gastrointestinal blood loss as determined by ^{51}Cr-labeled erythrocytes or whole body ^{59}Fe elimination rates has been used to gauge the sensitivity of chemical tests dependent upon the pseudoperoxidase activity of hemoglobin. The mean daily blood loss in normal human subjects as determined by ^{51}Cr label assays was found to be 0.5 ± 0.4 ml. A concentration of 2 mg of hemoglobin per gram of stool is considered to be the upper limit of normal (Morris *et al.*, 1976). Stroehlein *et al.* (1976b) found that with a fecal blood loss of 0–2 ml/day, Hemoccult positivity was 7.4%. Only with a blood loss of at least 10 ml/day were the majority of Hemoccult reactions positive. In an analysis of patients with colorectal polyps, Herzog and associates (1982) noted a Hemoccult positivity of 86% for a fecal blood loss of 2–4 ml/day from adenomas in the descending colon and rectosigmoid. However, positivity was reduced to 26% for the same amount of blood loss from polyps in the ascending and transverse colons. Macrae and associates (1982) have investigated Hemoccult positivity for colorectal cancers and adenomas. As measured by ^{51}Cr assays, there was greater blood loss from proximal colonic carcinomas (9.3 ml/day from cecal and ascending colonic cancers) than from distal colorectal carcinomas (1.5–1.9 ml/day from the transverse, descending, and sigmoid colons and rectum). Only adenomas larger than 2 cm in diameter resulted in blood loss greater than 2 ml/day. In the range of blood loss for left-sided colonic cancers and large colonic adenomas, 40% of the nonrehydrated Hemoccult II slides were positive compared to 70% of the rehydrated slides.

It is important to emphasize the radioassays are not the "gold" standard against which to judge the merit of guaiac-impregnated slides. Potential technical problems such as failure to label red blood cells uniformly with the isotope, incomplete reduction of Na_2CrO_4 by hemoglobin, and the labeling of red blood cells debris in addition to intact cells containing hemoglobin may detract from the efficacy of the chromium radioassay. More importantly, radioassays measure total fecal blood, whereas the slide test is designed to sample a small portion of stool for blood that is of inhomogeneous distribution (Winawer and Fleisher, 1982).

V. STORAGE AND REHYDRATION

Stroehlein and associates (1976a) have shown that the intensity of the Hemoccult reaction significantly decreases with storage of the slide. In their study, approximately 8 mg of hemoglobin per gram of stool gave a faintly positive Hemoccult reaction, and higher concentrations of hemoglobin gave proportionally greater responses. A reduction in the intensity of the reaction was evident after 4 days of storage, and after 8 days, slides smeared with hemoglobin concentrations less than 26 mg per gram of stool gave trace or negative reactions. Fleisher and associates (1977) found that the stability and specificity of the Hemoccult slide were hemoglobin dependent. Specimens containing 0.2% whole blood remained unequivocally positive for only 48 hours. The precise reason for this time-dependent loss of sensitivity is not known, although it is assumed that catabolic events brought about by stool enzymes and bacteria on hemoglobin may produce this effect. Also important to the problem of stability is the effects of temperature and desiccation of the specimens. It has been recommended that all slide tests be developed within 1–5 days of specimen application in order to minimize the possibility of deleterious effects of storage.

Rehydration of the FOB test increases its sensitivity in part by the dissolution of desiccated hemoglobin before the addition of the alcohol developing agent. At the same time, the peroxidase present in bacteria, vegetable matter, and meats may also be reactivated by hydration and thereby reduce the specificity of the test. This issue is addressed by Macrae and associates (1982) in a study of optimal dietary conditions for Hemoccult testing. Young, healthy individuals adhering to diets with differing peroxidase contents had stool specimens tested by Hemoccult II slides with and without rehydration. In those patients on a high-peroxidase diet, the false positivity of the slide increased from zero without rehydration to 4.2% with rehydration. However, on a low-peroxidase diet, rehydration produced only 0.6% false-positive reactions.

VI. QUALITY CONTROL OF FECAL OCCULT BLOOD TESTS

Many factors appear to influence FOB tests (Table IV). In fact, most FOB tests are performed outside of the laboratory setting; hence, quality control

TABLE IV

Fecal Occult Blood Testing: Factors that May Affect Accuracy

Specimen collection—improper sampling of stool specimen
Excessive delay between slide preparation and laboratory testing
Test conditions—rehydration may increase false-positive results
Nonhemoglobin interference by food or by bacterial peroxidase activity
Stool contamination due to menstruation or hemorrhoidal bleeding
Interference by medications such as salicylates and vitamin C
Variation in test senstivity from different manufacturers and from lot to lot
Differences in test methodology: guaiac or *O*-tolidine

considerations are not systematically pursued. For this reason, it is exceedingly important to follow standardized procedures, including quality control, in performing the FOB test. A reference laboratory for FOB testing was established at the Memorial Sloan-Kettering Cancer Center to serve as international reference laboratory for fecal occult blood testing. Investigations in the reference laboratory have centered on quality control, stability, sensitivity and reproducibility of the test (Fleisher *et al.*, 1980; Winawer *et al.*, 1982). The International Workgroup on Colorectal Cancer has developed specific guidelines and recommendations pertaining to FOB testing and quality control (Gnauck *et al.*, 1983). A key recommendation is for the establishment of quality control and proficiency test programs prior to the use of FOB tests in clinical screening programs. One element of the quality control program is the appropriate training of the personnel who perform the tests. The importance of training and its impact on interpretation of test results from this study clearly indicate an increase in test proficiency with training of individuals involved in performing the test (M. Fleisher, C. Smith, B. Diaz, S. J. Winawer, and M. K. Schwartz, unpublished data).

On-slide or "with-in" test quality control is available on two FOB test products. The Hemoccult test (SmithKline Diagnostics) contain test areas that are specially treated to yield negative (no color formation) and positive (blue color) test results following treatment with the developer reagent. Coloscreen (Helena Laboratories) also has a quality control monitor on each slide, as well as positive and negative quality control material (ColoCheck Monitors) supplied in a small plastic tube with the test slides. The quality control material is applied to separate, albeit attached, quality control test areas prior to treatment with the developer reagent. The main purpose of these quality control techniques is to verify the suitability of all aspects of the testing procedure, including the guaiac-impregnated test paper and developer reagent, and to provide the user with a color reference for positive and negative test results.

VII. AVAILABLE TESTS

The list of FOB procedures continues to grow at a rapid rate. Table V provides a list of the tests currently available. In addition to the Hemoccult slide, which has had its greatest clinical application in the United States, Europe, and Australia, the ColoScreen and Hema-Check FOB tests are the most widely used in the United States. The Hemoccult test has been replaced almost entirely by the Hemoccult II test. The two tests are similar, with the exception of some increased sensitivity and different packaging of the Hemoccult II. In Europe, notably in West Germany, Haemoscreen, Hemofec, and Colo-Rect are also tests of choice. The Quik-Cult and FeCult tests appear to be used more regionally in the United States; only minimal data are available on the effectiveness of these procedures. The Detecatest and Fecatest/Fecatwin procedures are new; the latter test is not currently distributed in the United States.

In 1979, Songster and associates (1980) introduced an immunochemical test for the detection of FOB. The test employs a high titer of monospecific antisera to intact human hemoglobin in a radial immunodiffusion assay. The assay is specific for human hemoglobin, 5–10 times more sensitive than the Hemoccult test, and stable for up to 3 days. In a study of 150 patients with colorectal carcinoma, test positivity was 65% with the immunochemical disc as compared

TABLE V

Currently Available Tests for Detecting Fecal Occult Blood

Hemoccult and Hemoccult II
SmithKlein Diagnostics, Sunnyvale, California
ColoScreen
Helena Laboratories, Beaumont, Texas
Hema-Chek
Miles Laboratories, Elkhart, Indiana
HemoFec
Boehringer-Mannheim, Mannheim, West Germany
Quik-Cult
Laboratory Diagnostics, Morganville, New Jersey
Colo-Rect
Roche Laboratories, Nutley, New Jersey
Haemoscreen
E. Merck Diagnostics, Darmstadt, West Germany
Detecatest
C. B. Fleet, Lynchburg, Virginia
FeCult
Gamma Diagnostics, Houston, Texas
Fecatest/Fecatwin
Labsystems, Finland

to 40% with the Hemoccult slide. A disadvantage of the immunochemical method is its lengthy and complex processing.

Currently under investigation is Hemoquant, a fluorescent assay based on hemoglobin-derived porphyrin in stool (Ahlquist *et al.*, 1983; Schwartz *et al.*, 1983). This quantitative test determines both fecal hemoglobin and the fraction of hemoglobin converted to porphyrin by intestinal bacteria. In the study of Ahlquist *et al.* (1983), Hemoquant had a median value in control patients of 1.19 mg of hemoglobin per gram of stool and 0.22 mg/g in control patients who were not taking aspirin and who were abstaining from rare meat. By this technique, FOB was found to be greater than or equal to 2.0 mg per gram of stool in 76% of the patients with polyps greater than or equal to 2 cm in size ($n = 12$), 93% of patients with colon cancer ($n = 30$), and 100% of patients with asymptomatic colon cancer ($n = 7$). In comparison to the *quantitative* measurement of hemoglobin-derived porphyrins, the *qualitative* FOB test gave a positive response in 17, 69, and 43% of these respective groups. It was suggested that the hemoglobin-derived porphyrin fraction measured by fluorescent analysis (Hemoquant) was significantly higher for blood loss from the upper gastrointestinal tract than for that from the colon.

A quantitative procedure for the measurement of hemoglobin in stool involving the oxidation of tetramethylbenzidine has been proposed (Welch and Young, 1983). The reaction depends on the pseudoperoxidase activity of the heme moiety of hemoglobin. This procedure is not subject to the usual interferences that may effect the dye-oxidation–based tests for FOB.

If the FOB test is to be used successfully in screening programs along with the recommended methodology (Table VI), quality control and proficiency testing should be established. The "simple" slide test for FOB as a possible screening tool for colorectal cancer is, in reality, exceedingly complex. It is apparent, from the considerations presented above, that if the test is to be used successfully, it must be carefully controlled, monitored, and ultimately standardized. In addition to such questions as diet, rehydration, and sensitivity, there are considerations of

TABLE VI

Recommended Methodology for Fecal Occult Blood Testing

Dietary restriction	Meat free, High fiber, low peroxidase[a]
Number of smears	Six
Type of slide	Impregnated guaiac, immunochemical
Rehydration	Only if a strict low-peroxidase diet is used
Storage interval	4 days preferred
Quality control	Window or laboratory assay

[a] Unnecessary if a vegetable peroxidase inhibitor is used.

proper application of the test to asymptomatic patients at risk for colorectal cancer.

Although this test is being increasingly incorporated into clinical practice, its ultimate value will have to await data regarding the benefits from screening programs.

REFERENCES

Adler, O., and Adler, R. (1904). Ueber einige recktioner der Kohlehydrate. *Hoppe-Seyler's Z. Physiol. Chem.* **41,** 59–67.

Ahlquist, D. A., McGill, D. B., Owen, R. A., Young, D. S., Taylor, W. F., and Schwartz, S. (1983). A new quantitative assay for fecal hemoglobin, Hemoquant: Analyses in health and gastrointestinal disease. *Gastroenterology* **84,** 1089 (abstr.).

Bassett, M. L., and Goulston, K. J. (1980). False positive and negative Hemoccult reactions on a normal diet and effect of diet restriction. *Aust. N.Z. J. Med.* **10,** 1–4.

Boas, I. (1901). Uberokkulte magenblutungen. *Dtsch. Med. Wochenschr.* **27,** 315–321.

Caligore, P., Macrae, F. A., St. John, D. J. B., Rayner, L. J., and Legge, J. W. (1982). Peroxidase levels in food: Relevance to colorectal cancer screening. *Am. J. Clin. Nutr.* **35,** 1487–1489.

Fleisher, M., Schwartz, M. K., and Winawer, S. J. (1977). The false-negative Hemoccult test. *Gastroenterology,* **72,** 782–784.

Fleisher, M., Schwartz, M. K., and Winawer, S. J. (1980). Laboratory studies on the Hemoccult slide for fecal occult testing. *In* "Progress in Cancer Research and Theory" S. J. Winawer, D. Schottenfeld, and P. Sherlock, eds.), Vol. 13, pp. 181–187. Raven Press, New York.

Glober, G. A., and Peskoe, S. M. (1974) Outpatient screening for gastrointestinal lesions using guaiac-impregnated slide. *Dig. Dis.* **19,** 399–403.

Gnauck, R., Macrae, F. A., and Fleisher, M. (1984). How to perform the fecal occult blood test. *Ca—Cancer J. Clin.* **34,** 134–147.

Gregersen, J. P. (1919). Unterssuchungen uber okkulte blutungen. *Arch. Verdau.-Kr.* **25,** 269–295.

Herzog, P., Holtermuller, K.-H., Preiss, J., Fischer, J., Ewe, K., Schreiber, H.-H., and Berres, M. (1982). Fecal blood loss in patients with colonic polyps: A comparison of measurements with ^{51}chromium-labeled erythrocytes and with the Haemoccult test. *Gastroenterology* **83,** 957–962.

Lifton, L. J., and Kreiser, J. (1982). False-positive stool occult blood caused by iron preparations—a controlled study and review of literature. *Gastroenterology* **83,** 860–863.

Macrae, F. A., and St. John, D. J. (1982). Relationship between patterns of bleeding and Hemoccult sensitivity in patients with colorectal cancers or adenomas. *Gastroenterology* **82,** 891–898.

Macrae, F. A., St. John, D. J., Caligiore, P., Taylor, L. S., and Legge, J. W. (1982). Optimal dietary conditions for Hemoccult testing. *Gastroenterology* **82,** 899–903.

Morris, D. W., Hansell, J. R., Ostrow, J. D., and Chuan-Shue Lee, M. S. (1976). Reliability of chemical tests for fecal occult blood in hospitalized patients. *Am. J. Dig. Dis.* **21,** 841–844.

Ostrow, J. K., Mulvaney, C. A., Hanell, J. R., and Rhodes, R. S. (1973). Sensitivity and reproducibility of chemical tests for fecal occult blood with an emphasis on false positive reactions. *Dig. Dis.* **18,** 930–940.

Schwartz, S., Dahl, J., Ellefson, M., and Ahlquist, D. (1983). The "Hemoquant" test: A specific and quantitative determination of Heme (hemoglobin) in feces and other materials. *Clin. Chem. (Winston-Salem, N.C.)* **29,** 2061–2067.

Songster, C. L., Barrows, G. H., and Jarrett, D. P. (1980). Immunochemical detection of fecal occult blood - the fecal smear punch-disc test: A noninvasive screening test for colorectal cancer. *Cancer* **45,** 1099–1102.

Stroehlein, J. R., Fairbanks, V. F., Go, V. L., Taylor, W. F., and Thompson, J. H., Jr. (1976a). Hemoccult stool tests—false-negative results due to storage of specimens. *Mayo Clin. Proc.* **51,** 548–552.

Stroehlein, J. R., Fairbanks, V. F., McGill, D. B., and Go, V. L. (1976b). Hemoccult detection of fecal occult blood quantitated by radioassay. *Dig. Dis.* **21,** 841–844.

Van Deen, J. (1864). Tinture guaijaci und ein ozonträgu, als Reagens auf sehr geringe Blutmengen, namentlich in medico-forensischen Fälen. *Arch. Holland Beitr. Natura Heilkd.* **3,** 228–231.

Welch, C. L., and Young, D. S. (1983). Spectrophotometry of occult blood in feces. *Clin. Chem.* **29,** 2022–2025.

Winawer, S. J., Fleisher, M., Baldwin, M., and Sherlock, P. (1982). Current status of fecal occult blood testing in screening for colorectal cancer. *Ca—Cancer J. Clin.* **32**, 3–15.

Winawer, S. J., and Fleisher, M. (1982). Editorial—Sensitivity and specificity of the fecal occult blood test for colorectal neoplasia. *Gastroenterology* **82,** 986–991.

Wu, H. (1922). Studies on hemoglobin—an ultra-micro-method for the determination of hemoglobin as a peroxidase. *J. Biochem. (Tokyo)* **2,** 189–194.

14

Sigmoidoscopy and Other Tests for Colorectal Cancer

F. A. MACRAE AND C. B. WILLIAMS

I.	Choice of Techniques: Risk Evaluation	250
	A. Average-Risk Groups	250
	B. Higher-Risk Groups	252
II.	Technical Aspects	256
	A. Proctosigmoidoscopy	256
	B. Colonoscopy	259
	C. Double Contrast Barium Enema	261
III.	Sensitivity and Specificity	262
	A. Rigid Proctosigmoidoscopy and Flexible Sigmoidoscopy	262
	B. Colonoscopy and Double Contrast Barium Enema	263
IV.	Logistics	264
V.	Training	265
	References	265

Screening tests for colorectal cancer need to be sensitive and specific. There are limitations to fecal occult blood testing that suggest that other techniques should be considered for screening, especially in higher-risk groups. These techniques may be used either instead of, or in addition to, screening for occult blood.

Rigid sigmoidoscopy, flexible sigmoidoscopy, colonoscopy, and barium enema are established techniques for detecting colorectal neoplasia, all of which involve a degree of discomfort and possible hazard to the patient. This compromises their application to screening programs. At present, the skills required to perform these investigations rest largely in the hands of doctors, and are thus relatively scarce and expensive. Nevertheless, each has an important role in

ISBN 0-12-496720-5

screening, particularly if there is an indication of increased risk for colorectal cancer.

Available serological tests for colorectal cancer have to date proved disappointing for screening because of lack of either specificity or sensitivity for early cancer. A highly specific and sensitive serological marker for localized bowel cancer would be an important development in screening. This chapter will concentrate on endoscopy and radiology in screening for asymptomatic neoplasms.

I. CHOICE OF TECHNIQUES: RISK EVALUATION

Consideration of screening tests for early detection of colorectal cancer cannot be divorced from an evaluation of risk and the circumstances that determine the risk (Table I). In general, the higher the risk, the more frequent the need for surveillance and the greater the need for some form of endoscopic screening. Since cancer can occur in any part of the large bowel, screening should potentially be capable of detecting tumors at any colonic site.

A. Average-Risk Groups

The majority of colorectal cancers (sporadic cancers) occur in individuals in whom no risk factors are currently identifiable. Fecal occult blood testing has received the widest attention for such average-risk screening. However, because

TABLE I

Suggested Screening Techniques According to Risk

	Fecal occult blood test	Sigmoidoscopy	Colonoscopy
Age > 45 years	*	*	
First-degree relative with colorectal cancer	*	*	
Inherited non-polyposis colon cancer syndrome	*		*
History of colorectal cancer	*		*
History of adenoma	*		*
Polyposis family members		*	
Ulcerative colitis		*	*
Ureterosigmoidostomy		*	
Colitis after subtotal colectomy		*	

there is an appreciable false-negative rate for colorectal cancers, particularly in the distal colon (Macrae and St. John, 1982), endoscopic screening must be considered as a complementary screening strategy.

Rigid sigmoidoscopy has long been recommended (American Cancer Society, 1980) as a screen for colorectal cancer. There is reasonable evidence from trials of sigmoidoscopic screening that detection and removal of adenomas and pathologically early cancers benefits the patient (Dales *et al.*, 1973a; Gilbertsen *et al.*, 1978).

Although this procedure remains a cornerstone of colorectal cancer prevention when regular health checks are made (Hertz *et al.*, 1960), there are wide international differences in its use for average-risk screening. In Europe, proctosigmoidoscopy is rarely done by general practitioners (Crespi *et al.*, 1983). In Australia, only 4% of general practitioners screen asymptomatic subjects with rigid protosigmoidoscopy (Macrae *et al.*, 1982). Just how widely such screening is practiced in the United States is unknown, although in 1961, 22.4% of physicians declared sigmoidoscopy to be one of their screening tests (McHardy *et al.*, 1968).

Flexible sigmoidoscopy using the *60-cm scope* yields a greater number of tumors than rigid sigmoidoscopy (Bohlman *et al.*, 1977; Winawer *et al.*, 1979; Leicester *et al.*, 1982; Vellacott and Hardcastle, 1981). Despite its increased cost, there is evidence that it is more cost effective than rigid proctosigmoidoscopy (Eddy, 1980, personal communication, 1983). This is underlined by data from several centers showing a trend in recent decades for colorectal cancers to be more proximally located than in the past, with proportionately fewer rectal tumors (Axtell and Chiazze, 1966; Cady *et al.*, 1974; Snyder *et al.*, 1977; Morgenstern and Lee, 1978; Abrahams and Reines, 1979; Rosato and Marks, 1981).

Flexible sigmoidoscopy using the *30-cm scope* has been advocated for screening because of its potential safety, even in inexpert hands, and the lack of need for formal training (Winawer *et al.*, 1982). The sigmoid colon is more consistently viewed with this instrument compared with a rigid proctosigmoidoscope, but the yield would presumably be lower than with the 60-cm endoscope. The cost of all flexible fiberoptic instruments remains a serious barrier to their widespread application for screening (Winawer *et al.*, 1982).

Whatever type of sigmoidoscope is used, patient compliance with proctosigmoidoscopic screening remains the single most important limiting factor in its ability to influence the incidence and mortality of cancer of the distal colon. Physicians have a powerful influence over their patients where health matters are concerned. Sigmoidoscopy with polypectomy is a technique proven to be of benefit in the prevention of rectal cancer. Its inclusion in the periodic health check is thus well justified and should be encouraged.

B. Higher-Risk Groups

1. First-Degree Relatives

First-degree relatives of patients with colorectal cancer carry a three- to four-fold increased risk for colorectal cancer (Woolf, 1958; Macklin, 1960; Lovett, 1974), giving them a lifetime risk of approximately 10%. Providing they are not members of an inherited nonpolyposis colon cancer syndrome (Lynch and Krush, 1967), the distribution of their cancers is indistinguishable from that of sporadic colorectal cancer. Because of the large number of first-degree relatives of patients with colorectal cancer in most Western communities, realistic screening programs for first-degree relatives can offer, at most, fecal occult blood testing and flexible sigmoidoscopy. Controlled trials point to the value of selecting relatives for screening programs (Rosen *et al.*, 1981). There is no information on the frequency with which screening should be performed in first-degree relatives.

2. Relatives in the Inherited Nonpolyposis Colon Cancer Syndromes

Pedigrees with these cancer family syndromes show autosomal dominant inheritance. Thus, the risk to unaffected first-degree relatives—either siblings or children—is about 50%. The risk seems maximal at 25–50 years of age and may dissipate as family members grow older. In this syndrome, there are classically no polyps associated with the cancers, and there is a recognizable tendency for cancers of the cecum and ascending colon to predominate (Lynch and Krush, 1967). Thus, in these circumstances, colonoscopic screening at reasonably frequent intervals between the ages of 25 and 50 years seems prudent. Although clinical experience with these patients indicates that their tumors may be less aggressive than sporadic cancers (Albano *et al.*, 1982), this should not be taken as an indication to relax surveillance measures. Fecal occult blood testing may be considered as offering protection between points of colonoscopic surveillance in an overall screening strategy. Proctosigmoidoscopy does not cover the at-risk region of the bowel. There is no information on the frequency with which such screening should be carried out, although a 2- to 3-year interval for colonoscopy would seem reasonable.

3. Familial Polyposis Coli

Familial polyposis coli, including Gardner's syndrome (Bussey, 1975), is an exception to the general rule that the entire colon needs surveillance. The appearance of adenomas is a recognizable marker for cancer potential in family members. In the St. Mark's registry of over 200 families, macroscopic adenomas were invariably present in the rectum in patients with familial polyposis coli (H.

J. R. Bussey, personal communication). There were no family members under surveillance who had annual rigid proctosigmoidoscopy in whom a colorectal cancer developed before the diagnosis of familial polyposis.

Flexible sigmoidoscopy, however, allows better and more extensive views of the distal colon with detection of smaller polyps. Dye spray enhancement will detect polyps only 1–2 mm in size—histopathologically microadenomas (Cotton and Williams, 1982). Adenomas in familial polyposis, at least as judged after subtotal colectomy with ileorectal anastomosis, grow slowly. It may therefore be reasonable to screen polyposis family members with flexible sigmoidoscopy at less frequent intervals, particularly in subjects whose compliance can be assured.

Several centers (Watanabe *et al.*, 1978; Ranzi *et al.*, 1981; Jarvinen *et al.*, 1983) have reported the findings of screening of the upper gastrointestinal tract for polyps in affected family members. The rationale for this is that patients with familial polyposis have an increased risk of small bowel cancer, particularly at the papilla of Vater (Bussey, 1972). Studies in which duodenal and gastric biopsy specimens have been taken from polypoid lesions of any size in patients with familial polyposis suggest that 50–60% of such patients have adenomas, particularly in the duodenum (Jarvinen *et al.*, 1983). It is certainly not clear, however, that detection of such adenomas in the asymptomatic phase is helpful in the overall management of these patients. There seems to us to be little indication for routine surveillance and detection of upper gastrointestinal polyps in patients with familial polyposis.

4. Other Familial Polyposis Syndromes

In Peutz-Jegher syndrome, endoscopic screening of both the upper and lower gastrointestinal tracts with therapeutic polypectomy is advisable, mainly to prevent recurrent bleeding or iron deficiency anemia (Williams, 1982). There is also a small risk of malignancy, particularly in the stomach and duodenum of these patients. This may result from adenomatous tissue which is occasionally intricately associated with Peutz-Jegher hamartomatous polyps. Prophylactic polypectomy may thus also be useful in cancer prevention. Particular care needs to be taken in evaluating Peutz-Jegher polyps for malignancy; the displacement of normal glandular tissue into the muscularis propria makes histological assessment of malignancy notoriously difficult.

Juvenile polyposis (10 or more juvenile hamartomatous polyps), as distinct from isolated juvenile polyps, has malignant potential. About 10% of juvenile polyposis patients develop cancer in their lifetime (H. J. R. Bussey, personal communication). The condition is rare but probably merits subtotal colectomy, or, if this is not accepted, endoscopic surveillance with multiple polypectomies. Malignancies, however, are not always colonic and may occur in the small intestine. There is also evidence that relatives of patients with juvenile polyposis, regardless of whether they have polyps present, have an increased risk of colorectal cancer (Stemper *et al.*, 1975). Juvenile polyposis-cancer families are reported.

5. *Patients with a History of Resected Adenomas*

Follow-up studies show that adenomas and cancers occur in these patients throughout the colon, with an incidence of 30–50% over 3–9 years (Kirsner *et al.*, 1960; Bonetti *et al.*, 1979; Waye and Braunfeld, 1982; Macrae and Williams, 1982). The relative risk compared with that of subjects without adenomas is about threefold, according to the very limited data available (Brahme *et al.*, 1974). The risk is highly age dependent. The number and size of previous adenomas are also predictive, and male sex may be important (Macrae and Williams, 1982). There is, therefore, a need for total colonic surveillance, possibly at intervals related to risk. Colonscopy is the preferred investigation, since it offers an opportunity for therapeutic intervention and is more accurate in follow-up (Williams *et al.*, 1982a). Fecal occult blood testing with guaiac tests may reliably detect early (asymptomatic) cancers, although this is unproven. The dynamics of adenoma formation in individual patients may be relevant to surveillance frequency. This is the basis of follow-up schedules that increase surveillance intervals after the finding of a colon free of adenomas during follow-up (Minopoulos *et al.*, 1983).

6. *Patients with a History of Resected Cancers*

The risk of a second (metachronous) cancer occurring within 25 years of resection of a first cancer is approximately 4% (Bussey *et al.*, 1967). This is close to the average lifetime risk of cancer in the general population, suggesting that such screening may not be more rewarding than the screening of unselected subjects over the age of 60 years. Radiological follow-up studies have generally had a low yield of neoplasms during surveillance (Tornqvist *et al.*, 1981). However, there is a substantial enhancement of risk if adenomas are associated with the cancer, either before the patient presents with cancer, in the original operative specimen, or during follow-up. Colonoscopic screening is technically easier after resection of the sigmoid colon and is the method of choice.

7. *Extensive Ulcerative Colitis*

The relative risk of cancer in extensive ulcerative colitis is difficult to determine because of the multitude of selection biases that influence almost all studies assessing the risk (Sackett and Whelan, 1980). Nevertheless, it seems clear that there is an increased risk beginning at 8–10 years after onset of the disease, which is enhanced with time (Lennard-Jones *et al.*, 1983). One series claims that the cumulative risk reaches 50% in patients surviving 25 years after the onset of colitis (Greenstein *et al.*, 1979). The risk is pancolonic and is not necessarily heralded by a premalignant change in the rectum. In our experience, severe dysplasia is identifiable by the endoscopist in only about 30% of cases, underlining the need for random biopsies. Polypoid dysplasia, or "dysplasia-associated masses" (Blackstone *et al.*, 1981), is well recognized by pathologists in operative specimens and should be visible on double contrast barium enema. Barium enema alone is, however, clearly not an adequate screening procedure for these patients, since only the minority have polypoid dysplasia, whereas postinflammatory polyps are common and may confuse the radiologist. The tendency of uncomplicated colitis to bleed makes fecal occult blood screening for neoplasia inappropriate.

8. Patients with Ureterosigmoidostomies

Cancer of the sigmoid colon has been reported with untoward frequency in patients with ureters implanted into the colon in infancy because of congenital abnormalities or in adulthood because of bladder tumors. A prevalence survey of relatively young patients with ureterosigmoidostomies showed that 17% had adenomas and, taking into account those who had adenomas and cancers removed in the past as well, a cumulative risk of 29%. The risk appears specific to the site of the urinary stoma, which is usually in the sigmoid colon, and becomes significant 8 or more years after implantation. The localized colonic tendency to neoplasm formation appears to persist for a long period even if the ureters are subsequently reimplanted into an isolated ileal conduit (Stewart *et al.*, 1982).

Flexible sigmoidoscopy provides adequate surveillance. Normal stomas can appear polypoid, or can become enlarged by inflammatory or granulation tissue, and may be indistinguishable from tumors. Stomatectomy is a catastrophe to be avoided. Preliminary biopsy of any apparent polyp is important to avoid this complication (Williams and Gillespie, 1979). Frusemide (5 mg IV) with or without methylene blue is helpful when trying to locate stomas, especially if they are deformed or difficult to identify. Flexible sigmoidoscopy every 2 years appears to provide reasonable surveillance for patients with ureterosigmoidostomies.

9. Patients Who Have Had Subtotal Colectomies for Ulcerative Colitis or Familial Polyposis Coli

Although these operations remove the majority of the colon and eliminate the potential for its malignant transformation, the rectal stump remains at risk for cancer. Rigid proctosigmoidoscopy has its most clearly defined screening role in these patients.

II. TECHNICAL ASPECTS

The quality of the investigation of the colon and rectum depends to a large extent on the availability of interested endoscopists and radiologists. Attention to the details of preparation, equipment maintenance, and posturing of patients during the examination is important in achieving optimal results.

A. Proctosigmoidoscopy

1. Equipment

The average distance of insertion of the proctosigmoidoscope is about 19 cm from the anal margin (Nivatvongs and Fryd, 1980). Most instruments are 25 cm long and 2 cm in diameter, although the shorter pediatric instruments of narrower caliber are adequate for most clinical purposes and more comfortable for the patient. Light that is transmitted fiberoptically to the head, or distal end, of the sigmoidoscope greatly improves the efficiency and brilliance of illumination compared to battery-operated light sources using conventional bulbs. Good suction facilities should be available. A variety of biopsy forceps are used; for mucosal biopsies, small cups are adequate and minimize the risk of perforation or bleeding. The recently introduced St. Mark's biopsy forceps are quick and easy to use, with cups that retract within a metal flange, obtaining a small biopsy specimen (Preston *et al,* 1983). These forceps are particularly appropriate for taking three to four rectal mucosal biopsy specimens when screening for dysplasia in ulcerative colitis.

For mass lesions, larger forceps allow more representative biopsies without significant risk. Stalked polyps are normally removed by snare polypectomy. Biopsies are inadequate to exclude cancer and may introduce artifact, which confuses eventual interpretation. Some sigmoidoscopes have magnification lenses incorporated at their eye piece, which can help to identify small polyps.

The 60-cm flexible sigmoidoscopes (Fig. 1) vary in their torsional and flexibility characteristics, width of field of view, and size of biopsy channels. In general terms, a relatively thin, flexible ''floppy'' instrument is best accepted for screening of the sigmoid colon. A moderately wide biopsy channel (3.7 mm) allows for better aspiration of residue and use of larger biopsy forceps. The new pediatric colonoscopes have many properties that are useful for screening; they are relatively flexible, easy to introduce, and easy to negotiate through tight regions of the sigmoid colon, often to the splenic flexure. They are generally less robust than the marketed flexible sigmoidoscopes.

Flexible sigmoidoscopes should replace rigid sigmoidoscopes for most screening purposes. The potential for complications is low, and the time taken is usually only 2–3 minutes longer than with the rigid instrument. Most patients have little or no discomfort (Winawer *et al.,* 1982).

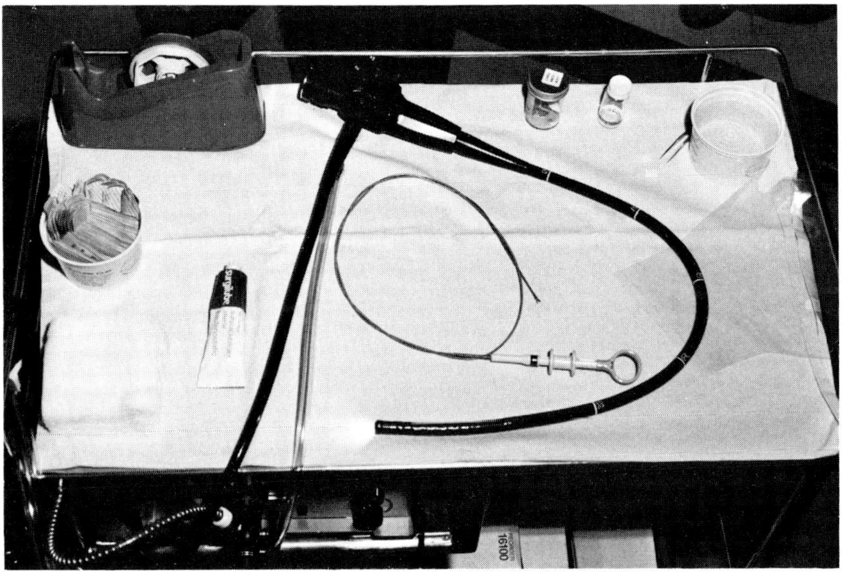

Fig. 1. Flexible sigmoidoscope with accessories. Note the micropore filter for mounting specimens. An external polythene suction tube avoids blockage in the umbilicus of the endoscope.

2. The Procedure

Ideally, proctosigmoidoscopy should be done initially without preparation, looking particularly for blood. If there is stool present, a phosphate enema should then be administered. With the 60-cm flexible sigmoidoscope, a routine preparatory enema is probably best, since the chance of the left colon being entirely clean without preparation is more remote.

Rigid sigmoidoscopy can be performed in either the left lateral or knee-chest (jackknife) position. Correct positioning of the patient and proper performance of the technique (Thomson *et al.*, 1981) are important if lesions are not to be missed and complications are to be avoided. Adequate training in proctosigmoidoscopy should be an important part of medical education.

3. Flexible Sigmoidoscopy

The use of flexible sigmoidoscopy in screening for colorectal cancer rests on the knowledge that the rectum and sigmoid colon are the regions of the colon at highest risk for neoplasia. A description of its use may be helpful in understanding both its potential and the skill required for optimal performance.

Posturing of the patient for flexible sigmoidoscopy is not as critical to obtain good views of the rectum. The patient is comfortably placed in the left lateral position. After digital examination, the lubricated endoscope is inserted under the protective cover of the endoscopist's index finger. The instrument is not advanced unless there is a clear view of the lumen more proximally. Sufficient air or carbon dioxide is insufflated to keep the walls of the bowel apart; overinsufflation is painful, makes the examination more difficult, and may lead to pressure injuries to the colon. Movement of the tip using the controls at the head of the endoscope, augmented by rotational movements of the shaft with the examiner's right hand, enables the more proximal lumen to be identified at all levels in the colon. Keeping the instrument straight in the sigmoid colon not only makes the procedure more comfortable for the patient but also enables the fibersigmoidoscope to reach the splenic flexure more consistently. Judging the location of the tip of the instrument within the colon by distance markers on the side of the endoscope is notoriously difficult. Loops frequently form within the patient and may not be discernible to the examiner without the aid of fluoroscopy (Lehman *et al.*, 1983).

Whether electrosurgery should be used during fibersigmoidoscopy remains a contentious issue. A bowel prepared only for flexible sigmoidoscopy may harbor explosive mixtures of methane and hydrogen. This hazard is avoided by fully exchanging the sigmoid colon gas with air or, preferably, carbon dioxide prior to electrosurgery. Nevertheless, many would argue that finding a single adenoma is an indication for total colonoscopy, which would then need to be performed at another sitting. Generally, during colonoscopy, facilities for polypectomy and hot biopsy destruction of small polyps are more readily available and, since full bowel preparation has been done, there is no risk of explosion. However, many colonoscopists have spent much time trying to identify 5-mm polyps seen at a preceding flexible sigmoidoscopy. It would seem reasonable to biopsy and destroy them by the hot biopsy technique at the time of flexible sigmoidoscopy, taking care to exchange carbon dioxide through the endoscope. Small polyps in the rectum are often metaplastic (hyperplastic) and do not indicate a need for total colonoscopy.

4. Complications

Perforation and bleeding are the main complications of proctosigmoidoscopy, but occur infrequently—in approximately 0.01% of cases (Katon, 1979).

Bacteremias with aerobic or anaerobic fecal flora can be induced by sigmoidoscopy or colonoscopy (LeFrock *et al.*, 1973; Pelican *et al.*, 1976). In patients with known valvular heart disease, prophylaxis with an aminoglycoside, metronidazole, and penicillin has been advocated, although there are no clear data to suggest that the low risk of endocarditis warrants prophylaxis. An argument can be made for antibiotic use in cirrhotic patients with ascites to prevent spontaneous bacterial peritonitis which also probably stems from bacteremia (Macrae and St. John, 1980).

With flexible sigmoidoscopy, about 11 complications have been reported among the 10,000 examinations reported in the literature (Crespi *et al.*, 1983). However, to date, flexible sigmoidoscopy has generally been done only by skilled endoscopists, whereas rigid proctosigmoidoscopy is practised more widely. Use of the flexible sigmoidoscope by untrained personnel could lead to more complications.

B. Colonoscopy

Colonoscopy is assuming increasing importance as a screening examination in high-risk individuals. It is now the procedure of choice for surveillance of many of the high-risk groups mentioned in previous sections. Accuracy in trained hands, access for tissue biopsy and therapeutic intervention, and lack of irradiation all favor its use for high-risk screening. It is a relatively safe procedure. Well-trained, competent colonoscopists experience only 2–5 significant complications in every 1000 diagnostic examinations (Macrae *et al.*, 1982). There are virtually no contraindications to colonoscopy in the context of well-person screening. Most of the usual contraindications (recent myocardial infarction, peritonism, acute inflammatory bowel disease, suspicion of an infectious cause of colitis) should normally not be encountered in well-person surveillance. Surveillance should wait until after pregnancy; a menstrual history should be taken if fluoroscopy is likely to be needed.

1. Equipment

All of the major endoscope manufacturers make good fiberoptic instruments. The choice of instruments and their attributes is now large. The variables to be considered are instrument length, torsional stability, degree of flexibility, channel size, and angle of view. For screening examinations, an intermediate-length (1300–1550 cm) scope may be advisable. An exceptionally redundant colon that proves to be difficult to examine endoscopically may be better surveyed by X ray. When used with a split overtube (Williams, 1983), the medium-length scope should cope with almost all problems of length and colonic redundancy.

The wide angle of view (110–120 degrees) of modern instruments has made "blind spots" around flexures less troublesome. A standard channel width (2.8 mm) is adequate, although wider channels (3.0–3.7 mm) allow better suction, larger biopsy specimens, and aspiration retrieval of many snared polyps.

2. Bowel Preparation

For surveillance examinations, patient-administered bowel preparations (oral or oral plus enema) for colonoscopy are desirable and help the endoscopy unit nursing staff to cope with mounting work loads (Davis *et al.*, 1980).

However, mannitol bowel preparation is now inadvisable, if not contraindicated, due to the hazard of explosion (Bond *et al.*, 1976; Bigard *et al.*, 1979;

LaBrooy *et al.*, 1981; Raillat *et al.*, 1982). Any residual pocket with an explosive mixture of hydrogen might be ignited if electrosurgery is used. Since electrosurgery is frequently used in adenoma or cancer follow-up, mannitol is inappropriate.

3. Sedation

There are many reasons to aim for little or no sedation in well-person follow-up. To encourage compliance and minimize inconvenience, a walk-in, walk-out follow-up service is desirable. This means avoiding parenteral administration of sedating drugs since traveling unaccompanied after their use is dangerous.

Sedation is needed if the examination becomes uncomfortable. A small (2.5–5.0 mg) dose of diazepam and a larger (25–75 mg) dose of pethidine (meperidine) is a reasonable choice. The narcotic can be reversed with naloxone (0.2 mg IV and 0.2 mg IM), arousing the patient. Greater reliance on pethidine also allows a greater margin for safety in elderly patients whose central cardiorespiratory centers may respond precipitously to even small doses of diazepam and/or pethidine.

Antispasmodics (hyoscine-*n*-butyl bromide, glucagon) aid visualization in patients with spastic colon. However, double blind trials have shown that glucagon is not associated with shortened insertion times (Foster *et al.*, 1981).

4. Technique

The technique of colonoscopy for screening in high-risk groups does not differ from that in routine applications (Cotton and Williams, 1982). The approach to well persons in surveillance differs from that in patients who present with symptoms. The procedure needs to be as comfortable as possible so that the patient will not be discouraged from attending for further surveillance. Thus, a lower threshold of discomfort may need to be accepted for well-person follow-up and alternate techniques employed in persons who are difficult to examine by endoscopy. For subsequent examinations of difficult patients, we schedule a combination of flexible sigmoidoscopy (using CO_2) and immediate double contrast barium enema at the same visit. The CO_2 is absorbed within 15 minutes and does not interfere with the X ray.

5. Complications

Colonoscopy is not without hazard (Berci *et al.*, 1974; Fruhmorgen and Demling 1979; Macrae *et al.*, 1983). Oversedation, vasovagal effects, septicemia, and perforation may occur during diagnostic colonoscopy, and hemorrhage is the main risk when polypectomy is performed. Perforations can occur unexpectedly, and delayed perforations have been reported. Undue force should never be employed, and patients with any abdominal pain that persists after the examination should be observed closely for any sign of deterioration and peritonism. Most small perforations can be managed conservatively, although with careful clinical observation. Indeed, a finding of air in the peritoneal cavity is not infrequent after an uncomplicated colonoscopy and, in itself, is benign (Ecker *et al.*, 1977).

Septicemia is a risk in immunosuppressed patients, particularly children. Prophylaxis (using an aminoglycoside, pencillin, and metronidazole) should be considered for such patients and for cirrhotic patients with ascites. A survey of infectious disease specialists and endoscopists in 1981 brought together six cases of bacterial endocarditis in which colonoscopy was implicated as the initial cause of bacteremia (Meyer, 1981).

C. Double Contrast Barium Enema

Although the double (air) contrast barium enema (DCBE) is notably more accurate than the single contrast examination, it is significantly less accurate than colonoscopy (see Chapter 18). Nevertheless, DCBEs are indicated in adenoma and cancer follow-up if colonoscopic facilities and/or expertise are scarce. In addition, radiological evaluation of the right colon, where colonoscopy is least accurate, is the method of choice where previous colonoscopy has for some reason been difficult. If it is combined with flexible sigmoidoscopy to check the overlapping sigmoid loops where radiological misses most frequently occur, overall accuracy of a technically satisfactory DCBE is acceptable. The use of CO_2 insufflation during the flexible endoscopic examination enables a perfect DCBE to be performed almost immediately, since the CO_2 is quickly resorbed through the colonic mucosa (Hussein and Williams, 1984). Air distention makes proper manipulation and coating of barium almost impossible.

In very-high-risk patients (those with an inherited non-polyposis colon cancer syndrome or with multiple adenomas), a combination of colonoscopy (with CO_2) and DCBE, either at the same time or on alternating screening schedules, is useful. The procedures are complementary: the blind areas proximal to acute flexures are well seen radiologically, and adenomas within a diverticular segment, frequently difficult to see on X ray, stand out clearly for the endoscopist (Williams *et al.*, 1982a).

Preparation for barium enema examination is similar to that of colonoscopy, but preparatory enemas are more important than for colonoscopy, since the radiologist has no access to aspirate fluid residue from the colon.

The technical aspects of barium enema examination have been well described in textbooks (Marshak *et al.*, 1980; Bartram and Kumar, 1982). Only double contrast examinations should be performed in screening, since they provide penetrating views of overlying colonic loops and the fine detail needed to detect small polyps. Clear views of all mucosal surfaces need to be obtained before the examination can be called satisfactory. Dense barium in overlying loops, especially with suboptimal coating, may mask even large lesions.

It is important to emphasize the care needed in the interpretation of X ray films. There is a significant additional diagnostic pickup if the films are reviewed on two occasions, particularly if a second radiologist is involved.

Complications

Perforation may occur because the tip of the inflatable catheter used to introduce barium or its balloon damages the full thickness of the rectal wall. Barium peritonitis from perforation above the peritoneal flexure is particularly serious. In general, barium enemas should not be performed after biopsy of the colon. This is undoubtedly true for sigmoidoscopic biopsies. With the small biopsies taken during flexible fibreoptic examinations, animal studies have shown that perforation is much less likely to occur under pressure (Harned *et al.*, 1982). Although the radiologist should be aware that such biopsies have been taken, it cannot be said that DCBE is contraindicated immediately after flexible endoscopy with biopsy. The overall risk of perforation in large series of barium enema examinations was approximately 0.01% (Lorinc and Brahame, 1959).

III. SENSITIVITY AND SPECIFICITY

A. Rigid Proctosigmoidoscopy and Flexible Sigmoidoscopy

The sensitivity of rigid proctosigmoidoscopy has never been closely evaluated, since it was considered the yardstick and standard diagnostic procedure for lesions of the rectum. The yield is only about one-third of that achieved with the 60-cm flexible sigmoidoscope, but this is mainly due to lesions found beyond the reach of the more limited instrument. Many gastroenterologists familiar with the use of flexible fiberoptic instruments feel that the yield of lesions, even within the rectum, is higher with flexible fiberscopes, compared with rigid instruments, since the optical systems and magnification that enable the flexible endoscopist to view the bowel from the tip of the instrument enhance its sensitivity for small lesions. Certainly, rigid sigmoidoscopes have more blind areas within the distal colon and rectum; low rectal lesions and distal sigmoid lesions around the rectosigmoid junction may be overlooked.

There are some data suggesting limitations in the accuracy of rigid sigmoidoscopy, even within the rectum. Of five neoplasms at least 1 cm in diameter in the rectum that were detected by flexible sigmoidoscopy in an adenoma follow-up study, two were missed at rigid sigmoidoscopy at the same sitting (Williams *et al.*, 1982a). In another study, rigid sigmoidoscopy detected only 6 of the 20 polypoid lesions located within 20 cm of the anal verge (Bohlman *et al.*, 1977). The sensitivity of flexible sigmoidoscopy within the rectum and sigmoid colon seems high, at least insofar as it can be compared with DCBE (Williams *et al.*, 1982a).

The specificity of endoscopy for the diagnosis of cancers and adenomas approaches 100%, since biopsy is an integral part of the technique when a possible lesion is seen. Even without biopsy, the direct view with color imaging makes the specificity high. Adenomas or cancers over 1 cm in size can usually be readily distinguished from nonneoplastic lesions. Polyps 5 mm or less, however, may look identical, whether they are neoplastic or not. In practice, the question of endoscopic specificity is academic, since the endoscopist electrocoagulates or removes by snare polypectomy all polyps seen, except for lipomas and wormlike postinflammatory tags.

B. Colonoscopy and Double Contrast Barium Enema

The sensitivity and specificity of colonoscopy and DCBE are clearly operator dependent, and the choice of procedure may be determined as much by local interest and expertise as by any other factor. Colonoscopy can miss lesions

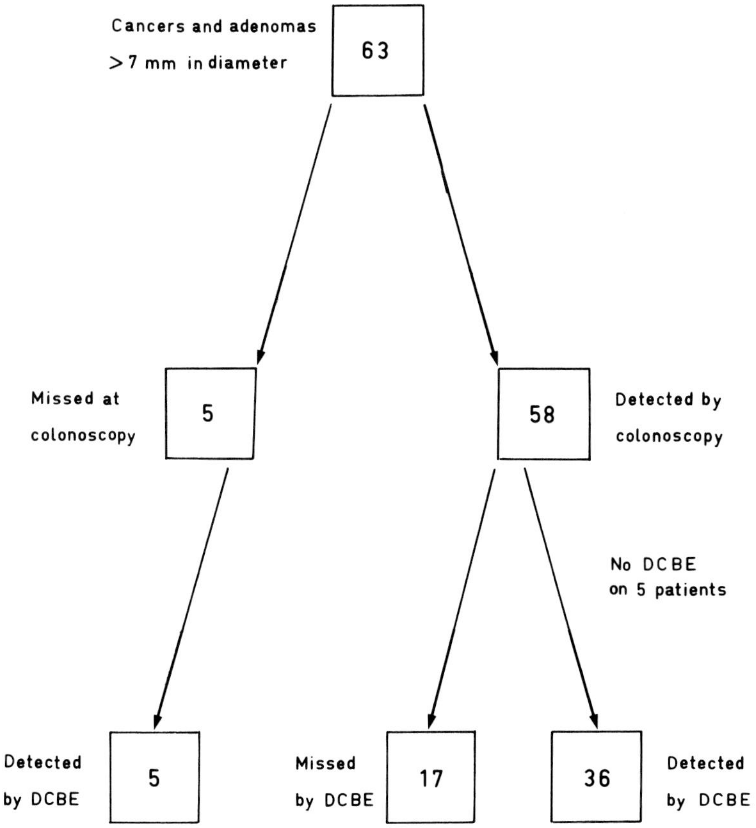

Fig. 2. Comparison of colonoscopy and DCBE for detection of cancers and large adenomas (From Williams *et al.*, 1982a).

shown on DCBE (Laufer *et al.*, 1976; Leinicke *et al.*, 1977), and vice versa. The radiologist reports on black-and-white shadows, and may misinterpret retained fecal matter, bubbles or diverticula for polyps, or even circular muscle spasm for cancer.

Most studies comparing DCBE and colonoscopy (or flexible sigmoidoscopy) have significant biases built into their design that invalidate their comparison of accuracy; all suffer from the lack of a final arbiter of accuracy (e.g. a colectomy specimen). Frequently, comparisons are made when only selected patients are referred for both investigations. Many patients with radiologically normal barium enemas do not even enter the comparative studies. Thus, the false-negative estimate of DCBE is underestimated. On the other hand, if the colonoscopist is not blinded to the results of DCBE, the sensitivity of colonoscopy may be overestimated.

In a study designed to avoid these biases (Williams *et al.*, 1982a), we found that DCBE missed 17 of 63 neoplasms over 7 mm in size and the colonoscopist missed 5 (Fig. 2). There were, however, only four false-positive DCBEs for polyps over 7 mm in size, confirmed by later multiple endoscopic views of the area of interest on the DCBEs. Over half of the radiologically missed lesions had another lesion demonstrated that would have indicated total colonoscopy, although the main lesion was missed. These data have caused us to rely more heavily on endoscopy in well-person surveillance.

Quality control or auditing, performed either blindly or with knowledge of the prior findings at the complementary examination, is important to maintain high diagnostic standards.

IV. LOGISTICS

Proper organization of surveillance is essential if well-person screening is to be supported by the higher-risk people concerned. The administration of such programs needs careful attention.

Computers can facilitate many of the secretarial tasks of routine surveillance, saving considerable time by producing word-processed individual letters, address stickers, listings, etc. Scheduling can be done by recalling those patients required each month. Ongoing data collection allows immediate analysis of results.

The choice of methodology is logical in most higher-risk groups because of the nature of their disease and the degree of risk. The frequency of surveillance is more problematical, since we know little of the natural history of asymptomatic colorectal neoplasia. Prospective controlled trials of adenoma follow-up are currently evaluating this problem, such as ours at St. Mark's Hospital, London, and the larger multicenter polyp follow-up study in the United States (Winawer *et al.*, 1981).

Risk profiles have been suggested using the results of laboratory *in vitro* tests. At the Memorial Sloan-Kettering Cancer Center, a profile of risk is generated in higher-risk groups utilizing results of carcinoembryonic antigen studies in colonic lavage, abnormalities of cell proliferation kinetics, actin patterns of skin fibroblasts in cell culture systems, metabolic derangements of fecal cholesterol and bile acids, and mixed leukocyte responses.

V. TRAINING

Sigmoidoscopy requires some training both in technique (for safety) and for lesion identification (for sensitivity and specificity). A questionnaire survey of interns in several teaching hospitals in Australia may be typical of the experience of most doctors graduating through medical school and internship (Speer *et al.*, 1984). Most (62%) had had bedside training in performing sigmoidoscopy, usually as interns. Most of this training had been done by their peers, who were only slightly more experienced than they themselves. Two-thirds considered their training in technique and lesion recognition poor. After training for several years in hospitals, less than half felt confident about their ability to perform proctosigmoidoscopy.

Just how widely sigmoidoscopic skills are distributed among primary care practitioners in the United States and Europe is uncertain. There may well be a need to improve teaching in sigmoidoscopy. In many centers, rigid sigmoidoscopy remains the cornerstone of investigation of symptomatic diseases of the distal colon and rectum and, where flexible sigmoidoscopy is not available, has an important place in the evaluation of positive stool guaiac tests. Training sessions in flexible sigmoidoscopy have been implemented successfully (McCray, 1981). Colonic models like the Shinya or St. Mark's models are of some help. Electronic training aids in fiber endoscopy are currently undergoing feasibility studies and appear promising. Concerted efforts may also be needed to train clinicians or paramedical personnel in the use of flexible endoscopes, of any length, if flexible endoscopy is to have an important part in colorectal cancer prevention at the primary care level (Johnson *et al.*, 1982).

REFERENCES

Abrahams, J. S., and Reines, H. D. (1979). Increasing incidence of right-sided lesions in colorectal cancer. *Am. J. Surg.* **137,** 522–526.

Albano, W. A., Recabaren, J. A., Lynch, H. T., Campbell, A. S. Mailliard, J. A., Organ, C. H., Lynch, J. F., and Kimberling, W. J. (1982). Natural history of hereditary cancer of the breast and colon. *Cancer* **50,** 360–363.

American Cancer Society (1980). Guidelines for the cancer-related check-up. recommendations and rationale. *Ca—Cancer J. Clin.* **30,** 208–215.

Axtell, L. M., and Chiazze, L. (1966). Changing relative frequency of cancers of the colon and rectum in the United States. *Cancer* **19,** 750–754.

Bartram, C. I., and Kumar, P. (1982). "Clinical Radiology in Gastroenterology." Blackwell, London.

Berci, G., Panish, J. F., Schapiro, M., and Corlin, R. (1974). Complications of colonoscopy and polypectomy. *Gastroenterology* **67,** 584–585.

Bigard, M. A., Gaucher, P., and Lasalle, C. (1979). Fatal colonic explosion. Colonic explosion during colonoscopic polypectomy. *Gastroenterology* **77,** 1307–1310.

Blackstone, M. O., Riddell, R. H., Rogers, B. H. G., and Levin, B. (1981). Dysplasia associated masses detected by colonoscopy in long-standing ulcerative colitis. *Gastroenterology* **80,** 366–374.

Bohlman, T. W., Katon, R. M., Lipshutz, G. R., McCool, M. F., Smith, F. W., and Melnyk, C. S. (1977). Fibreoptic pansigmoidoscopy. An evaluation and comparison with rigid sigmoidoscopy. *Gastroenterology* **72,** 644–649.

Bond, J. H. Levy, M. and Levitt, M. D. (1976). Explosion of hydrogen gas in the colon during proctosigmoidoscopy. *Gastrointest. Endoscopy* **23,** 41–42.

Bonetti, A., Buhler, H., Neusch, H. J., Kobler, E., Schapfer, H., and Deyle, P. (1979). Polypectomie in Dickdarm. Spatergebrisse. *Gastroenterol.* **17,** 791–794.

Brahme, F., Ekelund, G. R., Norden, J. G., and Wenekert, A. (1974). Metachronous colorectal polyps: Comparison of development of colorectal polyps and carcinomas in persons with and without histories of polyps. *Dis. Colon Rectum* **17,** 166–171.

Bussey, H. J. R. (1972). Extracolonic lesions associated with polyposis coli. *Proc. R. Soc. Med.* **65,** 294.

Bussey, H. J. R. (1975). "Familial Polyposis Coli." Johns Hopkins Univ. Press, Baltimore, Maryland.

Bussey, H. J. R., Wallace, M. H., and Morson, B. C. (1967). Metachronous carcinoma of the large intestine and intestinal polyps. *Proc. R. Soc. Med.* **60,** 208–210.

Cady, B., Persson, A. V., Morson, D. O., and Maunz, D. L. (1974). Changing patterns of colorectal carcinoma. *Cancer* **33,** 422–426.

Cotton, P. B., and Williams, C. B. (1982). "Practical Gastro-intestinal Endoscopy," 2nd ed. Blackwell, Oxford.

Crespi, M., Sherlock, P., Gilbertsen, V. A., Weissman, G. S., and Winawer, S. J. (1984). The role of proctosigmoidoscopy in screening for colorectal neoplasia. *Ca—Cancer J. Clin.* **34,** 158–166.

Dales, L. G., Friedman, G. D., and Collen, M. F. (1979). Evaluating periodic multiphasic health check-ups; a controlled trial. *J. Chronic Dis.* **32,** 385–404.

Davis, G. R., Santa Ana, C. A., Morawski, S. G., and Fordtran, J. S. (1980). Development of a lavage solution associated with minimal water and electrolyte absorption or secretion. *Gastroenterology* **78,** 991–995.

Ecker, M. D., Goldstein, M., Hoexter, B., Hyman, R. A., Naidich, J. B., and Stein, H. L. (1977). Benign pneumoperitoneum after fibreoptic colonoscopy. A prospective study of 100 patients. *Gastroenterology* **73,** 266–230.

Eddy, D. M. (1980). Computer models and the evaluation of colon cancer screening programmes. *In* "Colorectal Cancer: Prevention, Epidemiology and Screening" (S. J. Winawer, D. Schottenfeld, and P. Sherlock, eds.), pp. 285–298. Raven Press, New York.

Foster, G. E., Vellacott, K. D., Balfour, T. W., and Hardcastle, J. D. (1981). Outpatient flexible fibreoptic sigmoidoscopy, diagnostic yield and the value of glucagon. *Br. J. Surg.* **68,** 463–464.

Fruhmorgen, P., and Demling, L. (1979). Complications of diagnostic and therapeutic colonoscopy in the Federal Republic of Germany. Results of an inquiry. *Endoscopy* **11,** 146–150.

Gilbertsen, V. A., and Nelms, J. M. (1978). The prevention of invasive cancer of the rectum. *Cancer* **41,** 1137–1139.

Greenstein, A. J., Sachar, D. B., Smith, H., Pucillo, A., Papatestas, A. E., Kneel, I., Geller, S. A., Janowitz, H. D., and Aufses, A. H. (1979). Cancer in universal and left-sided colitis: Factors determining risk. *Gastroenterology* **77,** 290–294.

Harned, R. K., Consigny, M. P., Cooper, N. B., and Williams, S. M., Woltjen, A. J. (1982). Barium enema examination following biopsy of the rectum or colon. *Radiology* **145,** 11–16.

Hertz, R. E., Deddish, M. R., and Day, E. (1960). Value of periodic examinations in detecting cancer of the rectum and colon. *Postgrad. Med.* **27,** 290–294.

Hussein, A. M., Bartram, C. I. and Williams, C. B. (1984). Carbon dioxide insufflation for more comfortable colonoscopy. *Gastrointest. Endoscopy* **30,** 68–70.

Jarvinen, H., Nyberg, M., and Peltokallis, P. (1983). Upper gastrointestinal tract polyps in familial adenomatosis coli. *Gut* **24,** 333–339.

Johnson, R. A., Quan, M., and Rodney, W. M. (1982). Flexible sigmoidoscopy in primary care. The procedure and its potential. *Postgrad. Med.* **72,** 151–156.

Katon, R. M. (1979). Sigmoidoscopy (rigid and flexible). *In* "Proceedings of the Consensus Development Conference: Screening and Early Detection of Colorectal Cancer," NIH Publ. 80-2075, p. 115. Natl. Inst. Health, Washington, D.C.

Kirsner, J. B., Rider, J. A., Moeller, H. C., Palmer, W. W., and Gold, S. S. (1960). Polyps of the colon and rectum. Statistical analysis of a long-term follow-up study. *Gastroenterology* **39,** 178–182.

LaBrooy, S. J., Avgerinos, A., Fendick, C. L., Williams, C. B., and Misciewicz, J. J. (1981). Potentially explosive colonic concentrations of hydrogen after bowel preparation with Mannitol. *Lancet* **1,** 634–636.

Laufer, I., Smith, N. C. W., and Mullens, J. E. (1976). The radiological demonstration of colorectal polyps undetected by endoscopy. *Gastroenterology* **70,** 167–170.

LeFrock, J., Ellis, C. A., Turchick, J. B., and Weinstein, L. (1973). Transient bacteriaemia associated with sigmoidoscopy. *N. Engl. J. Med.* **289,** 467–471.

Lehman, G. A., Buchner, D. M., and Lappes, J. C. (1983). Anatomical extent of fibreoptic sigmoidoscopy. *Gastroenterology* **84,** 803–808.

Leicester, R. J., Hawley, P. R., Pollett, W. G., and Nicholls, R. J. N. (1982). Flexible fibreoptic sigmoidoscopy as an outpatient procedure. *Lancet* **1,** 34–35.

Leinicke, J. L., Dodds, W. J., Hogan, W. J., and Stewardt, E. T. (1977). A comparison of colonoscopy and roentgenography for detecting polypoid lesions of the colon. *Gastrointest. Radiol.* **2,** 75.

Lennard-Jones, J. E., Morson, B. C., Ritchie, J. K., and William, C. B. (1983). Cancer surveillance in ulcerative colitis. Experience over 15 years. *Lancet* **2,** 149–152.

Lorinc, P., and Brahame, F. (1959). Perforation of the colon during examination by the double contrast method. *Gastroenterology* **37,** 770–773.

Lovett, E. (1974). Familial factors in the aetiology of carcinoma of the large bowel. *Proc. R. Soc. Med.* **67,** 21–22.

Lynch, H. T., and Krush, A. J. (1967). Heredity and adenocarcinoma. *Gastroenterology* **53,** 517–527.

McCray, R. S. (1981). A fibreoptic sigmoidoscopy training programme for cancer screening physicians. *Gastrointest. Endoscopy* **27,** 137.

McHardy, G., Brown, C. H., and Kauvar, A. J. (1968). Proctosigmoidoscopy. *GP* **37,** 98–111.

Macklin, M. T. (1960). Inheritance of cancer of the stomach and large intestine in man. *J. Natl. Cancer Inst.* (*U.S.*) **24,** 551–571.

Macrae, F. A., and St. John, D. J. B. (1980). Spontaneous bacterial peritonitis. Reversible cause of deterioration in patients with cirrhosis. *Med. J. Aust.* **2,** 209–211.

Macrae, F. A., and St. John, D. J. B. (1982). Relationship between patterns of bleeding and Hemoccult sensitivity in patients with colorectal cancers or adenomas. *Gastroenterology* **82,** 891–898.

Macrae, F. A., and Williams, C. B. (1982). A prospective colonoscopic follow-up study of 500 adenoma patients with multivariate analysis to predict risk of subsequent colorectal tumors. *Gastroenterology* **82,** 1122.

Macrae, F. A., Hill, D. J., Dent, O., Goulston, K. J., and St. John, D. J. B. (1982). Colorectal cancer. Knowledge and attitudes of doctors in Victoria. *Aust. N.Z. Med.* **12,** 278–283.

Macrae, F. A., Tan, K. G., and Williams, C. B. (1983). Towards safer colonoscopy: A report on the complications of 5000 colonoscopies. *Gut* **24,** 376–383.

Marshak, R. H., Linder, A. E., and Maklansky, D. (1980). "Radiology of the Colon." Saunders, Philadelphia, Pennsylvania.

Meyer, G. W. (1981). Prophylaxis of infective endocarditis during colonscopy: Report of a survey. *Gastrointest. Endoscopy* **27,** 58–59.

Minopoulos, G. J., McIntyre, R. L. E., Lee, E. C. G., and Kettlewell, M. G. W. (1983). Colonoscopic polypectomy in a regional teaching hospital. *Br. J. Surg.* **70,** 51–53.

Morgenstern, L., and Lee, S. E. (1978). Spatial distribution of colonic carcinoma. *Arch. Surg. (Chicago)* **113,** 1142–1143.

Nivatvongs, S., and Fryd, D. S. (1980). How far does the proctosigmoidoscope reach? A prospective study of 1000 patients. *N. Engl. J. Med.* **303,** 380–382.

Pelican, G., Hentages, D., Butt, J., Haag, T., Rolfe, R., and Hutcheson, D. (1976). Bacteraemia during colonoscopy. *Gastrointest. Endoscopy* **23,** 33–35.

Preston, D. M., Butt, J. H., Lennard-Jones, J. E., Morson, B. C., and Williams, C. B. (1983). New rectal mucosal biopsy forceps. *Lancet* **1,** 157.

Raillat, A., deSaint-Julien, J., and Abgrall, J. (1982). Explosion colique au cours d'une electrocoagulation endoscopique aprés préparation au mannitol. *Gastroenterol. Clin. Biol.* **6,** 301–302.

Ranzi, T., Castagnone, D., Veleo, P., Bianchi, P., and Polli, E. E. (1981). Gastric and duodenal polyps in familial polyposis. *Gut* **22,** 363–367.

Rosato, F. E., and Marks, G. (1981). Changing site distribution of colorectal cancer at Thomas Jefferson University Hospital. *Dis Colon Rectum* **24,** 93–95.

Rosen, P., Fireman, Z., Terdiman, R., Hellerstein, M., Rattan, J., and Gilot, T. (1981). Selective screening for colorectal tumors in the Tel-Aviv area: Relevance of epidemiology and family history. *Cancer* **47,** 827–831.

Sackett, D. L., and Whelan, G. (1980). Cancer risk in ulcerative colitis: Scientific requirements for the study of prognosis. *Gastroenterology* **78,** 1632–1635.

Snyder, D. N., Heston, J. F., Meigs, J. W., and Flannery, J. T. (1977). Changes in site distribution of colorectal carcinoma in Connecticut, 1940–73. *Am. J. Dig. Dis.* **22,** 791–797.

Speer, A. G., Eaves, E. R., Gijsbers, A. J. and St. John, D. J. B. (1984). Training in sigmoidoscopy. An assessment in three teaching hospitals. *Med. J. Aust.* **141,** 223–225.

Stemper, T. J., Kent, T. J., and Summers, R. W. (1975). Juvenile polyposis and gastrointestinal carcinoma. A study of a kindred. *Ann. Intern. Med.* **83,** 639–646.

Stewart, M., Macrae, F. A., and Williams, C. B. (1982). Neoplasia and ureterosigmoidostomy; a colonoscopy survey. *Br. J. Surg.* **69,** 414–416.

Thomas, G., Brozinsky, S., and Isenberg, J. I. (1982). Patient acceptance and effectiveness of a balanced lavage solution. (Golytely) versus the standard preparation for colonoscopy. *Gastroenterology* **82,** 435–437.

Thomson, J. P. S., Nicholls, R. J., and Williams, C. B. (1981). ''Colorectal disease. An introduction for surgeons and physicians.'' p. 4. Heinemann, London.
Tornqvist, A., Ekelund, G., and Leandoer, L. (1981). Early diagnosis of metachronous colorectal carcinoma. *Aust. N.Z. Surg.* **51,** 442–445.
Vellacott, K. D., and Hardcastle, J. D. (1981). An evaluation of flexible fibreoptic sigmoidoscopy. *Br. Med. J.* **283,** 1583–1586.
Watanabe, J., Enjoji, M., Yao, T., and Ohsato, K. (1978). Gastric lesions in familial adenomatosis coli their incidence and histologic analysis. *Hum. Pathol.* **9,** 269–283.
Waye, J. D., and Braunfeld, S. (1982). Surveillance intervals after colonoscopic polypectomy. *Endoscopy* **14,** 79–81.
Williams, C. B., (1983). Split overtube for easier colonoscopy. *Gut* **24,** A492.
Williams, C. B., and Gillespie, P. E. (1979). Accidental removal of ureteral stoma at colonoscopy. *Gastrointest. Endoscopy* **25,** 109–110.
Williams, C. B., Macrae, F. A., and Bartram, C. I. (1982a). A prospective study of diagnostic methods in adenoma follow-up. *Endoscopy* **14,** 74–78.
Williams, C. B., Goldblatt, M., and Delaney, P. V. (1982b). 'Top and tail endoscopy' and follow-up in Peutz-Jeghers Syndrome. *Endoscopy* **14,** 82–84.
Winawer, S. J. Leidner, S. D., Boyle, C., and Kurtz, R. C. (1979). Comparison of flexible sigmoidoscopy with other diagnostic techniques in the diagnosis of rectocolon neoplasia. *Dig. Dis. Sci.* **24,** 277–281.
Winawer, S. J., Stewart, E., Gottlieb, L., and Andrews, M. (1981). National polyp follow-up study: organization and statement of purpose. *Gastroenterology* **80,** 1316.
Winawer, S. J., Cummins, R., and Baldwin, M. P. (1982). A new flexible sigmoidoscope for the generalist. *Gastrointest. Endoscopy* **28,** 233–236.
Woolf, C. M. (1958). A genetic study of carcinoma of the large intestine. *Am. J. Hum. Genet.* **104,** 42–47.

15

Physical Examination of the Breast and Breast Self-Examination

ALAN A. BASSETT

I.	Introduction	271
II.	The Technique of Physical Examination of the Breast	272
	A. Examination in the Upright Position	274
	B. Examination in the Supine Position	279
	C. Examination in the Oblique Position	282
III.	Breast Self-Examination	284
	A. First You Look	286
	B. Then You Feel	286
IV	Conclusion	290
	References	290

I. INTRODUCTION

In this chapter, the *technique* of performing physical examination of the breast and breast self-examination will be emphasized. Personal observation in a large referral practice, and in the Mount Sinai Hospital Centre of the National Breast Screening Study, Toronto, suggest that clinical examination of the breast is generally performed in a suboptimal manner. This must be the result of inadequate undergraduate emphasis, which carries over into clinical practice at all levels. It would be appropriate to emphasize the technique of clinical breast examination more thoroughly in the final medical year and reinforce it at the postgraduate level. This is best done by individualized instruction in a consulting office setting. The inexperienced or improperly taught physician will continue to perform an inadequate examination forever until a comprehensive and systematic method is demonstrated repeatedly on dozens of patients who present with normal and abnormal findings.

ISBN 0-12-496720-5

II. THE TECHNIQUE OF PHYSICAL EXAMINATION OF THE BREAST

There are many ways to do a proper breast examination, and the technique and sequence of movements are the preference of the examiner. The method to be described is the one practiced at the National Breast Screening Centre, Mount Sinai Hospital, Toronto.

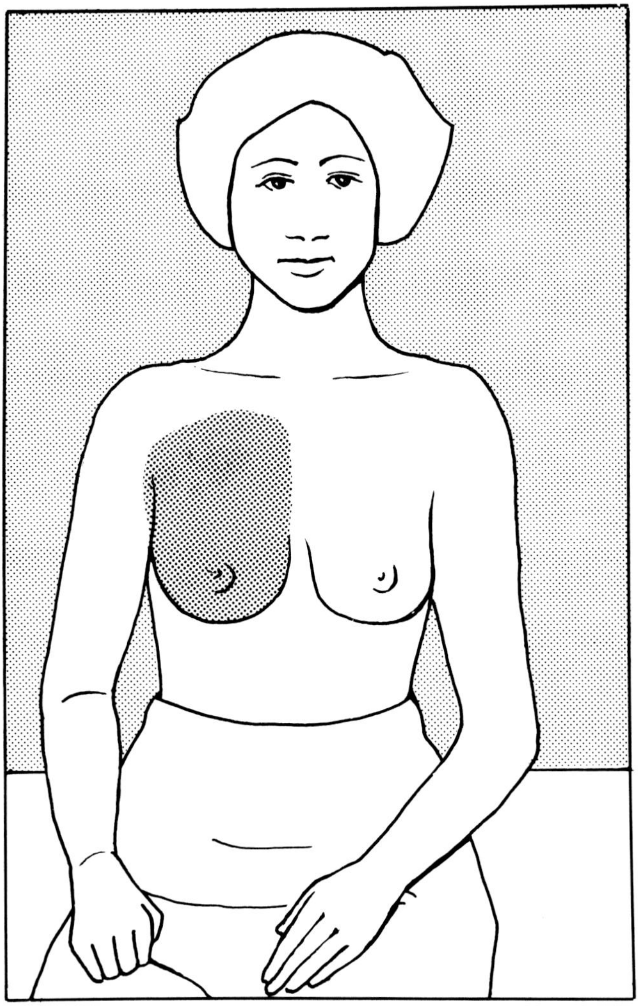

Fig. 1. Position of patient for inspection. The shaded area indicates the surface anatomy of the right breast.

It is thought by some (Mahoney and Csima, 1982) that in an annual clinical screening for breast cancer, certain steps in the physical examination can be eliminated, since they unnecessarily complicate the procedure. In fact, in a screening examination for breast cancer, it is necessary to be more thorough than when a patient comes to the physician with a lump. In the second instance a problem has already been detected, but in the first instance there is no perceived problem, and the examination must be more thorough to rule out an abnormality (Bassett, 1983). Because of the higher incidence and severity of fibrocystic disease in the premenopausal female, clinical assessment can prove to be more difficult, and extra care is required. The sequence of the examination is such that duplication of movement is avoided where possible, thus making the procedure efficient without sacrificing accuracy.

It is essential to be systematic and use the same method every time. The diagnostic harvest will be directly proportional to the thoroughness of the examination.

Examination of the breast encompasses an area that is beyond the mammary prominences (Fig. 1). The surface anatomy is from the second to the sixth ribs and from the lateral border of the sternum to the midaxillary line. In addition, the supraclavicular fossae and axillae are examined for evidence of abnormal lymph nodes.

The breast is examined in segments, in a radial pattern, along imaginary vectors, from periphery to nipple (Fig. 2). The flat surfaces of the distal phalanges of the middle three fingers (the finger pads) are used for palpation (Fig. 3). The fingers are kept extended, but slight flexing occurs at the metacarpophalangeal joints, as pressure is applied firmly but gently against the underlying chest wall. If palpation is done by sliding over the skin, underlying masses are easily missed. When palpation is done by picking up breast tissue and examining it between the thumb and fingers, false masses are felt and true tumors may be missed.

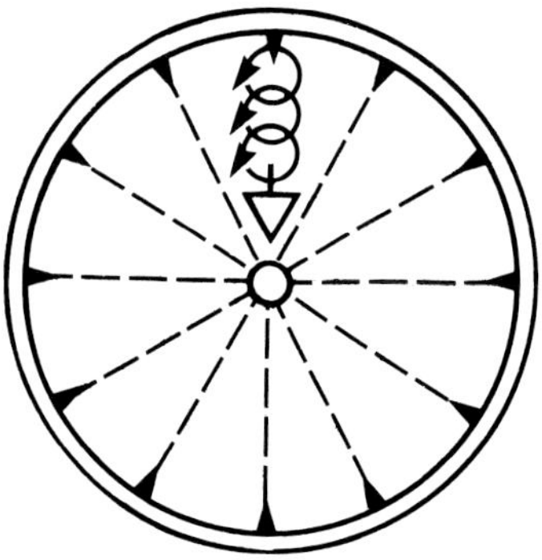

Fig. 2. Vectors for examination of the breast (radial pattern).

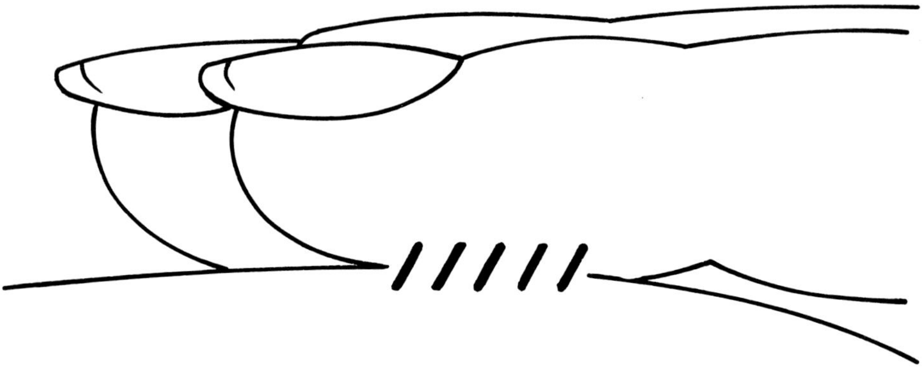

Fig. 3. The finger pads of the middle three fingers are used for palpation.

Small, tight, circular movements are made, moving toward the nipple, one to two circles for each area palpated, slightly lifting the finger pads from the skin each time before moving them into position for the next overlapping circle. Use whichever hand feels more comfortable for a particular position. Rotate the fingers clockwise when using the left hand and counterclockwise when using the right hand. After reaching the nipple, return to the periphery and repeat the procedure along the next vector until the entire breast has been examined. The examination is done in a deliberate and unhurried manner.

Other methods are practiced, such as along concentric circles, or following transverse or vertical lines. Our experience with the radial method has found acceptance with nurse examiners and medical students. The nipple is the end-point for each vector and helps to keep the examiner ''on course.'' The relatively short distance of each segment also assists in maintaining accuracy of coverage and minimizes the possibility of skipped areas. The radial method is also helpful in indicating on a chart the distance of a lesion from the nipple on a specific vector (e.g., 1 o'clock).

Three positions are used—the upright, the supine, and the slightly oblique. Good lighting is essential, and the examining table should be accessible from both sides. The examination will take about 3 minutes, and must be done systematically with attention to detail. To avoid duplication of illustrations, features of palpation in the upright and supine positions can be interchanged.

A. Examination in the Upright Position

1. Inspection

The patient is seated on an examining table, facing the examiner, disrobed to the waist, and hands relaxed on the thighs (Fig. 1). Look for asymmetry. A slight difference in the size of the breasts is not abnormal. Note any change in contour, such as a bulge, flattening, or dimpling. Look for eczema of the nipple and areola and evidence of nipple retraction. If there is nipple inversion, is it of recent onset? Note any edema, redness, or abnormal vascularity of the skin. Next, ask the patient to raise her arms straight up (Fig. 4). This will exaggerate any previously noted or suspected skin dimpling. Elevate the breasts (Fig. 5) so that the inferior surfaces can be visualized. If this is not done, a large portion of

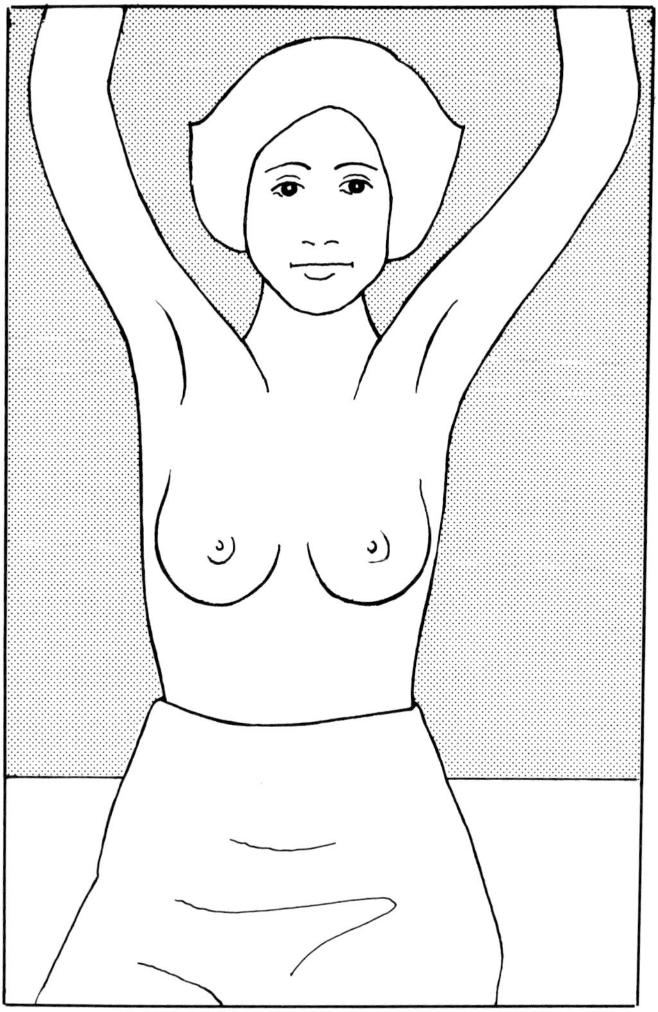

Fig. 4. Inspection with the patient's arms raised straight up.

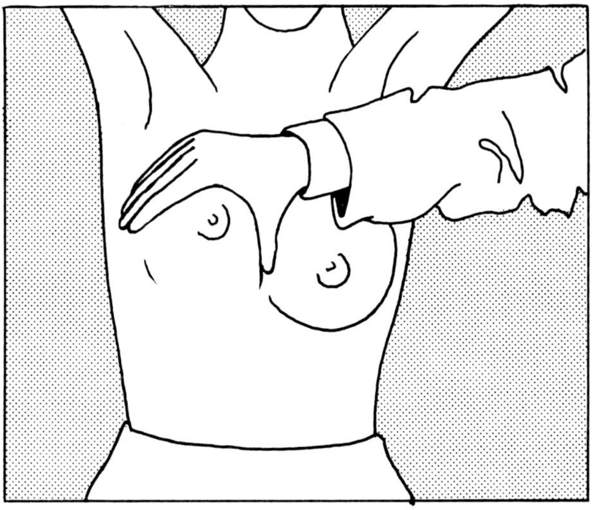

Fig. 5. Breast elevated to visualize the inferior surface.

the breast will be unobserved, particularly in women with large or pendulous breasts.

The patient now places her hands on her iliac crests (Fig. 6) and presses firmly inward, causing the pectoral muscles to contract. This will further accentuate what may have previously been subtle skin dimpling or detect skin dimpling not previously noted. A small underlying mass lesion may be missed on palpation if one's suspicion is not directed to an abnormality noted on inspection.

2. *Palpation*

The supraclavicular fossae (Fig. 7) and axillae (Fig. 8) are examined in the upright position. The axilla is examined by partly abducting and supporting the arm on the side to be examined; the examiner then examines the right axilla with the left hand and vice versa. Palpation of the axilla is done with the fingertips and pads, aiming toward the apex, pressing against the chest wall and gradually sweeping inferiorly with small rotary motions. The lymph nodes are best felt in the upright position, probably because of the effect of gravity.

The patient now places her hands behind the head, elbows out (Fig. 9), and palpation is performed. Although most lesions can be palpated in the supine position, a small percentage are best felt in the upright position, and some are missed entirely if palpation in the upright position is omitted.

Palpation begins at the periphery in the 12 o'clock position (Fig. 10) just

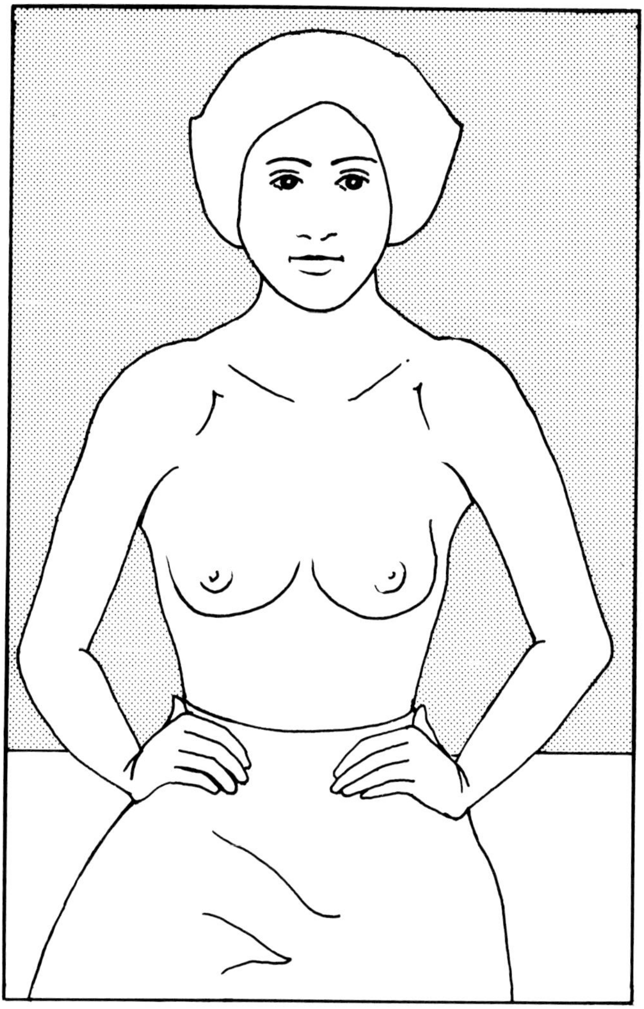

Fig. 6. Inspection with the patient pressing firmly on the iliac crests.

below the clavicle, examining the medial half first and then the lateral half, until the starting point is reached. The inferior portion of the breast is retracted upward and the lateral portion is retracted medially, so that the breast can be palpated firmly against the chest wall (Figs. 11 and 12). In a patient with very large, pendulous breasts, palpation in the upright position is not satisfactory, and is omitted.

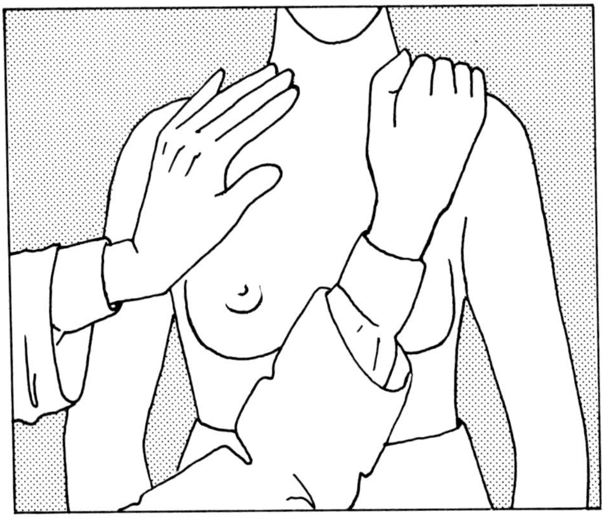

Fig. 7. Palpation of the supraclavicular fossae.

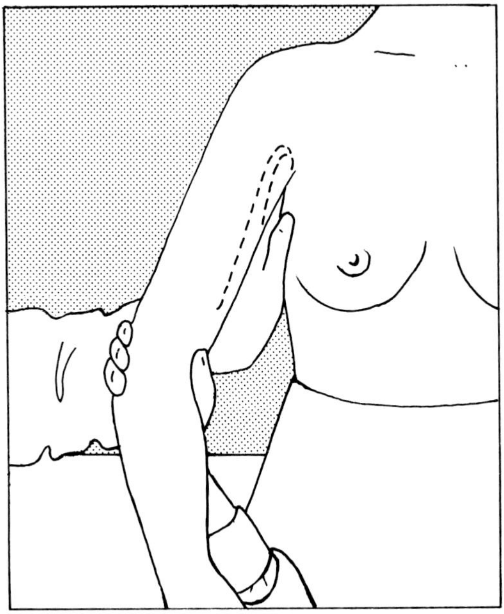

Fig. 8. Palpation of the axilla.

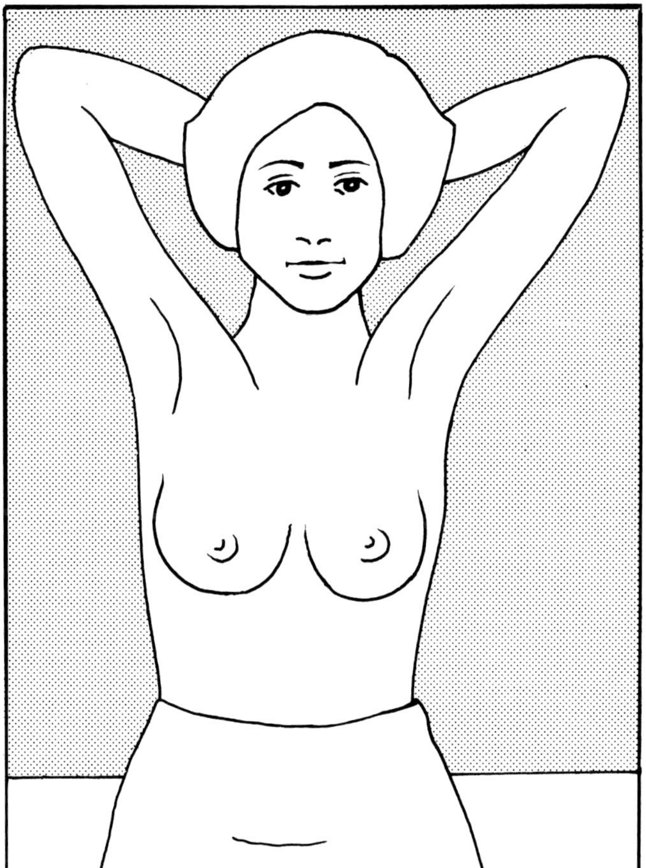

Fig. 9. Position of the patient for palpation in the upright position.

B. Examination in the Supine Position

Each breast should be palpated from the corresponding side of the examining table. The patient lies on a pillow that extends to just below the shoulders. In a clinical examination, it is not necessary to place a towel under the side being examined in order to distribute the breast tissue more evenly over the chest wall. It is more precise to shift the breast in relation to the area of examination, as previously described in palpation in the upright position.

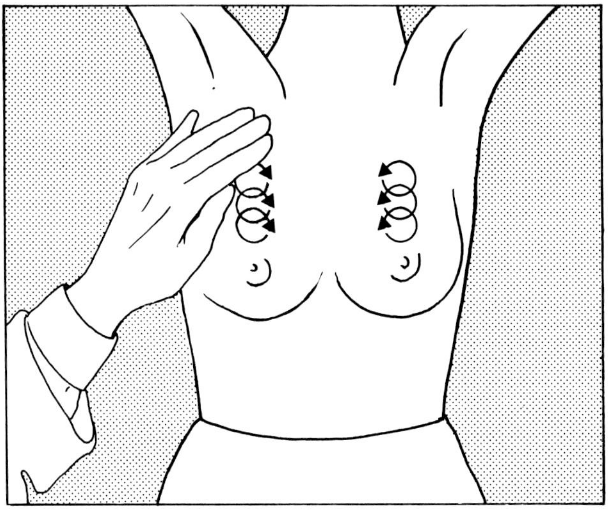

Fig. 10. Commencement of palpation in the upright position.

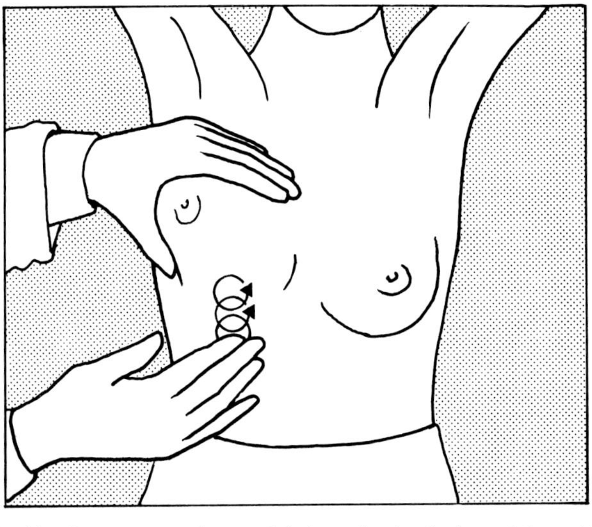

Fig. 11. Breast retracted upward during palpation in the upright position.

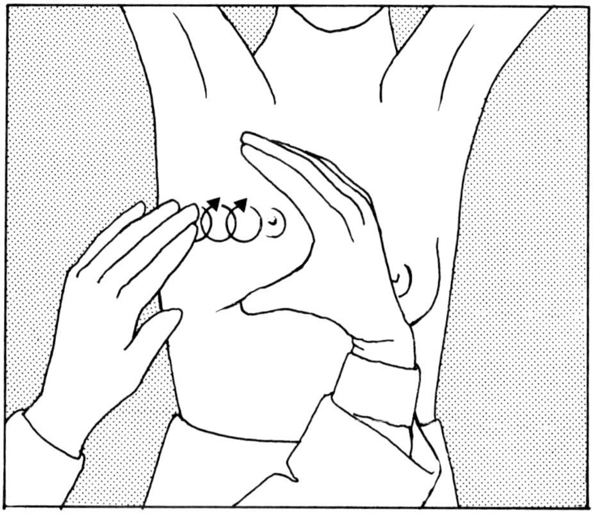

Fig. 12. Breast retracted medially during palpation in the upright position.

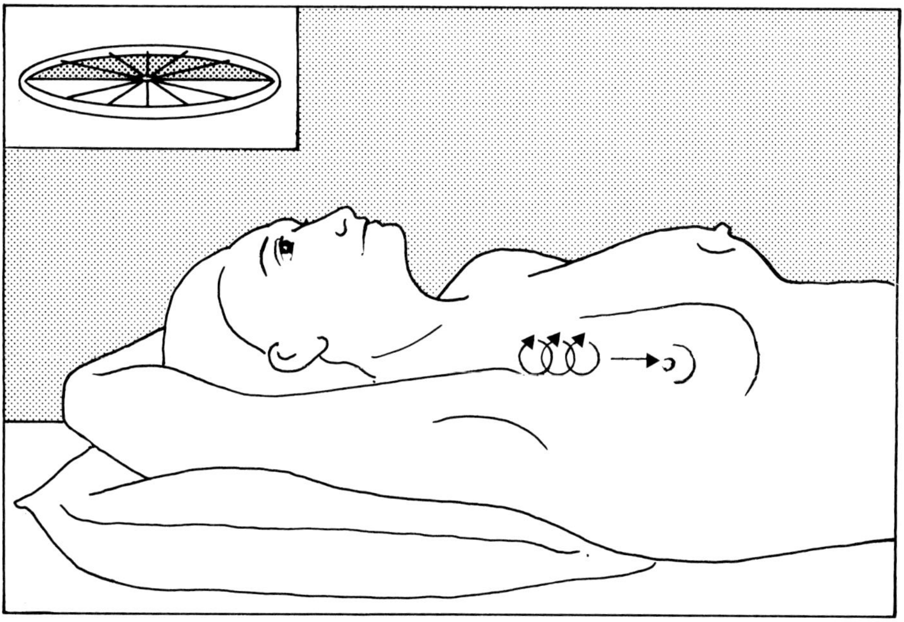

Fig. 13. Position of the patient for examination of the right breast in the supine position.

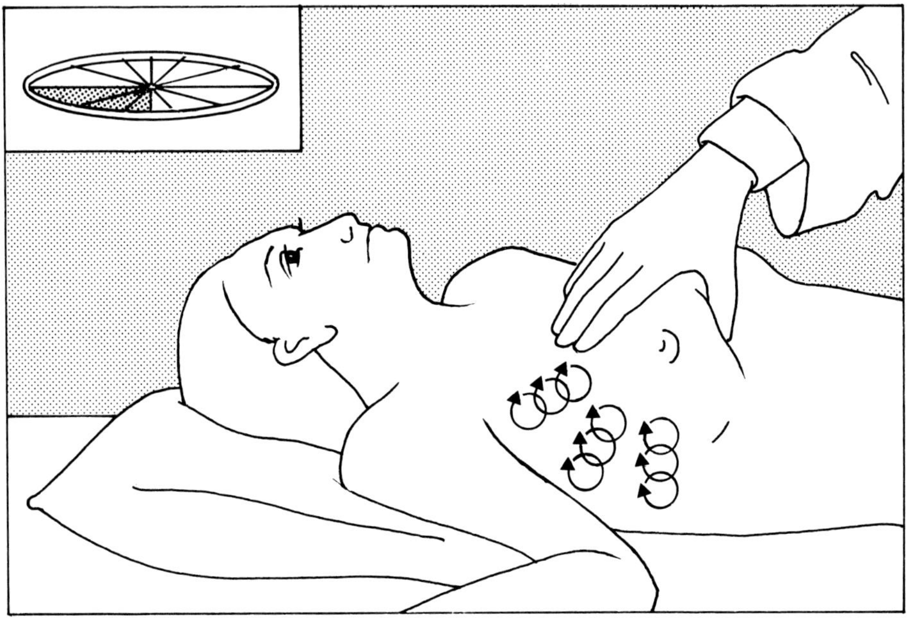

Fig. 14. Breast retracted medially for examination of the lateral half in the supine position.

To examine the right breast, the patient's right hand is placed under the neck (Fig. 13). This flattens the medial half of the breast against the chest wall. As in palpating in the upright position, the examination begins at the 12 o'clock position and the medial half is examined. At the 6 o'clock position, the patient's arm is brought down partly to the side, and the breast is retracted upwards so that, on palpation, the breast can be more readily compressed against the chest wall. The breast is retracted medially while the lateral half is examined (Fig. 14). The nipples are now gently compressed between the thumb and index fingers to note any discharge or thickening in the nipple. The subareolar area is assessed for any abnormal thickening or mass.

C. Examination in the Oblique Position (Fig. 15)

The patient rotates 10–15 degrees away from the examiner, with her forearm resting on the forehead. The lateral half of the breast is reexamined, with particular attention to the axillary tail of Spence. This is the best position to examine the tail of the breast.

This completes the physical examination of the breast. If the examination has not detected the area of concern to the patient, have her point it out and reassure her if it is not clinically significant.

During palpation, differentiation is made between three-dimensional masses and areas of ill-defined plaque-like thickening, nodular or granular areas. Three-dimensional masses are solid or cystic, and the differentiation is made by fine needle aspiration. One of the most grateful and relieved patients is a woman who has just had her breast lump disappear completely into a syringe. Fine needle aspiration can also be used to assess two-dimensional thickenings and nodularities.

The use of fine needle aspiration is now fairly well established in North America, having first been popularized in Europe (Zajicek *et al.*, 1970; Russ *et al.*, 1978; Salter and Bassett, 1981; Strawbridge *et al.*, 1981). An occasional complication of fine needle aspiration is hematoma and ecchymosis. Very rarely, pneumothorax may occur, either immediately or delayed.

Nipple discharge is frequently a source of concern to patients, particularly since it is listed as a symptom of breast cancer by cancer societies (personal communication Dr. James E. Devitt). Usually nipple discharge that is produced only on manipulation is bilateral and multiductal and is not significant. Many patients strip their nipples and produce a discharge that is usually milky, green, yellow, or brown to black. Sometimes such stripping can produce a tiny amount of blood. Patients frequently become quite concerned because of their finding. After clinical examination and mammography have revealed no abnormality, we

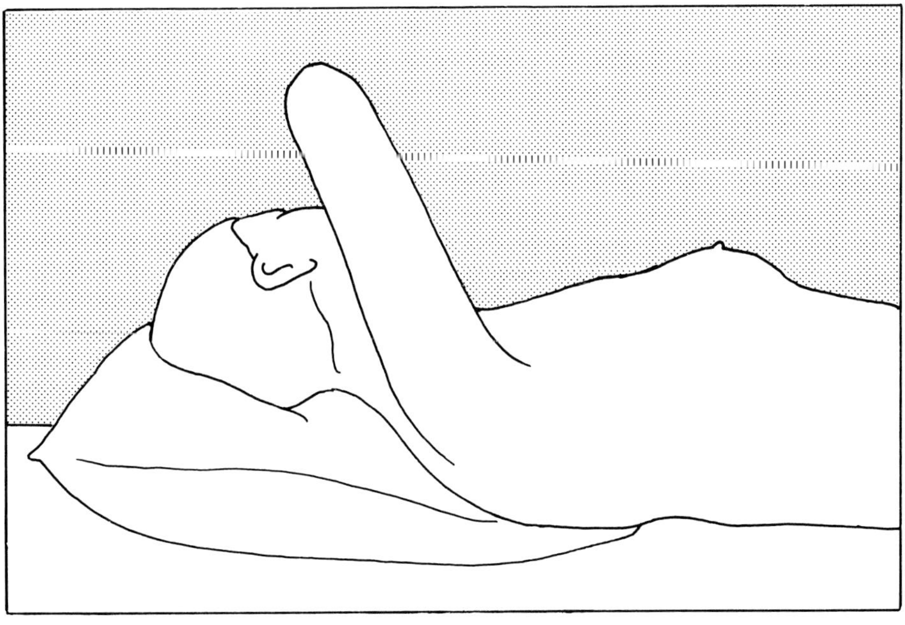

Fig. 15. Position of the patient for examination in the oblique position.

tell these patients that such a discharge is of no significance and advise them to stop the practice of nipple stripping.

A spontaneous nipple discharge in a nonlactating woman, which is usually detected by stains on a bra or nightgown, should be surgically explored, particularly if it is unilateral, whether bloodstained or not.

A prolactin level is obtained, especially if the discharge is milky and bilateral, and cytology is done. However, a negative clinical examination, cytology, and mammogram should not influence the decision for surgical excision of the duct system, although where these findings are negative, carcinoma is rarely the cause.

Differences of opinion in the interpretation of findings can be expected even where very experienced personnel are involved. This observer variability was noted in a small study done by Boyd *et al.* (1981). Fortunately, the variation arose largely from differences of opinion about the findings in patients who did not have breast cancer. Where breast cancer was found on subsequent biopsy, there was relatively little variation among them in the frequency with which biopsy was recommended.

The true-positive rate for breast carcinoma in the Cincinnati Breast Cancer Detection Center detected by physical examination alone was 38%, and the false-positive rate was 4% (Moskowitz, 1983). The omission of physical examination would have missed 16% of the minimal breast cancers.

In a summary of the experience in the U.S. Breast Cancer Detection Demonstration Projects, Baker (1982) noted that physical examinations alone detected 13.1% of the breast cancers in the 40–49 group age and 6.7% of the breast cancers in the 50–59 group age compared to 61.3% and 40% in the Hospital Insurance Plan of Greater New York (HIP) study. This marked difference might possibly by partly explained by the use of better clinical examiners in the HIP study.

We are in agreement with others (Moskowitz, 1979; George *et al.*, 1980) that nurse examiners can perform very efficiently as primary screeners. Our experience in the Mount Sinai Hospital Centre of the National Breast Screening Study indicates that they can perform breast examinations and determine the presence of significant clinical findings better than most physicians. Their performance is under constant review, and their expertise is used in teaching medical students and making teaching films.

III. BREAST SELF-EXAMINATION

An abnormality of the breast is, in most instances, first detected by the patient. Early detection is considered an important factor in reducing the mortality from breast cancer (Shapiro, 1977). The possible benefits of breast self-examination

(BSE) have not yet been properly evaluated, although indirect evidence suggests that it leads to increased discovery of small tumors with no nodal involvement. Current trials may eventually show the extent to which BSE reduces mortality from breast cancer (Miller and Bulbrook, 1982; also see Chapter 17). It would therefore seem appropriate for as many women as possible to become proficient in BSE. Although BSE is not a substitute for breast examination by a competent examiner, it detects lesions that may become physically evident between professional examinations.

In a survey sponsored by the American Cancer Society (1980), it was noted that although a majority of women performed BSE in the past year, the method left much to be desired.

Although women frequently complain that they don't know what they are feeling, the fact is that they frequently detect lumps so small that they must be pointed out even to a trained examiner. It would seem, therefore, that just as in teaching physicians, nurses, and other professionals, the "how-to" part of the examination (motor component) is easier to master than the interpretation of a finding (sensory component). For this reason, Baines (1983) advances the interesting thought that campaigns to increase the skill of physicians in breast examination might be more appropriate than campaigns to persuade women to practise BSE. One might also infer that improved physician skills in breast examination could translate into better patient instruction.

The most appropriate time to teach BSE is at the completion of a breast examination in the physician's office. It can also be taught by a trained nurse examiner, and this instruction has been incorporated into the Canadian National Breast Screening Study. In fact, such nurse examiners will become more proficient in doing a clinical breast examination and in instructing in BSE than most physicians. Compliance appears to be better when a woman is individually taught than when she receives instruction by group lectures or pamphlets (Miller and Bulbrook, 1982).

Pennypacker *et al.* (1982) have developed a complex model for teaching BSE. They indicate that a training technique involving both the model and the woman's own breast tissue is the method of choice for instruction in BSE. This method has not yet been scientifically evaluated.

BSE should be performed about a week after the beginning of each menstrual cycle. If the periods have stopped, either naturally or as the result of surgery or for other reasons, the first day of each calender month can be chosen.

The manual component of BSE is best taught by holding the woman's hand on her own breast, taking her through all the palpatory maneuvers in the proper systematic sequence, and then having her repeat the precedure under supervision. Her skills should be tested and reinforced where necessary at subsequent visits to the office or screening center. The method used at the Breast Screening Centre, Mount Sinai Hospital, Toronto, is shown and explained in the following photographs, and the narrative is set out as if a physician were teaching a woman how to do BSE.

A. First You Look

Undress to the waist in a well-lit room and sit or stand in front of a mirror, with your arms resting relaxed on your thighs if sitting (Fig. 16A) and at your sides if standing. Look in the mirror and observe your breasts carefully. One breast may be a bit larger than the other, but this is not abnormal. Look for any change in the nipple, such as eczema or an indrawing. Note any swelling or puckering of the skin. Look for other skin changes, such as redness or a change in texture such as an orange-peel appearance.

Raise the arms straight up over the head, and look for the same things as in Fig. 16A, also observing carefully for any subtle dimpling of the skin (Fig. 16B). Turn your body slightly from side to side.

Elevate each breast so that you can see the undersurface, and again look for the same changes (Fig. 16C). This is particularly important if your breasts are large or drooping.

With your hands on your hips, press firmly inward so as to tense the chest muscles (Fig. 16D). This will exaggerate any subtle skin dimpling and any abnormal nipple deviation.

B. Then You Feel

While still sitting, examine your armpit area for lumps (Fig. 16E). Then lie flat on your bed or on a carpeted floor. Lie on a pillow and place a folded bath towel under the side to be examined. Examine the right breast with the left hand, and vice versa. Examination is done with the pads of the middle three fingers (Fig. 3). Do not use the fingertips. Press the breast firmly but gently against the ribs, Examine by using small, overlapping circular movements from the periphery to the nipple—the radial method (Fig. 2). The fingers are kept straight, and there is a slight flexion at the knuckle joints in the hand. The area examined is roughly from just below the collar bone to about 3 cm below the lower breast margin, and from the breast bone to the outer side of the rib cage. Ensure that no part is missed.

Place the hand of the side being examined under the head (Fig. 16F) and examine the upper midportion followed by the inner half (Fig. 16G).

To examine the outer half, bring the arm down partly to the side (Fig. 16H). As you near completion of the examination, having come all around the breast, examine the armpit area again.

Now raise the arm over the head, so that the forearm rests on the forehead (Fig. 16I). Rotate the body slightly and reexamine the outer part, especially that

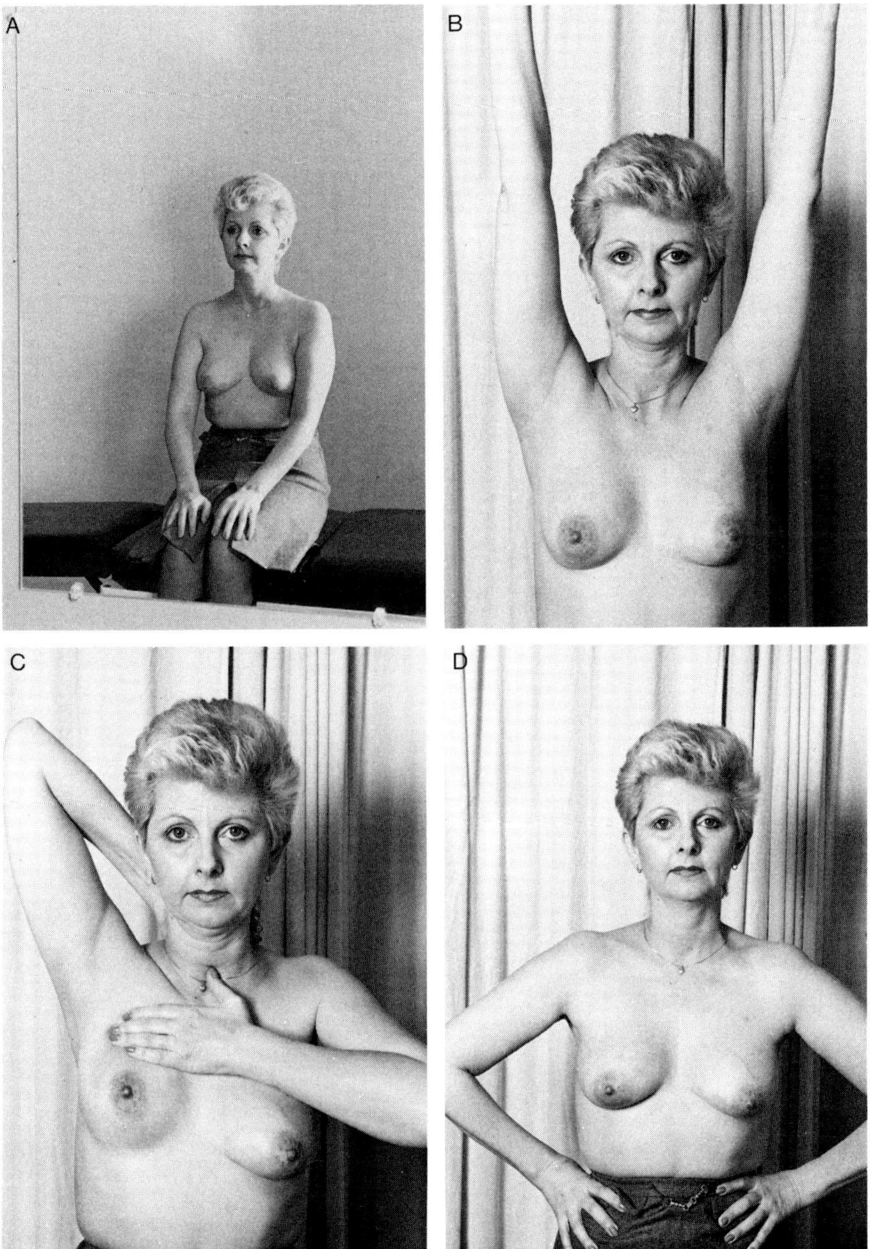

Fig. 16. Breast self-examination. (A) Woman in front of a mirror for visual inspection during BSE. (B) Inspection during BSE with the arms above the head. (C) Inspection of the undersurface of the breast during BSE. (D) Inspection during BSE with the hands pressed firmly on the hips.

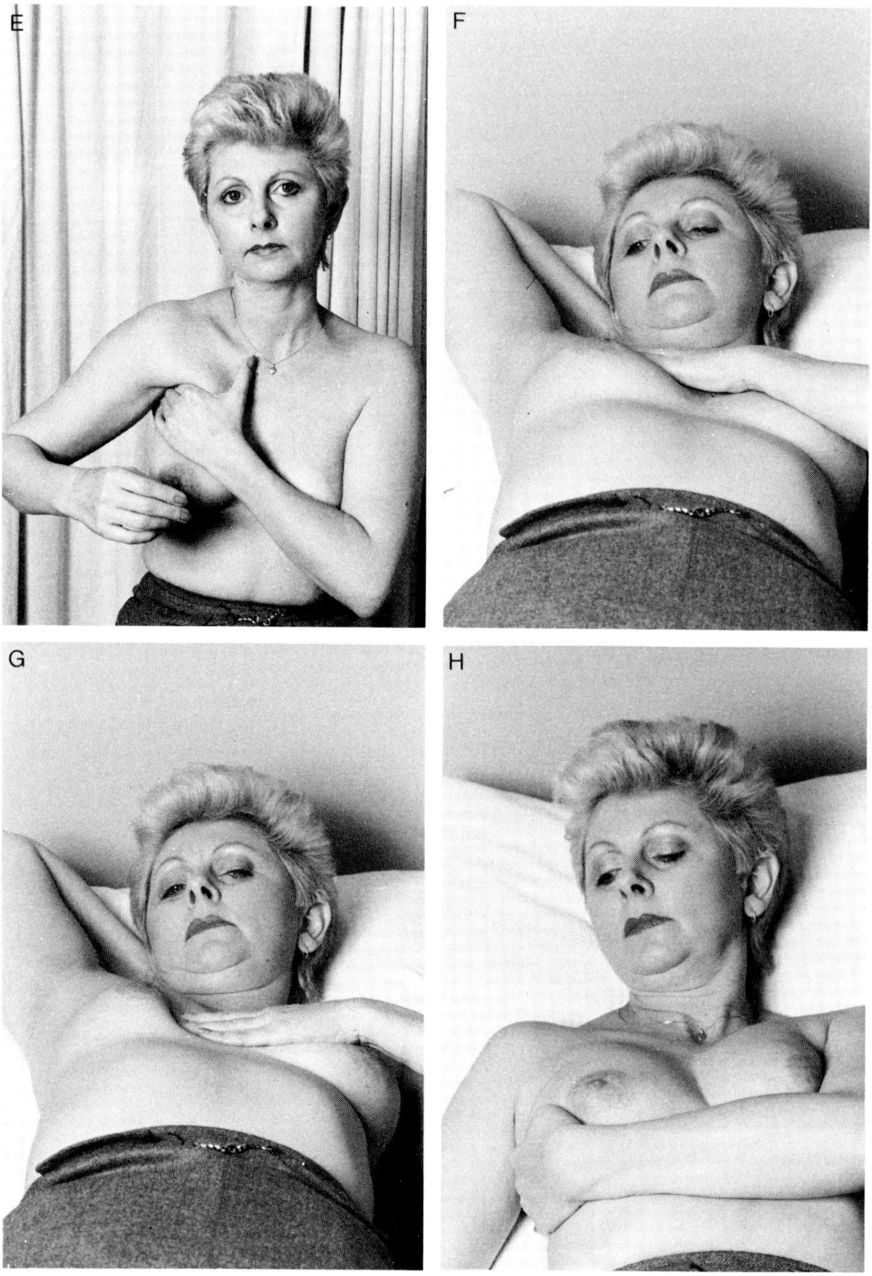

Fig. 16. (*Continued*) (E) Examination of the axillae during BSE. (F) Examination of the upper midportion of the breast, with the subject supine, during BSE. (G) Examination of the inner half of the breast, with the subject supine, during BSE. (H) Examination of the outer half of the breast, with the subject supine, during BSE.

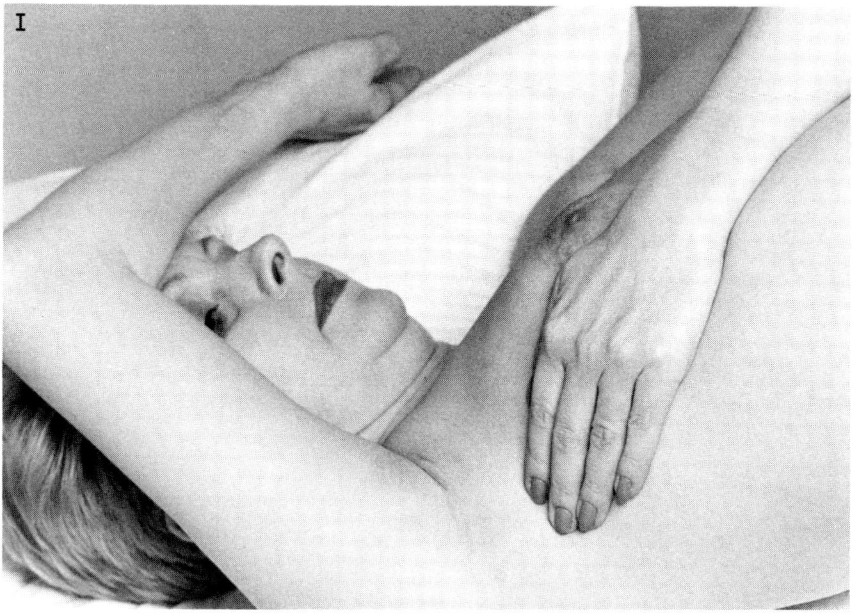

Fig. 16. *(Continued)* (I) Examination of the axillary tail of the breast, with the subject supine, during BSE.

portion of the breast that extends up to the armpit area. This part of the breast is called the *tail*, and is best examined in this slightly turned position.

Repeat the manual procedure for the other breast.

Now examine your breasts again manually while standing in the shower or sitting in the bathtub. The soaped, wet skin enhances the sensitivity of the examination. If your breasts are pendulous, it will be necessary to elevate the breast with one hand while examining it with the other. This is essential so that no areas are missed. Remember always to press the breast against the rib cage.

Great care is needed to perform BSE properly. Do it regularly and without haste. Become aware at the first examination what your breasts look and feel like normally, so that you will know if a change occurs. It is normal to have some lumpiness, especially until you reach menopause, and you should know what is normal for you. Any spontaneous nipple discharge is considered abnormal.

Report to your physician if there are abnormal signs noted on visual examination or changes from the norm on palpation, such as new lumps (especially if they are dominant) and thickenings not noted before.

IV. CONCLUSION

Physical examination of the breast by physicians or physician surrogates (e.g., nurse examiners), performed on a regular (annual) basis, can potentially play an important role in screening for breast cancer. BSE performed on a regular monthly basis also has the potential for reducing mortality from the disease, since it can detect abnormalities developing between regular screens, as has already been demonstrated in the National Breast Screening Study. However, as pointed out by Miller in Chapter 17, the role of both examinations needs careful evaluation.

Such evaluations have to be tempered by the fact that the procedures need to be performed by skilled practitioners, requiring careful teaching and subsequent reinforcement by physicians and nurse examiners, and of the woman herself for BSE. The purpose of this chapter has been to describe appropriate techniques, which although they require attention to detail, are not excessively time-consuming, and fall within the capabilities of physicians and nurses and, for BSE, of women themselves.

REFERENCES

American Cancer Society (1980). Public attitudes toward cancer and cancer tests. *Ca—Cancer J. Clin.* **30,** 92–98.

Baines, C. J. (1983). Editorial. Some thoughts on why women don't do breast self-examination. *Can. Med. Assoc. J.* **128,** 255–256.

Baker, L. H. (1982). Breast cancer detection demonstration project: Five-year summary report. *Ca—Cancer J. Clin.* **32,** 194–225.

Bassett, A. A. (1983). Reply to Mahoney and Csima. Letter to the Editor. *Can Med. Assoc. J.* **128,** 366.

Boyd, N. F., Sutherland, H. J., Fish, E. B., Hiraki, G. Y., Lickley, H. L., and Maurer, V. E. (1981). Prospective evaluation of physical examination of the breast. *Am. J. Surg.* **142,** 331—334.

George, W. D., Sellwood, R. A., Asbury, D., and Hartley, G. (1980). Role of non-medical staff in screening for breast cancer. *Br. Med. J.* **1,** 147–149.

Mahoney, L., and Csima, A. (1982). Efficiency of palpation in clinical detection of breast cancer. *Can Med. Assoc. J.* **127,** 729–730.

Miller, A. B., and Bulbrook, R. D. (1982). Screening, detecting and diagnosis of breast cancer. *Lancet* **1,** 1109–1111.

Moskowitz, M. (1979). Clinical examination of the breasts by non-physicians—a viable screening option? *Cancer* **44,** 311–314.

Moskowitz, M. (1983). Screening for breast cancer: How effective are our tests? A critical review. *Ca—Cancer J. Clin.* **33,** 26–39.

Pennypacker, H. S., Bloom, H. S., Criswell, E. L., Neelakantan, P., Goldstein, M. K., and Stein, G. H. (1982). Toward an effective technology of instruction in breast self-examination. *Int. J. Ment. Health* **11,** 98–116.

Russ, J. E., Winchester, D. P., Scanlon, E. F., and Christ, M. A. (1978). Cytologic findings of aspiration of tumors of the breast. *Surgery, Gynecol. Obstet.* **146,** 407–411.

Salter, D. R., and Bassett, A. A. (1981). Role of needle aspiration in reducing the numbers of unnecessary breast biopsies. *Can J. Surg.* **24,** 311–313.

Shapiro, S. (1977). Evidence on screening for breast cancer from a randomized trial. *Cancer* **39,** 2772–2782.

Strawbridge, H. T. G., Bassett, A. A., and Foldes, I. (1981). Role of cytology in management of lesions of the breast. *Surgery, Gynecol. Obstet.* **152,** 1–7.

Strawbridge, H. T. G., Bassett, A. A., and Foldes, I. (1981). *Surgery, Gynecol. Obstet.* **152,** 1–7.

Zajicek, J., Caspersson, T., Jakobsson, P., Kudynowski, J., Linsk, J., and Us-Krasovec, M. (1970). Cytologic diagnosis of mammary tumors from aspiration biopsy smears. *Acta Cytol.* **14,** 370–376

III

Screening for Specific Cancer Sites

16

Screening for Cancer of the Cervix

ANTHONY B. MILLER

I. Introduction ... 295
II. Natural History ... 296
A. Early Studies ... 296
B. The British Columbia Cohort Study ... 298
C. Dysplasia as a Possible Precursor ... 301
III. Evaluation of the Outcome ... 303
A. Effect of Screening on the Incidence of Cancer of the Cervix ... 303
B. Effect of Screening on Mortality from Cancer of the Cervix ... 306
C. Other Evaluation Approaches ... 311
IV. Risk Groups for Screening ... 312
V. Optimal Screening Schedules ... 313
VI. Research Issue ... 319
VII. Conclusion ... 319
References ... 320

I. INTRODUCTION

In this chapter, I shall concentrate on two different types of studies related to screening for cancer of the cervix. The first is epidemiological studies in which information was sought on the natural history of carcinoma *in situ* and other precursors of clinical invasive cancer. The second is studies of the outcome of screening specifically relating incidence and mortality trends to the intensity of screening in different areas or to comparisons between areas. These observational studies have their own particular difficulties but are the only ones available that enable us to assess the effectiveness of screening in view of the absence of any controlled trials of screening for cancer of the cervix. I shall then consider the appropriate approaches used to determine screening frequency in order to achieve maximal impact with the most efficient use of resources.

ISBN 0-12-496720-5

II. NATURAL HISTORY

A. Early Studies

Screening programs for cancer of the cervix are largely based on the assumption that individuals found to have a confirmed histological diagnosis of dysplasia, carcinoma *in situ,* carcinoma *in situ* with microinvasion, or occult invasive carcinoma of the cervix will progress to clinical invasive carcinoma unless detected and successfully treated. Nevertheless, the idea that carcinoma *in situ* could regress arose once it was appreciated that the cumulative incidence of carcinoma *in situ* exceeded the expected cumulative incidence of clinical invasive carcinoma. Dunn (1953) indicated the importance of determing the proportion of cases of carcinoma *in situ* that were destined to become invasive, the proportion of invasive cervical cancers that began as carcinoma *in situ,* the average duration of carcinoma *in situ,* and the variation around that mean in understanding the natural history of carcinoma of the cervix. Dunn analyzed data derived from screening programs in San Diego County, California (Dunn *et al.*, 1959), and in Shelby County, Memphis, Tennesee (Kashagarian and Dunn, 1970). He produced estimates of the average duration of carcinoma *in situ* of 5 years (Dunn, 1960) 8.1 (Dunn and Martin, 1967) and 11 years (Kashagarian and Dunn, 1970) and, for dysplasia, 3.8 years (Dunn and Martin, 1967). He pointed out the discrepancy in some of these studies between the amount of disease that appeared to be occurring in the area under the curve of age-specific incidence, and suggested that the combination of dysplasia and carcinoma *in situ* exceeded the needs for invasive cancer and that some cancers would terminate in regression (Dunn and Martin, 1967). The maximum incidence of carcinoma *in situ* occurred in women age 25–29, with a decrease to a low level after age 35 (Dunn and Martin, 1967). The incidence of dysplasia rose rapidly and at an earlier age than that of carcinoma *in situ.* Not all new disease developing from a population that has been repeatedly negative cytologically is found in the carcinoma *in situ* stage; 10–15% of the cases of carcinoma of the cervix appear to become invasive early in their development. However, in Memphis, Dunn and Martin (1967) did not find excess rates for intraepithelial cancer, but rather a deficit possibly made up by the beginning of invasive cancer in stages other than the intraepithelial stage.

Barron and Richart (1968) studied the rates of progression from cytological dysplasia to carcinoma *in situ* in 557 American women with abnormal cytology and assessed the general validity of these estimates by comparing them with the prevalence of dysplasia in a cross-sectional study of 11,814 women screened in Barbados, West Indies (Barron and Richart, 1970). Only a small proportion of these women regressed to normal cytology, and the authors estimated that 66% would progress from cytological dysplasia to carcinoma *in situ* over a 10-year follow-up period. In these studies, cytological sampling and diagnosis was used because of the destructive and potentially curative nature of histologic diagnosis.

Barron *et al.* (1978) used data from the Barbados screening program and from British Columbia (Fidler *et al.*, 1968), and compared the observed incidence and prevalence rates for carcinoma *in situ* based on an assumption of no regression of disease. They estimated that the duration of carcinoma *in situ* ranged from 3 to 10 years.

Kasper *et al.* (1970) from Alberta, Canada, analyzed the prevalence and incidence of gynecologic cancer detected cytologically in 175,767 women. They concluded that the generation of new cases of carcinoma *in situ* begins in the 20–24 age groups at a very significant rate and that carcinoma *in situ* develops six times more frequently in age groups under 45 years than in older women. They estimated that in the average case, detectable carcinoma *in situ* was present 8–10 years before the development of the disease.

Coppleson and Brown (1974), using a mathematical modeling approach and data from a number of sources, estimated false-negative error rates for carcinoma *in situ* on initial examination ranging from 20 to 45%, stepping down on subsequent screenings. They could not explain the prevalence of dysplasia and carcinoma *in situ,* and the incidence of invasive cancer determined in cross-sectional data by Bibbo *et al.* (1971), without postulating substantial regression of carcinoma *in situ* to dysplasia (Coppleson and Brown, 1975).

In the Task Force (1976) report on cervical cancer screening in Canada, cross-sectional data from the British Columbia Screening Program were interpreted to suggest a somewhat longer natural history than was suspected previously. However, this interpretation was dependent on an assumption of the progressive nature of the natural history.

The dilemma in interpretation was illustrated by Knox (1973) using computer simulation, which indicated the substantially different impact of screening policies depending on whether a purely progressive or a "dynamic" natural history was postulated. The dynamic natural history modeled by Knox involved two components: the probability that cases of carcinoma *in situ* as well as dysplasia regress, and the probability that a proportion of cases progress to invasive cancer after so short a preclinical phase that any reasonable screening program would be incapable of detecting abnormalities in the stage of dysplasia or carcinoma *in situ*. The second group was postulated from theoretical considerations. If a proportion of lesions regress, and if a number persist unchanged in women without progression, estimates of the mean duration of dysplasia and carcinoma *in situ* must encompass some with a rapid progression to clinically invasive cancer.

This problem is important because if a high proportion of lesions identified by screening would never have progressed if left alone, a substantial effort may be required to identify those women with a high probability of developing progressive disease. Some have postulated two types of cancer of the cervix: those with a slowly progressive preclinical stage with little contribution to eventual mortality, and those with a very rapid preclinical phase with a low probability of detection but a high probability of becoming progressive invasive cancer and ending in death (Ashley, 1966; Bailar, 1961; Pedersen *et al.*, 1971). Without further information on the natural history of the disease, screening programs might be wrongly concentrating on women at the lowest risk of developing disease and allowing those likely to die to slip through.

B. The British Columbia Cohort Study

It was against this background that the British Columbia Cohort Study was designed (Boyes *et al.*, 1982). If there is a wholly progressive natural history from *in situ* carcinoma to clinical invasive carcinoma, the cumulative incidence of preclinical carcinoma should coincide with the sum of the cumulative incidence of invasive carcinoma and the prevalence of preclinical carcinoma. Most previous studies had shown a substantial discrepancy, called by Cochrane the "yawning gap." However, regression is not the only explanation for the gap. Other factors that could explain it include denominator error, and a cohort effect.

Various sources of denominator error affect the calculation of rates of preclinical disease in a screened population. They include problems of identification, such as misspelling of names or change of names following marriage, which result in a failure to identify women as having been previously screened when they return for reexamination. Thus, they do not contribute to the denominator for incidence rates of preclinical disease, but instead falsely appear in the denominator for prevalence. This tends to lower the estimated prevalence and raise the estimated cumulative incidence.

False-negative cytological diagnoses (negative error) have an important effect in increasing the yawning gap, since they result in an estimated prevalence that is lower lower than reality and an increase in the estimated incidence of preclinical carcinoma.

The third factor is a cohort effect. If the incidence of preclinical cancer in younger women is on the increase, rates from young cohorts, which largely contribute to the cumulative incidence of preclinical cancer, result in an artificial gap because the cumulative incidence rates of invasive cancer are largely derived from older cohorts and thus provide a lower expected incidence than might be anticipated in the younger cohorts in the absence of a screening program.

In the British Columbia Cohort Study (Boyes *et al.*, 1982), the two cohorts studied were women born in 1914–1918 and 1929–1933, comprising 52,452 and 66,701 women, respectively, who entered the screening program during the period 1949–1969. These cohorts were selected so that the older ones would approach the maximum incidence of invasive carcinoma and the younger ones would pass the maximum incidence of carcinoma *in situ*.

Considerable effort was devoted to minimizing denominator errors, including corrections for duplication, migration away or into the population, hysterectomies, and deaths from other causes. A cohort effect was not seen, presumably because the younger cohort had reached the age of maximum operation of risk factors for cancer of the cervix before the recent changes in sexual habits that have affected the incidence of carcinoma *in situ* and dysplasia in more recent cohorts.

There are two components of false negatives on cervical cytology. The first, or laboratory component, is the failure to identify an abnormality even though it is present on the smear. In British Columbia, a review of previous smears when abnormalities were detected on second or subsequent examinations enabled us to identify lesions that were present, although initially missed on the first examination.

The second component of false negatives we called the *biological* or *taker error*. This refers to abnormalities that were present at the time the smear was taken but were missed either because cells were not exfoliating at the time of the examination or because the examination was inadequate and cells that were present were not picked up on the smear. An estimate of the size of this component was obtained indirectly by a comparison of incidence rates on reexamination by smear rank and interval. As a result of these combined approaches, we estimated that the proportion of false negatives on initial examination approximated 25%.

One additional difficulty was in dating the actual point of occurrence of an abnormality. A normal approach would be to assume that a lesion occurred in the interval between the last normal smear and the first abnormal one. However, because the number of persons accessioned into the cohorts was growing as the period of observation increased, attribution of event times to the midpoint between a normal and an abnormal observation may be in error. We therefore adopted two approaches to dating, one to the midpoint and the other to the first abnormality.

A further difficulty arose in developing an expectation of rates of invasive cancer in the absence of a screening program. One approach is to use the estimates derived from unscreened women found to have invasive cancer, either without a screening examination or on the first examination, which is often conducted for diagnostic purposes. However, the unscreened proportion of the population became smaller as time went on, and the rates grew progressively out of line with those expected from the rates previously operating in the province—for example, in 1955–1957, before the screening program could have had much impact (Table I). This is probably because high-risk women tend to be less well

TABLE I

Incidence of Invasive Cancer of the Cervix (per 100,000 Women)[a]

Age	British Columbia (1955–1957)	Cohort: unscreened 2	Cohort: unscreened 1
20–24	0.8	1.0	—
25–29	5.6	6.8	—
30–34	9.9	22.7	6.7
35–39	22.7	53.1	20.3
40–44	27.4	—	42.3
45–49	40.2	—	56.5
50–54	45.5	—	141.5

[a] From D. A. Boyes, B. Morrison, E. G. Knox, G. J. Draper, and A. B. Miller, "A cohort study of cervical cancer screening in British Columbia," copyright 1982, Pergamon Press.

screened and thus are selectively concentrated in the unscreened group. We decided to use both sets of clinical invasive cancer rates. Even if the British Columbia rates for 1955–1957 were also too high, this would underestimate the extent to which regression was occurring and thus would be a conservative approach. By whatever approach used, the ratio of the prevalence of carcinoma *in situ* plus the cumulative incidence of clinical invasive cancer to the cumulative incidence of carcinoma *in situ* was less than 1, as expected on the basis of the postulated regression (Table II). We concluded that regression is an important part of the natural history of cancer of the cervix, especially in younger women.

The implication of this conclusion is that we are dealing with a dynamic natural history. With regression occurring, there is always a possibility that identified abnormalities would not have progressed, whereas individuals whose disease happens to be going through a phase of regression, and recurs and progresses subsequently, may not be observed to have an abnormality at the time an examination is conducted. This would tend to increase the requirements for repeat smear examinations, whereas a purely static natural history would substantially reduce these requirements, particularly if one could predict that most abnormalities would have occurred by a certain age. Thus, we now face two conflicting requirements: first, the need to ensure that too many smears are not done, because otherwise we might just be detecting a great deal of disease that would not have progressed; and second, the need to ensure that the important disease does not slip through the screening net.

Whether or not an appreciable proportion of women with dysplasia or carcinoma *in situ* progress rapidly was not apparent from the British Columbia Cohort Study (Boyes *et al.*, 1982), largely because of the short follow-up period

TABLE II

British Columbia Cohort Study: Estimated Accumulated Incidence and Prevalence per 1000 Women for Carcinoma *in Situ* or Worse to Mean Age 53[a]

Accumulated incidence of carcinoma *in situ* or worse dated to the first abnormality	19.25
Accumulated incidence of carcinoma *in situ* or worse dated to the midpoint	24.02
Accumulated incidence of clinical cancer in unscreened women	10.29
Accumulated incidence of clinical cancer in the population of British Columbia, 1955–1957	6.24
Prevalence of carcinoma *in situ* or worse	8.12
Ratio of accumulated incidence of invasive carcinoma plus the prevalence of carcinoma *in situ* or worse to accumulated incidence of carcinoma *in situ* or worse	
Dated to the first abnormality using the unscreened clinical cancer rate	0.96
Dated to the midpoint using the unscreened clinical cancer rate	0.77
Dated to the first abnormality using the clinical cancer rate of British Columbia, 1955–1957	0.75
Dated to the midpoint using the clinical cancer rate of British Columbia, 1955–1957	0.60

[a] From D. A. Boyes, B. Morrison, E. G. Knox, G. J. Draper, and A. B. Miller, "A cohort study of cervical cancer screening in British Columbia," copyright 1982, Pergamon Press.

for the majority of the participants. Fidler *et al.* (1968) reported that 64 cases of clinical invasive carcinoma occurred in screened women during the years 1961–1966, a crude rate of 4.5 per 1000 screened. After the earlier cytological smears of these cases were reviewed, 36 were found to have had false-negative reports. Of the remainder, the time interval from the last negative smear to the diagnosis of clinical invasive carcinoma ranged from 1 to 10 years, with 15 having an interval of less than 4 years. At that time, therefore, it seemed that only a small proportion of cases progressed rapidly. More recently, however, it has been suggested that more rapidly progressive cases may be occurring, especially in younger women (Berkeley *et al.*, 1980). An extension of the British Columbia Cohort Study, already underway, may help to resolve this problem.

C. Dysplasia as a Possible Precursor

There is no unanimity of view as to whether or not dysplasia should be regarded as a precursor of carcinoma *in situ* or whether only certain subgroups, particularly lesions classified as severe dysplasia, should be so regarded. The findings from the British Columbia Cohort Study were related to carcinoma *in situ* or worse, conditional on dysplasia not having been already diagnosed. When we performed analyses for dysplasia or worse, we found that the estimated extent of regression was increased.

Johnson *et al.* (1968) studied 11,340 screenees, of whom 8000 had a repeat examination. They concluded that dysplasia is a precursor of carcinoma *in situ*, the course over 9 years being one of regression and recurrence. They postulated that carcinoma *in situ* develops from dysplasia during a period of recurrence; however, the number of patients they studied who developed carcinoma *in situ* was small.

Stern *et al.* (1977a) determined the cumulative probability of progression from dysplasia to carcinoma *in situ* over a 7-year period. Although the number of persons under observation toward the end of the period was rather small, over 7 years approximately 26% of women with dysplasia progressed to carcinoma *in situ*.

Thomas (1973) conducted a case control study of 324 women with cytological abnormalities and 302 controls drawn at random from those with negative smears in the laboratory. Of the cases, 104 had carcinoma *in situ*, 105 had dysplasia, and 25 had chronic cervicitis. He found that the women with carcinoma *in situ* differed from controls in the prevalence of trichomoniasis, a history of marital instability, and a history of a first child conceived before marriage. The women with dysplasia, however, differed from the controls only in the prevalence of trichomoniasis and in a history of vaginal discharge. Only women with severe dysplasia were epidemiologically similar to those with carcinoma *in situ*. Carcinoma *in situ*, however, appeared to be epidemiologiclly similar to invasive cancer. In a second paper, Thomas and Anderson (1974) suggested that most squamous dysplasia represents a nonspecific reaction of the cervical epithelium to inflammatory agents.

Berget (1975) and Terris *et al.* (1980) also concluded that women with dysplasia did not have the epidemiologic characteristics of women with carcinoma *in situ* and invasive cancer. Harris *et al.* (1980), however, found little difference in the expression of risk factors in patients with carcinoma *in situ* or dysplasia. They suggested that part of the explanation for the different findings in the various studies may be discrepancies in pathologic interpretation and nomenclature.

With a tendency to concentrate on cases of dysplasia with locally directed treatment following colposcopy, we need to know a great deal more about the natural history of these possible precursors of carcinoma *in situ* and of invasive cancer. We are currently collecting data in Toronto to throw light on the natural history of these lesions.

However, in the meantime, it is not desirable to assume that all abnormalities are part of a continuum even though there may be difficulty in adequately distinguishing them. I do not find it helpful to use the concept of cervical intraepithelial neoplasia. All authors should attempt to distinguish dysplasia from carcinoma *in situ* and to grade the severity of dysplasia using reproducible histologic criteria (Task Force, 1982; Alderson *et al.*, 1983).

III. EVALUATION OF THE OUTCOME

A. Effect of Screening on the Incidence of Cancer of the Cervix

A screening program directed to a precursor lesion should have two major effects: it should reduce the incidence of the fully developed symptomatic clinical lesion, and it should reduce mortality from the disease. Assessment of both of these effects involves difficulties, particularly if there appears to be an indication from prescreening data of changing incidence or mortality. In fact, the trends in cervical cancer may be changing in some countries in relation to particular birth cohorts (Adelstein *et al.*, 1971; Hill and Adelstein, 1967), and several countries experienced a reduction in mortality even before screening programs could have shown an effect (Adelstein *et al.*, 1971; Higgins, 1971; Miller 1973). Higgins (1971) failed to find evidence of the rise in mortality from cancer of the cervix in women under 60 years in the United States that had occurred in England and Wales (Hill and Adelstein, 1967). One possible explanation was that screening could have prevented a rise in mortality, since screening was more prevalent in the United States than in the United Kingdom.

Hill *et al.* (1983), after applying a log-linear model to data on the incidence of cancer of the cervix in Alberta, Canada, over the period 1953–1977, were able to separate age, secular, and cohort trends. They demonstrated a substantial reduction in the secular trend index for cancer of the cervix from 1968–1972 to 1973–1977, which was possibly attributable to screening. However, they also noted a substantial rise in the incidence of the disease for cohorts born since 1943, compared to a diminishing trend for cohorts born up to 1933.

A number of attempts have been made to assess changes in incidence in areas subjected to intensive screening. Burns *et al.* (1968) described the Toledo Community Program, initiated in 1947 with follow-up through 1963. More than two-thirds of the women 30 years or more of age in Lucas County, Ohio, were included, comprising 100,257 women with a total of 278,302 examinations. Although the rates of invasive cancer were reduced in this population, the prevalence of the disease on first examination also fell during the time period considered. Thus, it is not clear that the program was wholly responsible for the reduction in invasive cancer rates.

Kim *et al.* (1978) updated the follow-up of this program to 1974. A comparison of rates between 1955–1958 and 1971–1974 in metropolitan Toledo showed a 66% reduction in average annual incidence and a 61% reduction in deaths from cervical cancer. The decrease was more pronounced in women of age 50 or less and was greater in black than in white women.

One of the best-documented programs is that of Christopherson and his colleagues from Louisville, Kentucky. When the rates of invasive cervical cancer in

1963 were compared with those of the precytology period, 1953–1955, a 22.7% reduction was noted (Lundin *et al.*, 1965). The proportion of cases in stage 1 increased, and the cases of invasive cancer that occurred were associated with a low socioeconomic status.

Subsequently, Christopherson *et al.* (1976) reported on morbidity and mortality trends in Louisville over a 21-year period. They showed a rduction in both incidence and mortality rates for cancer of the cervix, with a 70.8% reduction of incidence in women aged 30–39, a 50% reduction of incidence in women aged 40–49, and a 69% reduction of mortality in women aged 50–59. They pointed out the difficulty in assessing the significance of these changes with the decrease in incidence of cancer of the cervix in the United States since 1949 and the almost universal application of cervical cytology screening in urban areas in the United States.

Dickinson *et al.* (1972a) evaluated the effectiveness of cervical cancer screening in Olmstead County, Minnesota, over the period 1955–1967. The incidence of cancer of the cervix had been increasing, but it fell by 40% after 1957. However, this is rather difficult to interpret, as the authors included carcinoma *in situ* in calculating the total incidence. The mortality for cancer of the cervix approximated 5 to 7 per 100,000 before 1960 and fell to 3 per 100,000 after 1960. The authors believed that this was probably due to early detection and treatment since the proportion of women screened who were age 21 or more increased from less than 10% in 1957 to 43% in 1967. Dickinson *et al.* (1972b) also estimated that patients treated during a period of screening gained at least an additional 3.23 years of total life after diagnosis.

In Canada, it was not possible to determine whether part of the observed decrease in the incidence of carcinoma of the cervix was due to screening (Task Force, 1976). A possible acceleration in the rate of decline due to the screening program observed up to 1973 in Saskatchewan was not confirmed by later data (Miller, 1978b).

The available data on the incidence of cancer of the cervix from the cancer registries in Canada were again reviewed by the reconvened task force on cervical cancer screening programs (Task Force, 1982). For each province with data available up to 1977, the rate of decline in incidence in women aged less than 65 had slowed. In some provinces, there was an indication of an increase in incidence in women aged 20–34 and/or 35–64. In recent years, the reported incidence of carcinoma *in situ* has also increased dramatically. An example of these trends is presented for Alberta in Fig. 1.

There can be major difficulties in interpreting incidence data from cancer registries. A cancer registry may not be able to distinguish cases diagnosed on screening from those that presented clinically, and cases of carcinoma *in situ* may be registered as invasive if the pathology report on which registrations are often based is not sufficiently specific. Although, with increasing *in situ* rates,

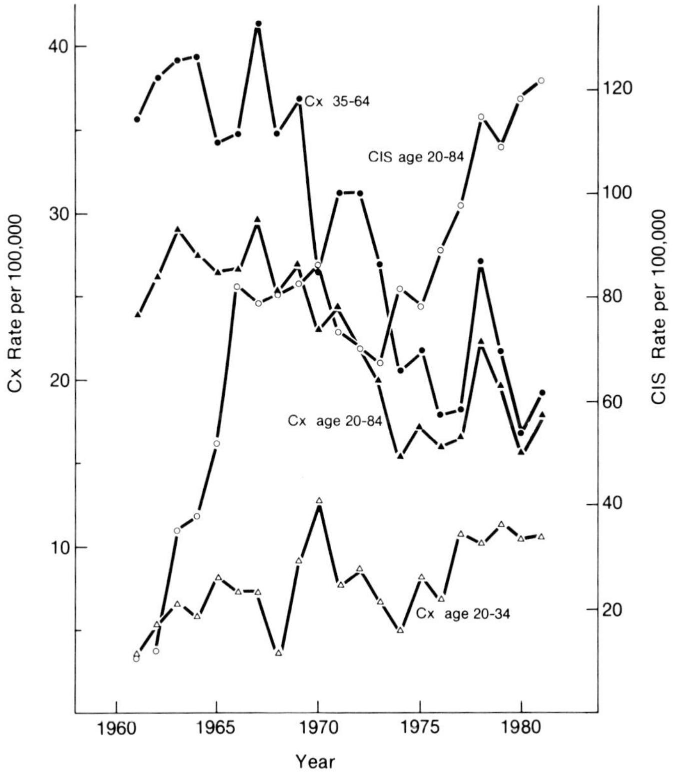

Fig. 1. Incidence of cancer of the cervix (cx) and of carcinoma *in situ* of the cervix (CIS) in Alberta, 1961–1981, age-standardized rates per 100,000.

recent changes in reported incidence could be partly due to such artifacts, it is difficult to explain all changes on such a basis, especially in well-screened areas such as Alberta and British Columbia, where, with continuation of screening, the incidence of abnormalities discovered on screening should be expected to fall rather than rise.

However, an additional factor has entered into the picture with the introduction of colposcopy on a provincial basis (Task Force, 1982). The multiple superficial biopsy specimens obtained on colposcopy may be difficult to interpret, and changes that might have been previously signed out as less advanced than carcinoma *in situ,* may now be so reported.

It is possible that were it not for the screening program in Canada, the incidence of invasive cancer would have risen. The rising registrations of carcinoma *in situ* might be regarded as supporting this contention. If, in the absence of screening, the incidence of invasive cancer were now rising, it might be anticipated that with this rise, there would be a rise in the absolute number (although not necessarily in the proportion) of those with rapidly progressive disease not likely to be detected in time to be preempted by screening. Hence, an increase in their number would be particularly noticeable because the proportion of these cases would be much greater in the presence of an effective screening program. Somewhat paradoxically, therefore, reports on a greater proportion of these lesions (e.g., Berkeley *et al.*, 1980) do *not* indicate that the screening program is ineffective in preventing a large majority of cases from progressing.

Perhaps the most convincing evidence of the effectiveness of screening programs arises from a comparison of trends in incidence between Norway and Denmark, Sweden, Finland, and Iceland (Hakama, 1982). Only Norway has so far failed to introduce a population screening program for cancer of the cervix, and no reduction in incidence has been noted. All of the other Nordic countries have introduced population screening programs, and all show a reduction in incidence. Previously, Denmark showed the highest incidence of cancer of the cervix, with the other four countries showing similar but much lower levels. This differential is believed to be due to a corresponding differential in the prevalence of risk factors for cancer of the cervix in the population. Now Norway has the same incidence as previously high-incidence Denmark. Studies in Denmark show that a reduction in incidence is greatest in areas with organized screening programs (Lynge, 1983).

B. Effect of Screening on Mortality from Cancer of the Cervix

Even if an effect of screening on incidence had been established, it would be necessary to be certain that the program had an effect on mortality. Not only is mortality the more important measure, but is is possible that lesions identified in screening programs are relatively benign biologically and unlikely to result in death, whereas those missed do result in death.

In Canada, there have been a number of attempts to assess trends in mortality from cancer of the uterus, either in comparisons within the country or with England and Wales (Ahluwalia and Doll, 1968; Sellers and McLerie, 1973). Most suggested that screening had little effect, although Kinlen and Doll (1973), who assessed age-specific mortality trends from 1955–1956 to 1970–1971 in British Columbia, Ontario, and the rest of Canada, noted that at ages 45–64 the mortality had declined more in British Columbia than in the rest of Canada. They suggested this might have been partially due to different hysterectomy rates in British Columbia compared to the rest of the country, as well as to screening.

Miller *et al.* (1976) correlated the extent of screening and the fall in mortality at the provincial and county or census district levels. We evaluated mortality from total uterine cancer in view of differences in death certification practices in varying parts of the country and a tendency toward progressive reduction in the proportion of cases certified to uterus unspecified. Having demonstrated a correlation at both levels, we endeavored to explain this by introducing, in a multivariate analysis, indices of income, education, housing, and sanitation from the 1961 and 1971 censuses that might be indirectly associated with mortality from cancer of the cervix. We were able to demonstrate a significant effect of the intensity of screening on the fall of mortality after taking account of these other factors.

Christopherson *et al.* (1970) compared death rates for Jefferson County with the rest of Kentucky over the period 1953–1967. The analysis indicated a reduction in death rates from cancer of the cervix and total uterine cancer that was significant in Jefferson County but not for the rest of Kentucky. The slopes were also significantly different.

Cramer (1974) also reported a significant positive correlation between the rate of cytologic screening determined from national surveys of cytologic facilities during the period 1953–1968 and the amount of decrease in morbidity and mortality from cervical cancer in various parts of the United States over the period 1950–1954 to 1965–1969. Gardner and Lyon (1977) reevaluated mortality trends in the United States and concluded that a causal association of cytologic screening with decreasing mortality and decreasing incidence of invasive cervical cancer could not be established using current data. However, this conclusion was drawn after fitting a quadratic curve for the decline in mortality for 1946–1955 and showing that this coincided with the subsequent decline. It is not clear, however, why they chose this particular curve or whether they evaluated alternative fits of the data prior to 1955. It seems possible that a simple linear regression might have been appropriate and that an alternative conclusion, namely, that there had been an acceleration in reduction in mortality attributable to screening, could have been drawn.

One explanation for mortality decrease in relation to screening programs could be the influence of the number and types of hysterectomies performed. Stern *et al.* (1977b) reported a shift from subtotal to total hysterectomies, thus raising the possibility that some of the mortality fall may be due to the fact that in earlier years a higher proportion of women retained the cervix. Data from British Columbia show that the proportion of subtotal hysterectomies dropped from 4.7% of 2490 hysterectomies in 1961 to 0.5% of 7580 hysterectomies in 1972. Thus, the proportion of subtotal hysterectomies in earlier years was low, and most of the acceleration in the number of hysterectomies has occurred in recent years. It therefore seems unlikely that this effect could have made more than a minor contribution to the mortality fall from cancer of the uterus in the decade 1961–1971. We were able, however, to obtain data at the provincial level on hysterectomies performed over the time period 1969–1976. Using earlier data from British Columbia and elsewhere, we determined the possible range of increase in the prevalence of hysterectomies over the preceding few decades and then corrected the observed reductions in mortality from women at risk to uteri at risk (Miller *et al.*, 1981). Figure 2 indicates the minor effect of this correction on trends of mortality from total uterine cancer, cancer of the cervix, and cancer of the endometrium in women aged 30–64. We incorporated this correction for hysterectomies in our analysis of the correlation of mortality falls from 1960–1962 to 1970–1972 at the provincial level with the intensity of screening. There was no evidence that correcting for the hysterectomy effect abolished the significant association between reduction in mortality and the intensity of screening that we reported in 1976. Indeed, if anything, the strength of the correlation in-

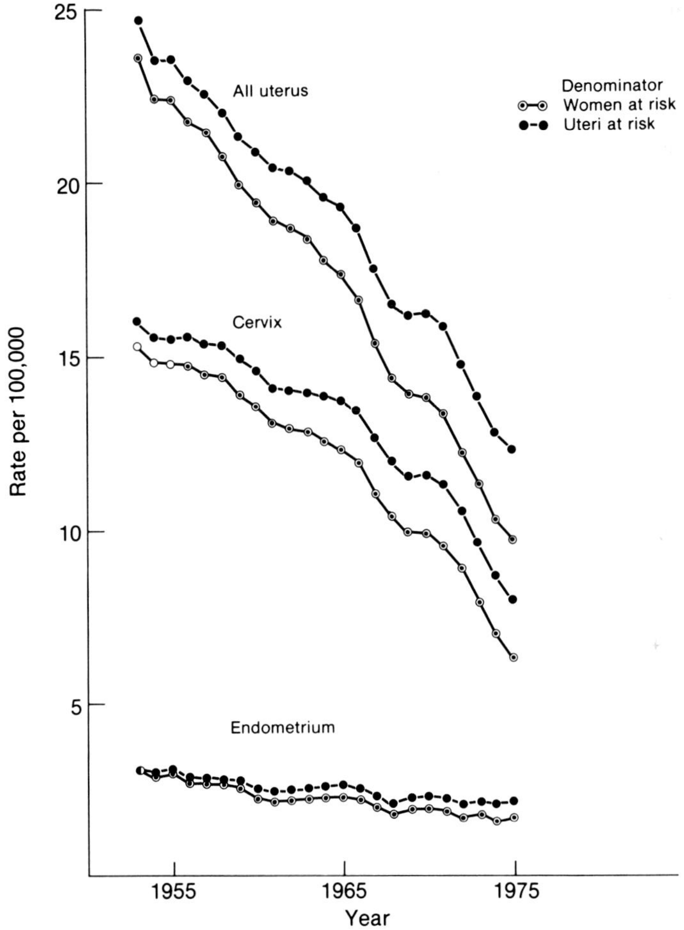

Fig. 2. Mortality from carcinoma of the uterus (all sites combined), cervix, and endometrium in Canada, 1952–1954 to 1974–1976. Three-year moving averages, women aged 30–64, aged-standardized rates per 100,000 with corrections for hysterectomies.

creased. This is perhaps not surprising, since women who have hysterectomies for nonmalignant conditions are more likely to be of higher socioeconomic status than the general population. Thus, they are probably at lower risk of death from cancer of the cervix than the general population.

Nevertheless, when the analysis of screening with reduction in mortality was extended to 1974–1976, the correlation disappeared. Part of the difficulty could be that correlation analysis may be an insufficiently powerful tool to detect small nonlinear changes in mortality resulting from increases in screening intensity. However, there are other explanations. Most plausible is that once population screening intensity reaches a certain level, further increases lead only to a marginal further reduction in mortality. This may reflect the fact that in most programs, an increase in the number of examinations is largely due to repeat smears of the same women rather than to initial examinations of previously unscreened women, many of whom will be at high risk of the disease.

However, it is the unscreened women who tend to be at highest risk in whom most of the mortality from the disease occurs. Hakama (1980) has pointed out that in Finland, with mass screening organized on a 5-year basis, it had been estimated that about 20% of frankly invasive cases had a preinvasive stage shorter than the time lag between the repeated screenings. Although part of this "escape from curability" could have been due to false-negative smears on first examination, the evidence from Finland, combined with data on attendance rates, enabled Hakama to estimate a final 60% reduction in the incidence of frankly invasive cancer, a prediction that was verified by the observed trends in cervical cancer in Finland. Hence, in Canada, within the context of the screening program as applied up to 1976, further reduction in mortality could possibly not have been expected.

Other possible explanations for the disappearance of the association between intensity of screening and mortality falls in Canada include an increase in mortality due to changes in the incidence of the disease commented on previously, especially in the young, a natural history of the preinvasive phases less amenable to influence by screening than had been assumed, and a reduction in the overall quality of detection by cervical cytology laboratories secondary to the increased load of largely repetitive normal examinations.

It is not possible, on the basis of the present evidence, to distinguish between these various explanations. All of them may contribute in part. However, the analysis of Miller *et al.* (1981) was not regarded by the Task Force (1982) as a justification for any relaxation of endeavors to control cancer of the cervix through screening using cervical cytology. Nevertheless, they emphasized the necessity to ensure that screening programs are conducted with adequate attention to screening at-risk women who have never been screened and on quality control in cytology laboratories.

The trends in mortality for women aged 20–34, 35–64, and 20-84 (standardized for age, but without correction for hysterectomies performed) from 1952 to 1982 for Canada are shown in Fig. 3. It is apparent that the reduction in mortality may have slowed from about 1975. Thus, it is possible that with changing sexual practices and a rising incidence of carcinoma *in situ* and dysplasia in younger people, were it not for cervical cancer screening programs, mortality from cancer of the uterus might begin to rise rather than remain static or continue to fall.

Several reports on the effectiveness of screening for cancer of the cervix have appeared from Europe. In Britain, MacGregor and Teper (1978) continue to report reduced mortality in Aberdeen compared to other areas of the United Kingdom. Yule (1978), however, commented on the increasing mortality from cancer of the cervix in women aged less than 35 in England and Wales in spite of screening programs that appear to concentrate on this age group. Draper (1982) noted that in England and Wales, the mortality rate in the 25–34 age group more than doubled from 11 per million in 1968–1970 to 27 per million in 1978–1980.

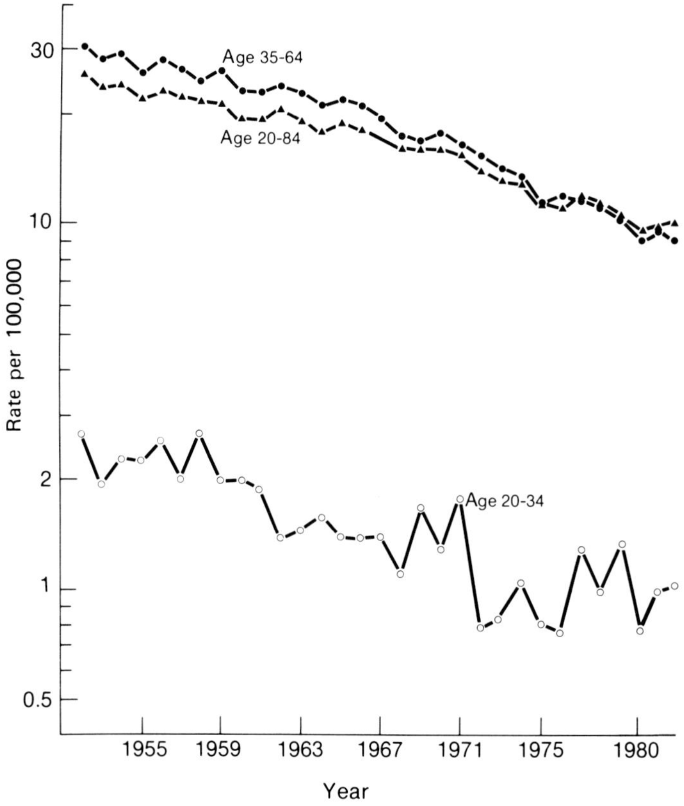

Fig. 3. Mortality from carcinoma of the uterus (all sites combined), Canada, 1952–1982, age-standardized rates per 100,000.

Draper and Cook (1983) and Parkin *et al.* (1985) pointed out that there continues to be evidence of marked cohort effects in the patterns of cervical cancer rates in England and Wales, making it difficult to identify an effect of screening. Nevertheless, it seems possible that some of the reduction in mortality at ages over 35 can be attributed to screening, and that screening may have resulted in a reduction in clinical cancer between the ages of 25 and 54. In the Nordic countries, reductions in mortality have been reported from Iceland (Johannesson *et al.*, 1978) and Finland (Hakama, 1978), which appear very likely to be consequential on the rapid impact of screening in these countries.

C. Other Evaluation Approaches

Clarke and Anderson (1979) evaluated screening by performing a case-control study of Toronto area residents aged 20–69 with newly diagnosed invasive cervical cancer. They interviewed 212 of 323 eligible patients ascertained and five controls per case matched within a 10-year age bracket and by neighborhood. They sought information on the Pap smear history as recalled by the woman in the 5 years preceding the diagnosis or interview, and for a sizeable proportion of those interviewed, they were able to validate this information through physicians' records. They found that 68% of the patients had a history of no screening Pap smears in the preceding 5 years compared to 44% of the controls, for a relative risk of 2.7. Control for age, income, education, and age at first intercourse did not appreciably change the relative risk. Controlling for other risk factors (marital history, smoking habits, employment status, access to medical care), either alone or in a multiple regression analysis, also failed to reduce the relative risk to nonsignificant levels. The authors concluded that the Pap smear is an effective screening procedure for invasive cervical cancer.

On aspect of this study is relevant to the application of cervical cytology. A total of 73% of the patients and 88% of the controls had visited a physician in the 5 years before the year of diagnosis, but only 44% of the patients had been screened compared to 63% of the controls. Thus, 32% of all of the interviewees had had at least one physician visit during the 5 years before the diagnosis of invasive cancer of the cervix, and the opportunity had *not* been taken to obtain a pap smear.

This was the first time that the case-control approach has been used to evaluate cervical cancer screening. Possibly the reason was concern over the almost certain socioeconomic status difference between the patients and controls and a possible inability to take note of this in the analysis, avoided by Clarke and Anderson by the collection of multiple matched controls.

The appropriateness of the case selection for this study was subsequently questioned (Morrison, 1982). In response, although admitting that their approach, in permitting the inclusion of asymptomatic screen-detected cases, may have reduced their estimate of the protective effect of screening, Clarke and Anderson (1983) pointed to the logistic difficulties of obtaining the screening histories of patients with advanced disease, otherwise the preferable group (Morrison, 1983).

Case-control studies evaluating screening for cancer of the cervix have also been conducted in Milan and Geneva (Berrino *et al.*, 1984). In general, these studies produced results similar to those of the Toronto study in showing the protective effect of the Pap smear.

The selection of both cases and controls for a case-control study designed to evaluate the effect of a screening program is further discussed in Chapter 1.

IV. RISK GROUPS FOR SCREENING

The possibility of identifying high-risk groups on whom screening should be concentrated is discussed by Hakama in Chapter 4. However, for cancer of the cervix, it is possible to identify a group of women who do *not* need to be screened. The two Canadian task forces (1976, 1982) decided that the female population can be classified into two different groups:

1. The group that is not at risk and should not be included in a screening program for cancer of the cervix.
   a. Women who have never had sexual activity.
   b. Women over 60 who have been screened in the past and have been found continuously negative. A woman over 60 who has been sexually active but has never been screened, however, should enter the screening program.
   c. Women who have had a hysterectomy for benign disease, with complete removal of the cervical epithelium.
2. The group at risk for cancer of the cervix.
   Women over 18 and under 60 who are or have been sexually active.

In the 1976 report, the Task Force identified a high-risk subgroup consisting of women with early sexual activity and women with multiple sexual partners. This subgroup also included women whose husband or other regular or only sexual partner had had multiple sexual partners. In the 1982 report, however, the Task Force recognized that there were questions as to how, in clinical practice women at high risk can be identified. Further, no data are available to indicate that women in the high-risk subgroup have a more rapid rate of progression from dysplasia or carcinoma *in situ* to invasive cancer (and death) than women at risk who develop the disease. Hence, selective screening based on the high-risk/at-risk distinction has only limited applicability.

The Task Force (1982) noted that there is a practical point that applies in the 1980s. The majority of women born from 1955 on can now be regarded as falling in the high-risk subgroup. Therefore, the policies on age at first screening and frequency of rescreening that should be applied to such women should be designed for all at-risk women, without subcategorization by degree of risk.

There is as yet no firm evidence that taking oral contraceptives places a woman in a special risk category, since oral contraceptives themselves do not increase the risk of developing cervical cancer (Miller and Rawls, 1981).

However, Vessey *et al.* (1983) reported a possible adverse effect of the pill in causing neoplasia of the cervix uteri. This was based on a 10-year follow-up of 6838 parous women who entered the Oxford Family Planning Association contraceptive study while using oral contraceptives (OC) and 3154 parous women who entered the study while using an intrauterine device (IUD). There were no invasive cancers of the cervix detected in the IUD group but 13 in the OC group, of whom 9 had more than 6 years' use of the pill. There were no major differences in the frequency of detection of precursors of cancer of the cervix according to the total duration of contraceptive use in the IUD group, but there was a significant increase in the detection rate with increasing duration of oral contraceptive use in the OC group. The women with invasive cancer detected following an abnormal Pap smear appeared to do well, but two deaths occurred in women diagnosed with symptoms, one of whom apparently had never been screened.

This study is somewhat difficult to interpret, since it was not possible to take adequate note of possible differences in sexual activity between the two groups, especially risk factors for the development of cancer of the cervix such as age at first intercourse. Further, the major reason for the difference in invasive cancer incidence is a deficiency of cases of invasive cancer in the IUD group. It is possible that the IUD group might have had delayed onset of sexual activity, since the authors had defined these women as never having used oral contraceptives, yet IUDs are usually not prescribed to women before the first pregnancy. Less than normal sexual activity could possibly explain the absence of invasive cancer in the IUD group; another reason, other than chance, could be that they were particularly well screened, having had regular cervical cytology. That they were screened is shown by the fact that they did not have a lower frequency of smears taken in the clinics than the OC group.

The authors recommended that women who have had more than 4 years of oral contraceptive use should have cervical smears regularly. This recommendation is appropriate for all at-risk women, including those who are on oral contraceptives or who have a past history or oral contraceptive use.

V. OPTIMAL SCREENING SCHEDULES

The Task Force (1976) recommended that a woman should enter a screening program when she became sexually active or at the age of 18, whichever is later, should have a repeat smear at an interval of 1 year, 3-yearly smears to age 35, and 5-yearly smears thereafter to age 60, always providing such smears are satisfactory and without significant atypia.

This proved to be one of the most controversial of all the Task Force's recommendations, although it was not greatly out of line with the practice in Europe. Thus, in the Nordic countries, mass screening programs have been introduced on a 4- or 5-yearly basis. In Britain, the recommendation of the Ministry of Health is to initiate screening at the age of 35 and continue it every 5 years up to the age of 70. Spriggs and Husain (1977) recommended initial screening at the age of 25 if resources permit, and stated that rescreening should occur initially every 5 years and then every 3 years from the age of 35.

A working party of the Department of Health and Social Security committee on gynecological cytology recommended a revised policy for England and Wales (Draper, 1982). They proposed an immediate publicity campaign to encourage all women aged 35 and over who had never had a cervical smear to attend for screening. They also recommended scheduled population screening, with all women invited to attend for smears to be taken at ages 35, 40, 45, 50, 55, 60, and 65. No further smears needed to be taken by women over age 65 who had had at least two recent negative smears (e.g., at ages 60 and 65) and who have never had a positive or doubtful smear. For younger women, ad hoc screening was recommended using attendance for other forms of medical care (especially for pregnancy, family planning, etc.). In practice, however, only two tests under the age of 35 were recommended, at ages 22 and 30.

Clearly, in making these recommendations, the working party was concerned about the high cost of screening women, especially at younger ages, with relatively minimal return. Many Pap smears are being taken in Britain in younger women, although most are in women at relatively low risk of the disease. The rising mortality rate in young women indicates a failure of the existing program to reach those at high risk of the disease. The working party therefore sought to redistribute the effort in the hope that the total population could be covered without any increase in resources.

In the United States, the American Cancer Society (1980) recommended 3-yearly screening starting after the onset of sexual activity. This recommendation was largely based on a mathematical model developed by Eddy (1980). The American Cancer Society's recommendation proved possibly even more controversial than the Canadian one. A statement by the International Academy of Cytology, criticizing the recommendation, defended annual Pap smears on the basis of its value in bringing in women for other gynecologic examinations, including a breast examination, the difficulty of identifying high-risk women, and the problems of sample preparation and quality control in laboratories. These issues were debated in a National Institutes of Health (NIH) Consensus Development Conference on Screening for Cancer of the Cervix. The report of the panel

(National Institutes of Health, 1980) recommended a 1- to 3-year frequency, presumably depending on the assessment by a woman's physician of her degree of risk and of the available evidence on frequency. However, it was accompanied by a minority report by Neuhauser, who argued for a reduced frequency on economic grounds.

The concern that moving from an annual Pap smear to a less frequent one would prevent women from having annual pelvic examinations is a paradoxical reversal of the philosophy that should underlie the application of screening tests. There is no evidence that annual pelvic examinations have made any impact on mortality from, for example, endometrial or ovarian carcinoma. It seems extremely unlikely that these examinations, even if performed by skilled gynecologists, would have much of an impact. Thus, what should be challenged is the concept of an annual pelvic examination, not the concept of a 3- or 5-yearly Pap smear.

The 1982 Canadian Task Force recognized that there was some evidence that physicians had not yet accepted the Task Force (1976) recommendations on frequency (Kassirer, 1980). They approached the reexamination of optimum screening schedules largely by an assessment of mathematical models of cancer screening, particularly through the application of inferences on natural history derived from the British Columbia Cohort Study (Boyes *et al.*, 1982) and Canadian trends in incidence and mortality to the model of Knox (1973). Full details of these simulations were given in Yu *et al.* (1982).

In this application of the model, a dynamic natural history involving regression of carcinoma *in situ* was assumed, but the effect of a component of the disease too rapid for the preinvasive lesions to be detectable in a screening program was evaluated independently. Strategies were evaluated on the basis of three alternative natural histories: one based on the incidence of invasive carcinoma in British Columbia in 1955–1957 and the mortality from cancer of the uterus in Canada in 1955; one based on a 5-year advancement and a doubling of the age-specific rates of onset of carcinoma *in situ* or worse and a 50% increase in the lifetime cumulative incidence and mortality over that previously used; and one based on a further doubling of the age-specific onset rates of carcinoma *in situ* or worse, with cessation of onset after age 35 and with more rapid progression to invasive cancer but no change in the other input parameters. Regression terms and hysterectomy rates for nonmalignant disease derived from Miller *et al.* (1981) were also incorporated. In practice, conclusions on ages of onset and cessation and frequency of screening did not differ using the first two natural histories. Where these conclusions should be modified for the third (younger and more rapidly progressive) natural history, comments can be found below.

The marginal return from increasing numbers of tests in a woman's lifetime becomes less and less. Lacking any valid method to distinguish adequately the women destined to develop and die from invasive cancer of the cervix from those who will develop curable invasive cancer or never develop disease, it becomes a matter of judgment as to how many resources should be invested. In the judgment of the Task Force (1982), programs should be designed that are capable of preventing at least 90% of mortality from the disease.

The results of the analyses of Yu *et al.* (1982) are summarized in Table III. Our conclusions on screening the at-risk woman were as follows:

1. As screening intensity increases, the marginal yield from additional tests is reduced. Optimal mortality reduction follows 9 or 10 tests applied at appropriate ages, although additional tests will result in further mortality reduction.
2. The optimum age to initiate screening is 25.
3. No gain follows from a repeat examination after 1 year, providing the first smear occurs no later than age 27.
4. Three-yearly examinations are appropriate up to age 40.
5. From age 40 on, 5-yearly examinations will suffice. However, if resources are available, 3-yearly examinations will provide additional benefit.

TABLE III

Summary of the Results of Computer Simulation of Screening Programs[a]

Screening schedule					
Onset age	Frequency	End age	Total tests	Mortality per 10,000	Reduction (%)
At-risk women					
None			0	108.3	—
28	3, 5 yearly[b]	55	8	9.4	91
25	3, 5 yearly[b]	60	10	7.1	93
22	3, 5 yearly[b]	65	12	6.4	94
20	3, 5 yearly[c]	60	11	7.8	93
25	3 yearly	59	12	5.4	95
25	1, 2 yearly[d]	61	22	1.7	98
High-risk women					
None			0	132.7	—
25	3, 5 yearly[b]	60	10	28.6	78
20	3, 5 yearly[c]	60	11	11.0	92
20	3 yearly	53	12	9.2	93
25	1, 5 yearly[c]	60	16	3.1	98
20	1, 5 yearly[c]	60	21	1.3	99
20	1, 3 yearly[c]	60	24	1.1	99

[a] From Yu *et al.* (1982).
[b] Change frequency at age 40.
[c] Change frequency at age 35.
[d] Change frequency at age 31.

6. Screening examinations need not be given after the age of 60 providing the woman has been previously screened.

7. If a screening examination is missed on a 3-yearly schedule, the woman should be called in for an examination as soon as possible.

8. If population acceptance falls below 80%, every effort should be made to correct this situation. This is more effective than more frequent screening at a lower acceptance level. (This conclusion was based on a simulated assumption that the distribution of level of acceptance is random. Since this is certainly not so, the conclusion that every effort should be made to bring in and maintain women in screening programs is reinforced.)

9. If the sensitivity of the screening test falls below 75%, it is more effective to rectify this situation than to attempt to compensate by a greater screening frequency.

When the younger and more progressive natural history was used for the simulations (an attempt to model the high-risk subgroup of women), our conclusions were as follows:

1. The optimal age for starting screening is 20.

2. A screening frequency of 3-yearly examinations, changing at age 35 to 5-yearly and continuing to age 60, can be regarded as satisfactory, but if resources permit, further benefit is obtained from annual examinations up to the age of 35.

3. The conclusions on population acceptance and sensitivity of the test were unchanged.

It is relevant that in an analysis of the duration of protection provided by a negative cervical cytological examination using data derived from the study of Clarke and Anderson (1979), it was apparent that maximum protection is provided by a negative smear for 1 year, somewhat less for negative smears after 1–5 years, and little or none after 5 years (E. A. Clarke and G. Eyssen, personal communication, 1981). Similar conclusions were derived from other case-control studies (Berrino *et al.*, 1984).

The Task Force (1982) interpreted the above considerations as reinforcing the general validity of their previous recommendations. Canadian women aged 35 years or more have, in general, entered screening programs and should require no more than 5 yearly screening. However, younger women belong to high-risk birth cohorts, and therefore annual screening is justifiable until age 35.

The Task Force (1982) emphasized that their recommendations on screening frequency over the age of 35 were based on the availability of appropriate registries to ensure that these recommendations are not translated into less frequent schedules by default. They require the availability of physicians or others who know how to take adequate smears and skilled cytological assessment in laboratories with adequate quality control programs. They also apply only to women who remain free from abnormal cytology indicating epithelial atypia. Whenever such changes are detected on a Pap smear, schedules of repeat examination should be dictated by the requirements of surveillance, diagnosis, treatment, and adequate follow-up of identified abnormalities.

In considering these revised recommendations, it is important to bear in mind that the Task Force (1982) was concerned that indications of a changing epidemiologic situation with an increase in the incidence of preinvasive lesions in young women in Canada and possibly of invasive cancer, and with the absence of a dramatic impact of their earlier recommendations on reduction in the frequency of screening, should not result over the next decade in an unacceptable increase in the incidence and mortality from cancer of the cervix. However, the fact remains that the Task Force may have been overcautious and that its recommendations on frequency could result in a concentration of resources on the wrong segment of the population. Table 3 indicates that a relatively modest investment in repeat smears, conducted as recommended earlier (Task Force, 1976) on a 3-year schedule in younger women, would result in approximately a 90% reduction in mortality even when a high-risk natural history is simulated. However, it is also necessary to recognize that the model assumed an 80% population coverage and that the 20% lack of compliance was random in the population. This we know not to be the case. It is this consistent failure of 20% of the population, often representing high-risk women, to enter screening programs that presumably explains why no country, even with intense endeavors, has yet achieved a 90% reduction in mortality. Much has been achieved, for example, in Finland using an organized approach to screening, reducing the proportion of the population who fail to attend by means of postal invitation letters. Letters of this type are feasible in Finland because of the population register, but they are also possible because the Finnish Cancer Society has accepted responsibility for sending them. The recommendations of the Task Force (1982) on the necessity of follow-up systems, coupled with invitations to women with negative smears to reattend for screening, would enable Canada to move toward the organized program approach that has been so successful in Finland. In Canada, within each province, health care insurance schemes basically provide sufficient identification information on all women in the province to permit an organized approach to invitations to attend for screening, whether or not the women have already entered the program. Many other countries have similar facilities, and such an approach has been advocated in the United Kingdom (Draper, 1982). Even though such registries would require an injection of resources, it seems likely that the total cost of a registry-based approach, with periodic screening more in keeping with reality such as 3-yearly examinations, would achieve the same or greater benefits than have yet been achieved in Canada at a substantially lesser cost than would follow if the recommendations of the Task Force (1982) were applied over the whole population.

In order to achieve this, it would be necessary to reassure the medical profession, and women, that registration schemes can be run with appropriate preservation of confidentiality. In this respect, the Task Force (1982) desires to recommend schedules that would be appropriate to all women, implicitly recognized the undesirability of attempting to identify risk categories of women in a central registry. What an organized program is capable of achieving, however, is a system to ensure that women attend at the appropriate schedule for those of average risk. If a woman's physician or the woman herself, through knowledge of her risk characteristics, decides that a more frequent schedule is appropriate, then it would be up to them to take the necessary steps to attain it.

VI. RESEARCH ISSUE

A research issue of the highest priority is the evaluation of different strategies for ensuring that women enter screening programs. It is necessary not only to determine the behavioral barriers to entrance, but also the mechanisms needed to overcome them. An appropriate comparison of strategies that might be developed would be with indirect approaches for bringing women into Pap smear programs. It is well recognized that most women at risk for cancer of the cervix do have physician contacts for other purposes. It is not yet clear whether an approach based on utilizing such physician contacts would be as efficient as or possibly even more efficient than direct approaches to the woman based on overcoming behavioral barriers. Such a study should be conducted in different racial and socioeconomic groups and might have as an endpoint the proportion of the test populations that have had, for example, their first Pap smear by age 25 or two Pap smears by age 30. It would have to be based on an area where it is possible to link the records of identified population groups with laboratories providing the necessary expertise and with appropriate strategies in place for follow-up. Since longer-term endpoints such as the reduction of invasive cancer incidence would be of interest, such a study should probably be based on an area with an ongoing efficient cancer registry.

VII. CONCLUSION

In conclusion, the available evidence supports a role for screening in the reduction of both morbidity and mortality from cancer of the cervix. However, it is still not clear whether deficiencies in the application of the process, or a problem that is less tractable than has been thought to exist up to now accounts for the failure of the approach to abolish mortality from cancer of the cervix in the areas in which it has been applied. If a proportion of the cases are not amenable to detection by screening because the women do not develop detectable preclinical disease, we need to recognize their existence, if only to ensure that overenthusiastic expectations do not lead us to such frequent (and unnecessary) rescreening as to make the whole process uneconomic.

REFERENCES

Adelstein, A. M., Hill, G. B., and Maung, L. (1971). Mortality from cancer of the uterus. An international cohort study. *Br. J. Prev. Soc. Med.* **25,** 186–191.

Ahluwalia, H. S., and Doll, R. (1968). Mortality from cancer of the cervix in British Columbia and other parts of Canada. *Br. J. Prev. Soc. Med.* **22,** 161–164.

Alderson, M., Correa, P., Ford, J., Jensen, O. M., Kupka, K., Miller, A. B., Muir C. S., Nectou, J., Waterhouse, J. A., and Young, J. L. (1983). Cervical intra epithelial neoplasia. *Lancet* **1,** 1166.

American Cancer Society (1980). ACS report on the cancer-related health check-up. *Ca—Cancer J. Clin.* **30,** 194–240.

Ashley, D. J. B. (1966). Evidence for the existence of two forms of cervical carcinoma. *J. Obstet. Gynaecol. Br. Commonw.* **73,** 382–389.

Bailar, J. C. (1961). Uterine cancer in Connecticut: Late deaths among 5-year survivors. *JNCI, J. Natl. Cancer Inst.* **27,** 239–257.

Barron, B. A., and Richart, R. M. (1968). A statistical model of the natural history of cervical carcinoma based on a prospective study of 557 cases. *JNCI, J. Natl. Cancer Inst.* **41,** 1343–1353.

Barron, B. A., and Richart, R. M. (1970). Statistical model of the natural history of cervical carcinoma: II. Estimates of the transition time from dysplasia to carcinoma in situ. *JNCI, J. Natl. Cancer Inst.* **45,** 1025–1030.

Barron, B. A., Cahill, M. C., and Richart, R. M. (1978). A statistical model of the natural history of cervical neoplastic disease. The duration of carcinoma in situ. *Gynecol. Oncol.* **6,** 196–205.

Berget, A. (1975). Epidemiologic characteristics in patients with epithelial dysplasi, carcinoma in situ and invasive carcinoma of the uterine cervix. The population screening for cervical carcinoma in Maribo amt (county) 1967-1969. *Dan. Med. Bull.* **22,** 252–259.

Berkeley, A. S., Li Volsi, V. A., and Schwartz, P. E. (1980). Advanced squamous cell carcinoma of the cervix with recent normal Papanicolau tests. *Lancet* **2,** 375–376.

Berrino, F., Gatta, G., D'Alto, M., Crosignani, P., and Riboli, E. (1984). Use of case-control studies in evaluation of screening programs. *In* "Screening for Cancer" (P. C. Prorok, and A. B. Miller, eds.), UICC Tech. Rep. Ser., Vol. No. 78, pp. 29–43. Int. Union Against Cancer, Geneva.

Bibbo, M., Keebler, C. M., and Weid, G. M. (1971). Prevalence and incidence rates of cervical atypia. A computerized file analysis on 148,735 patients. *J. Reprod. Med.* **6,** 79–83.

Boyes, D. A., Morrison, B., Knox, E. G., Draper, G. J., and Miller, A. B. (1982). A Cohort study of cervical cancer screening in British Columbia. *Clin. Invest. Med.* **5,** 1–29.

Burns, E. L., Hammond, E. C., Percy, C., Seidman, H., and Gorski, T. W. (1968). Detection of uterine cancer. Results of a community program of 17 years. *Cancer* **22,** 1108–1119.

Christopherson, W. M., Parker, J. E., Mendez, W. M., and Lundin, F. (1970). Cervix cancer death rates and mass cytologic screening. *Cancer* **26,** 808–811.

Christopherson, W. M., Lundin, F. E., Mendez, W. M., and Parker, J. E. (1976). Cervical cancer control. A study of morbidity and mortality trends over a twenty-one year period. *Cancer* **35,** 1357–1366.

Clarke, E. A., and Anderson, T. W. (1979). Does screening by "Pap" smears help prevent cervical cancer? *Lancet* **2,** 1–4.

Clarke, E. A., and Anderson, T. W. (1983). Re: "Case definition in case-control studies of the efficacy of screening." *Am. J. Epidemiol.* **117,** 518–519.

Coppleson, L. W., and Brown, B. (1974). Estimation of the screening error rate from the observed detection rates in repeated cervical cytology. *Am. J. Obstet. Gynecol.* **119,** 953–958.

Coppleson, L. W., and Brown, B. (1975). Observations on a model of the biology of carcinoma of the cervix: A poor fit between observation and theory. *Am. J. Obstet. Gynecol.* **122,** 127–136.

Cramer, D. W. (1974). The role of cervical cytology in the declining morbidity and morality of cervical cancer. *Cancer* **34,** 2018–2027.

Dickinson, L., Mussey, M. E., Soule, E. H., and Kurland, L. T. (1972a). Evaluation of the effectiveness of cytologic screening for cervical cancer: I. Incidence and mortality trends in relation to screening. *Mayo Clin. Proc.* **47,** 534–544.

Dickinson, L., Mussey, M. E., and Kurland, L. T. (1972b). Evaluation of the effectiveness of cytologic screening for cervical cancer: II. Survival parameters before and after inception of screening. *Mayo Clin. Proc.* **47,** 545–555.

Draper, G. J. (1982). Screening for cervical cancer: Revised policy. The recommendations of the DHSS committee on gynaecological cytology. *Br. J. Fam. Plann.* **8,** 95–100.

Draper, G. J., and Cook, G. A. (1983). Changing patterns of cervical cancer rates. *Br. Med. J.* **287,** 510–512.

Dunn, J. E. (1953). The relationship between carcinoma in situ and invasive cervical carcinoma. *Cancer* **6,** 873–886.

Dunn, J. E. (1960). The epidemiologic aspects of cervical carcinoma as revealed by cytologic study. *J. Int. Coll. Surg.* **34,** 720–725.

Dunn, J. E., and Martin, P. L. (1967). Morphogenesis of cervical cancer. Findings from the San Diego County cytology registry. *Cancer* **20,** 1899–1906.

Dunn, J. E., Slate, T. A., Merritt, J. W., and Martin, P. L. (1959). Findings for uterine cancer from one or more cytologic examinations of 33750 women. *JNCI, J. Natl. Cancer Inst.* **23,** 507–527.

Eddy, D. M. (1980). "Screening for Cancer: Theory, Analysis and Design." Prentice-Hall, Englewood Cliffs, New Jersey.

Fidler, H. K., Boyes, D. A., and Worth, A. J. (1968). Cervical cancer detection in British Columbia, a progress report. *J. Obstet. Gynaecol. Br. Commonw.* **75,** 392–404.

Gardner, J. W., and Lyon, J. L. (1977). Efficacy of cervical cytologic screening in the control of cervical cancer. *Prev. Med.* **6,** 487–499.

Hakama, M. (1978). Mass screening for cervical cancer in Finland. *In* "Screening in Cancer" (A. B. Miller, ed.), UICC Tech. Rep. Ser., Vol. 40, pp. 93–107. Int. Union Against Cancer, Geneva.

Hakama, M. (1980). Projection of cancer incidence: Experiences and some results in Finland. *World Health Stat. Q.* **33,** 228–240.

Hakama, M. (1982). Trends in the incidence of cervical cancer in the Nordic Countries. *In* "Trends in Cancer Incidence" (K. Magnus, ed.), pp. 279–292. Hemisphere Publ., Washington, D.C.

Harris, R. W., Brinton, L. A., Cowdell, R. H., Skegg, D. C., Smith, P. G., Vessey, M. P., and Doll, R. (1980). Characteristics of women with dysplasia or carcinoma in situ of the cervix uteri. *Br. J. Cancer,* **42**:359–369.

Higgins, I. T. T. (1971). Recent mortality from cancer of the cervix in the United States and United Kingdom. *Lancet* **2,** 1141–1143.

Hill, G. B., and Adelstein, A. M. (1967). Cohort mortality from carcinoma of the cervix. *Lancet* **2,** 605–606.

Hill, G. B., Burns, P. E., Koch, M., Lees, A. W., and Starreveld, A. A. (1983). Trends in the incidence of cancer of the female breast and reproductive tract in Alberta, 1953 to 1977. *Prev. Med.* **12,** 296–303.

Johannesson, G., Geirsson, G., and Day, N. (1978). The effect of mass screening on Iceland, 1965-74, on the incidence and mortality from cervical carcinoma. *Int. J. Cancer* **21,** 418–425.

Johnson, L. D., Nickerson, R. J., Easterday, C. L., Stuart, R. S., and Hertig, A. T. (1968). Epidemiologic evidence for the spectrum of change from dysplasia through carcinoma in situ to invasive cancer. *Cancer* **22,** 901–914.

Kashagarian, M., and Dunn, J. E. (1970). The duration of intra epithelial and preclinical squamous cell carcinoma of the uterine cervix. *Am. J. Epidemiol.* **92,** 211–222.

Kasper, T. A., Smith, E. S. O., Cooper, P., Clayton, J., and Todd, D. (1970). An analysis of the prevalence and incidence of gynecologic cancer cytologically detected in a population of 175,767 women. *Acta Cytol.* **14,** 261–269.

Kassirer, E. (1980). Impact of the Walton report on cervical screening programs in Canada. *Can. Med. Assoc. J.* **122,** 417–423.

Kim, K., Rigel, R. D., Patrick, J. R., Walters, J. K., Bennett, A., Nordin, W., Claybrook, J. R., and Parekh, R. R. (1978). The changing trends of uterine cancer and cytology. A study of morbidity and mortality trends over a twenty year period. *Cancer* **22,** 2439–2449.

Kinlen, L. J., and Doll, R. (1973). Trends in mortality from cancer of the uterus in Canada and in England and Wales. *Br. J. Prev. Soc. Med.* **27,** 146–149.

Knox, E. G. (1973). A simulation system for screening procedures. Computer simulations of cervical cytology screening programmes. *In* "The Future - and Present Indicatives," (G. McLachlan, ed.) Problems and Progress in Medical Care, 9th Ser., pp. 19–55. Nuffield Provincial Hospitals Trust, Oxford Univ. Press, London and New York.

Lundin, F. E., Christopherson, W. M., Mendez, W. M., and Parker, J. E. (1965). Morbidity from cervical cancer. Effects of cervical cytology and socio-economic status. *JNCI, J. Natl. Cancer Inst.* **35,** 1015–1025.

Lynge, E. (1983). Regional trends in incidence of cervical cancer in Denmark in relation to local smear-taking activity. *Int. J. Epidemiol.* **12,** 405–413.

MacGregor, J. E., and Teper, S. (1978). Mortality from carcinoma of the cervix uteri in Britain. *Lancet* **2,** 774–776.

Miller, A. B. (1973). Evaluation of screening for carcinoma of the cervix. *Mod. Med. Can.* **28,** 1067–1069.

Miller, A. B., ed. (1978a). "Screening in Cancer," UICC Tech. Rep. Ser., Vol. 40. Int. Union Against Cancer, Geneva.

Miller, A. B. (1978b). Screening for cancer of the cervix in Canada, post-Walton. *In* "Screening in Cancer" (A. B. Miller, ed.), UICC Tech. Rep. Ser., Vol. 40, pp. 73–92. Int. Union Against Cancer, Geneva.

Miller, A. B., and Rawls, W. E. (1981). Epidemiology of gynecologic cancer: I. Cervix. *In* "Gynecologic Oncology" (M. Coppleson, ed.), Vol. I, pp. 9–18. Churchill-Livingstone, Edinburgh and London.

Miller, A. B., Lindsay, J., and Hill, G. B. (1976). Mortality from cancer of the uterus in Canada and its relationship to screening for cancer of the cervix. *Int. J. Cancer* **17,** 602–612.

Miller, A. B., Visentin, T., and Howe, G. R. (1981). The effect of hysterectomies and screening on mortality from cancer of the uterus in Canada. *Int. J. Cancer* **27,** 651–657.

Morrison, A. S. (1982). Case definition in case-control studies of the efficacy of screening. *Am. J. Epidemiol.* **115,** 6–8.

Morrison, A. S. (1983). The author replies. *Am. J. Epidemiol.* **117,** 520.

National Institutes of Health (1980). "Cervical Cancer Screening: The Pap Smear," Nat. Inst.

Health Consensus Dev. Conf. Summ., Vol. 3, No. 4. U.S. Gov. Printing Office, Washington, D.C.

Parkin, D. M., Nguyen-Dinh, X., and Day, N. E. (1985). The impact of screening on the incidence of cervical cancer. *Br. J. Obstet. Gynaecol.* **93** (in press).

Pedersen, E., Hoeg, K., and Kolstad, P. (1971). Mass screening for cancer of the uterine cervix in Ostfold County, Norway: An experiment. Second report of the Norwegian Cancer Society. *Acta Obstet. Gynaecol. Scand., Suppl.* **11.**

Sellers, A. H., and McLerie, E. E. (1973). A note on trends in mortality from cancer of the cervix, Ontario and British Columbia. 1950-1971. *Can. J. Public Health* **64,** 364–367.

Spriggs, A. I., and Husain, O. A. N. (1977). Cervical smears. *Br. Med. J.* **1,** 1516–1518.

Stern, E., Forsythe, A. B., Youkeles, L., and Coffelt, C. F. (1977a). Steroid contraceptive use and cervical dysplasia. Increased risk of progression. *Science* **196,** 1460–1462.

Stern, E., Misczynski, M., Greenland, B., Damus, K., and Coulson, A. (1977b). "Pap" testing and hysterectomy prevalence: A survey of communities with high and low cervical cancer rates. *Am. J. Epidemiol.* **106,** 296–305.

Task Force (1976). Appointed by the Conference of Deputy Ministers of Health. Cervical cancer screening programmes. The Walton Report. *Can. Med. Assoc. J.* **114,** 1003–1033.

Task Force (1982). Cervical cancer screening programs: Summary of the 1982 Canadian task force report. *Can. Med. Assoc. J.* **127,** 581–589.

Terris, M., Wilson, F., and Nelson, J. H. (1980). Comparative epidemiology of invasive carcinoma of the cervix, carcinoma in situ and cervical dysplasia. *Am. J. Epidemiol.* **112,** 253–257.

Thomas, D. B. (1973). An epidemiologic study of carcinoma in situ and squamous dysplasia of the uterine cervix. *Am. J. Epidemiol.* **98,** 10–28.

Thomas, D. B., and Anderson, R. I. (1974). An epidemiologic and serologic comparison of uterine carcinoma in situ and squamous dysplasia. *Am. J. Epidemiol.* **100,** 113–123.

Vessey, M. P., Lawless, M., McPherson, K., and Yeates, D. (1983). Neoplasia of the cervix uteri and contraception: A possible adverse effect of the pill. *Lancet* **2,** 930–934.

Yu, S. Z., Miller, A. B., and Sherman, G. J. (1982). Optimizing the age, number of tests and test interval for cervical screening in Canada. *J. Epidemiol. Commun. Health* **36,** 1–10.

Yule, R. (1978). Mortality from carcinoma of the cervix. *Lancet* **1,** 1030–1032.

17

Screening for Cancer of the Breast

ANTHONY B. MILLER

I. Introduction 325
II. Problems in the Evaluation of Screening for Breast Cancer 326
III. The Health Insurance Plan (HIP) Study 328
IV. The Breast Cancer Detection Demonstration Projects (BCDDP) 330
V. The International Union Against Cancer (UICC) Workshop 332
VI. Further Studies on Breast Screening 332
  A. The Kaiser-Permanente Study 332
  B. Studies in The Netherlands 333
  C. The United Kingdom Study 333
  D. The Swedish Trials 334
  E. The Canadian National Breast Screening Study (NBSS) 334
VII. Other Modalities for Screening for Breast Cancer 337
VIII. Future Application of Breast Cancer Screening 338
  A. Evaluation Issues 338
  B. Barriers in Applying Advances in Screening Detection Technology to Everyday Practice 339
IX. Conclusion 342
  References 343

I. INTRODUCTION

Breast cancer is the most important cancer in women. In North America, in the absence of death from other causes, 1 out of 11 women will encounter breast cancer in their lifetime. In Canada it is the most important cause of death in women aged 35–54. In the absence of major advances in treatment, and with a potentially long delay before primary prevention of breast cancer can have a major impact, screening seems to have the most immediate potential for control of the disease (Miller, 1983a). Screening for breast cancer has, however, been controversial even though the approach to its evaluation has included one com-

ISBN 0-12-496720-5

pleted controlled trial. The controversies that have arisen have been influenced by the public's changing perception of risk and benefit. In order to understand them, it is important to consider the studies of breast cancer screening that have been conducted. However, largely because of these controversies, further controlled trials have been initiated. Until these have been completed, adequate guidance on policies for control of breast cancer based on screening will be lacking.

II. PROBLEMS IN THE EVALUATION OF SCREENING FOR BREAST CANCER

In screening for breast cancer, one is seeking the cancer as distinct from an identified precursor, as in screening for cancer of the cervix. However, the relatively inefficient nature of currently available screening tests for breast cancer result in detection of the cancer at a fairly late stage in its natural history. For a breast cancer to be detectable, it has to reach 0.5 cm in size or more. Therefore, it has already been through many cell divisions, may have become intimately related to the vasculature and lymph channels. Further, if it is invasive, it must have had many opportunities to metastasize.

The problems of lead time and length bias were discussed in Chapter 1. Another difficulty is related to self-selection for attendance at breast screening programs. The factors that cause people to volunteer for such programs are various. They include a perceived perception of increased risk for the disease (such as a positive family history) and some awareness of approaches they can take to improve their health care. These individuals may be more likely to present promptly for treatment if they develop symptoms. In the absence of screening, therefore, their outcome is likely to be better than that of the general population. Part of this effect is offset by the self-selection of individuals at increased risk. It has been well documented that women who accept invitations to attend breast screening programs are at higher risk of developing breast cancer but at lower risk of dying of other causes than those who decline the invitations (Beahrs *et al.*, 1979). Thus, there is great difficulty in assessing the effectiveness of breast screening unless a control group is an integral part of the design of the study.

It should be noted that surrogate measures that are known in the clinical situation to relate to outcome, such as distribution of cases by stage of disease, lymph node involvement, tumor size, and so on are all influenced by the same potential biases. The closest of these measures to mortality is the rate or absolute number of cases of advanced disease occurring in the total population to whom screening is offered (Miller and van Slooten, 1983). Evaluation of any approach to breast screening therefore has to be performed by a methodology that avoids these biases. No one has yet devised a method that takes note of the biases and corrects for them, although they are avoided in a controlled trial (Prorok *et al.*, 1984).

As part of their educational approach to the problem of cancer, the cancer societies of North America have provided information to the public on breast cancer in the hope that women will not delay seeing their physician if they find a lump in the breast. In addition they have urged women to practice breast self-examination (BSE) on a regular basis in the hope that if a change does occur, the woman will detect it promptly. Neither the educational messages to the general public nor BSE has ever been appropriately evaluated. Some investigators have evaluated the stage distribution of cases found on BSE, but for the reasons discussed in Chapter 1, it is impossible to equate these measures with eventual reduction in deaths from breast cancer. Cole and Austin (1981) concluded that BSE may contribute more in situations where women do not utilize other screening modalities, but this conclusion was based on a review of studies that used surrogate measures to assess the outcome. Further, no one has evaluated the extent to which regular physician examination of well women on an annual basis results in reduction of mortality from breast cancer. Hence this procedure, in common with many other routinely performed examinations by physicians (Task Force, 1979), still requires evaluation.

As will be apparent later in this chapter, there are no ongoing studies that will determine unequivocally the effectiveness of physical examination of the breast as a screening test for breast cancer. This is unfortunate, since there is some evidence that this has contributed to a reduction in mortality from breast cancer when fairly skilled examinations were conducted. Nevertheless, as emphasized by Bassett in Chapter 15, these procedures are often done poorly, or not at all, and it is conceivable that without extensive public and professional education, the potential benefits of these procedures, which are maximal under study conditions, may not be realizable in practice.

During the time period when these approaches to early diagnosis have been promulgated and increasingly used, it has not been possible to detect any impact on overall trends of mortality for breast cancer. Any trends that have been seen appear likely to be related to changes in fertility practices, which seem to have affected the incidence and hence the mortality from breast cancer at certain ages (Fabia *et al.*, (1977). In Canada in the last 20 years, there has been some reduction in mortality in women under 50, but a corresponding increase in mortality in women over 50, so that the overall mortality has hardly changed. This is so in spite of a substantial rise in the incidence of breast cancer, particularly in postmenopausal women (Miller, 1983a). Some of the increase might be caused by earlier diagnosis, but most of it is probably due to the diagnosis of cases that previously would not have been diagnosed and that would not have resulted in death from breast cancer—a diagnostic artifact, a situation in which women, physicians, and pathologists are searching more actively for cancers.

III. THE HEALTH INSURANCE PLAN (HIP) STUDY

This study, based on contributors to the Health Insurance Plan (HIP) of Greater New York, was the first randomized controlled trial to evaluate screening for cancer of any site (Shapiro *et al.*, 1973; Shapiro, 1977). The screening modalities evaluated were the combination of mammography, using the Eagan technique (Eagan, 1964), and physical examination of the breasts by skilled examiners. BSE was not taught. A total of 62,000 women were included in the study and were randomized to study or control groups by a pairwise allocation procedure. Of the 31,000 women allocated to the study group, 65% attended one or more of the four annual screening examinations scheduled. The investigators evaluated the outcome in the total study group in comparison to the control group, since they could not have identified within the control group those who would have refused screening if it had been offered to them. Hence, the policy of inviting women to attend for screening was evaluated. All women received the routine care available from HIP. Follow-up was through the plan and other mechanisms. The wisdom of the controlled trial approach, and, as a corollary, the difficulty of evaluating screening without an appropriate control group, were emphasized when it became apparent that mortality from causes other than breast cancer was substantially lower in those who accepted the invitation to attend for screening than in the control group (Beahrs *et al.*, 1979). Indeed, the percentage reduction in mortality from breast cancer in those screened compared to the controls was less than the reduction in mortality from all causes other than breast cancer. This apparent paradox was resolved when it was appreciated that the women who accepted the invitation to attend for screening had a higher incidence of breast cancer than those who refused (Beahrs *et al.*, 1979).

The controlled trial design avoids the biases discussed in Chapter 1 because mortality from breast cancer was assessed. There is bound to be a differential lead time between those cases identified on mammography, those identified on physical examination, and those identified on both modalities. Such a differential confounds attempts to use case fatality as a measure of outcome in determining the relative contribution of the modalities used in screening programs. Its presence has been largely confirmed in the long-term follow-up of the study by the increasing juxtaposition, after about a 5-year interval, of the survival of patients detected by mammography alone compared to those detected on physical examination alone or physical examination plus mammography (Shapiro, 1982).

Confining our attention, therefore, to comparisons of mortality between the study and control groups, two striking features emerged as a result of the analyses. The first was that although there were no differences between study and control groups in deaths from breast cancer in the first 2 years after the initiation of screening, a differential was seen from 3 years that became maximal at 7 years (Shapiro, 1982). This indicates that the effect of the screening program in producing a mortality reduction was not particularly delayed. This early impact of a screening modality must mean that relatively rapidly progressive cases were affected by the screening process. Walter and Day (1983) modeled the lead time distribution and found a best fit with an exponential distribution. This gave an estimate of a mean lead time of 1.7 years (20 months), corresponding to approximately 44% of cases having a duration of less than 1 year and 5% with a duration of more than 5 years. It seems unlikely that the cases with a longer than average lead time, many of which were probably identified by mammography, could have contributed to an early mortality reduction. The implication is that screening for breast cancer reduces the risk of death in patients whose disease is detected somewhat late in its natural history. Thus, the physical examinations offered in the study probably made a substantial contribution to the overall reduction in mortality. It has been calculated that this contribution might amount to as much as 70% of the mortality reduction (Bailar, 1976; Breslow *et al.*, 1977).

Two other observations support the inference that the reduction in mortality was due to the earlier detection of advanced disease, with a major contribution from the physical examination component of the screen. The first is that the survival of the stage II (involved node) patients in the study group was better than that of patients in the same stage in the control group. The second is the progressive erosion of the survival advantage of the patients detected by mammography alone in the study group with increasing duration of follow-up (Shapiro, 1982).

The other striking aspect of the study was the apparent differential in the effectiveness of screening at different ages. The initial analyses of the study were published according to the age of the women at death (Shapiro *et al.*, 1973). On this basis, all of the mortality reduction occurred in women over the age of 50 at death, there being no difference between the study and control groups in deaths at ages 40–49. However, interpretation of this age differential has been difficult. Various commentators have pointed out that in the study, by design, women were allocated to the two groups according to age at entry (Pasternack and Strax, 1979; Prorok *et al.*, 1981). When women are so categorized, an apparent benefit from screening for women aged 40–49 on entry is seen. Part of the explanation is that the differential in women under the age of 50 at entry is related to the patients first diagnosed over the age of 50 (Shapiro, 1977, 1979). Women who enter a screening program under the age of 50 and who continue to be screened as they age beyond this presumably artificial boundary appear to derive benefit from the screening examinations at the older ages. There is, however, a difficulty with this explanation: screening examinations will inevitably result in earlier diagnosis of cases in the screened group compared to the control group. Thus, if mortality is compared in terms of age at diagnosis, some of the cases that would have been diagnosed in the study group in the absence of screening have been transferred by the screening examinations from an older to a younger age. Some deaths classified by age at diagnosis are therefore being applied in the study group to younger ages than they would be in the absence of screening. Hence, in analyses with cases classified by age at diagnosis, there will be a deficit of deaths at older ages in the screened group but an excess at younger ages.

To some, the age differential was not surprising. The age of 50 roughly corresponds to the menopause, and it is known that premenopausal women have denser breasts than postmenopausal women, in whom much of the glandular tissue is replaced by fat. Fat is more radiolucent, and thus early cancers are easier to detect on mammography in postmenopausal than in premenopausal women (see Chapter 7). Mammography in the early 1960s was relatively inefficient compared to now, especially in younger women. Only 19% of the cases of breast cancer identified on screening in women aged 40–49 in the HIP study were found on mammography alone compared to 44% in women aged 50–59 (Shapiro *et al.*, 1973). However, an alternative explanation for differential effectiveness at younger compared to older ages is a difference in biological aggressiveness of breast cancer in premenopausal compared to postmenopausal women. Such a difference has been noted in response to therapy in early disease (Canellos *et al.*, 1982). Further, physical examination of the breasts was applied equally in the two age groups, and if it was effective at older ages, why not at younger ages? The growth rate of cancers may be faster in premenopausal than in postmenopausal women. Nevertheless, it has to be borne in mind that the HIP study was not designed to evaluate an age effect. Thus, the sample sizes were not able to exclude a beneficial effect of screening in the younger women with reasonable confidence. Hence, the age differential may have been due purely to chance.

The question of an age differential effect of screening must be regarded, therefore, as having been raised by the HIP study, but it must be answered by other investigations. However, any attempt to capitalize on the results of the HIP study should take into account the possibility of an age differential. One of the major difficulties in the history of breast cancer screening is related to the fact that this age differential was for a while ignored.

IV. BREAST CANCER DETECTION DEMONSTRATION PROJECTS (BCDDP)

In 1973 the American Cancer Society initiated the concept of centers designed to assess the extent to which women would attend for breast cancer screening.

This idea was taken up by the National Cancer Institute and was eventually extended to include 28 centers in 27 cities throughout the United States. In each city 10,000 women between the ages of 35 and 74 were to be recruited. They were to provide information on risk factors for breast cancer and to be screened using physical examination, thermography, and mammography.

In their recruitment drives, the centers were eminently successful. Recruitment was facilitated by the publicity surrounding the development of breast cancer in the wives of the then president and vice president of the United States.

Unfortunately, the organizers of this program did not take into account the age differential in the HIP study. However, even at the time the project was initiated, a number of people were advising caution. Thus, an ad hoc committee of the Canadian Association of Radiology concluded in 1973 that the implications then emerging from the HIP study would require its replication (Leger *et al.*, 1974). One of the concerns of the committee—namely, radiation-induced breast cancers in an age group in whom benefit had not yet been demonstrated, came to the fore when Bailar (1976) predicted that at the mammography dosage then used, the BCDDPs might be responsible for as many radiation-induced cancers as the number of deaths that might be prevented by the program. Eventually, mammography for women under the age of 50 was withdrawn in the BCDDPs unless these women had a history of breast cancer (Beahrs *et al.*, 1979; Breslow *et al.*, 1977). A special working group to review the BCDDPs concluded that in the absence of defined populations from which the women who volunteered for the projects were drawn, and because of the lack of a suitable control group, it would not be possible to determine the program's effectiveness in terms of mortality reduction (Beahrs *et al.*, 1979). However, there was one hopeful sign, namely, that the proportion of cancers identified on mammography alone at the first two screenings in younger women was the same as that in the older women, an apparently dramatic improvement on the earlier HIP study.

A further lesson was learned from the BCDDPs. A review of cancers classified as minimal by a special pathology panel suggested that a number of them might not have been cancer at all (Beahrs *et al.*, 1979). Although this conclusion was challenged (Beahrs and Smart, 1979), and possibly too high a false-positive rate was initially reported because of difficulties in collecting material, the specter was raised of women treated by mastectomy for noncancerous abnormalities. Further, there was always the possibility that some minimal cancers might never have progressed, and that in the absence of screening they might never have become clinically detectable.

However, to the extent that earlier diagnosis of abnormalities identified on screening results in less extensive treatment, the process can be regarded as beneficial. The increasing information that suggests the appropriatenes of conservative therapy for early breast cancer (Canellos *et al.*, 1982) suggests that women with screen-detected early cancer should in general be managed conservatively. At the same time, particular care should be taken by pathologists to ensure that overdiagnosis is avoided.

An analysis of the cancers identified over the 5 years of the BCDDPs (Baker, 1982) confirms the earlier one at 2 years (Beahrs *et al.*, 1979) in showing the greatly improved detection ability of mammography in women under the age of 50 compared to the HIP study. However, an attempt by Moskovitz and Gartside (1982) to assess the mortality benefits appears to be confounded by the predicted absence of deaths from breast cancer in the first few years after women enter a breast cancer screening program, because of the exclusion of women with preexisting breast cancer.

V. THE INTERNATIONAL UNION AGAINST CANCER (UICC) WORKSHOP

During a UICC workshop on screening held in 1978, the problem of the applicability of breast cancer screening was recognized (Miller, 1978b). Difficulties arise over the approach to be advocated for women over the age of 50. In a situation where mammography using film–screen combinations results in a cumulative radiation dose to breast tissue after five examinations of less than 1 Rad, conventional extrapolation of radiation effects suggests that the hazard in this age group is likely to be minimal, whereas the benefit could be substantial (Howe *et al.*, 1981). The American College of Radiology (1976) had endorsed the concept of annual mammography for women over the age of 50. However, recognizing the substantial logistic difficulties of population-wide mammography screening programs, the participants in the UICC workshop emphasized the desirability of assessing the independent contribution of mammography to breast cancer screening. The advocacy of mammography on a routine basis for women over the age of 50 requires the availability of facilities and personnel to conduct such examinations. These are costly. Thus, in the absence of proof that mammography really does contribute substantially to the mortality reduction that was noted in the HIP study, it is unlikely that routine mammographic screening for breast cancer in women over the age of 50 will be introduced. This consideration led directly to the design of one of the components of the Canadian randomized trial of breast screening.

VI. FURTHER STUDIES ON BREAST SCREENING

A. The Kaiser-Permanente Study

The use of mammography was evaluated as part of a controlled trial of multiphasic screening in the Kaiser-Permanente Program in California in women aged

45 or more, with follow-up from 1964 to 1975 (Dales *et al.*, 1979). The early results of this trial showed no mortality differential for breast cancer. Fourteen deaths from breast cancer were reported in each of the two groups compared. Nevertheless, three-quarters of the subjects were under the age of 50 when the study began. Thus, although this study does not have sufficient power to refute the HIP findings, it does reinforce the desirability of not extrapolating from the HIP findings without further study.

B. Studies in The Netherlands

Two screening projects have been initiated in the Netherlands. In Utrecht, all women over the age of 50 on the population register have been invited to attend a center at which they are offered mammography and physical examination, the latter being conducted by radiology technicians (de Waard *et al.*, 1984). With a high population coverage, there is a possibility that a mortality differential may be demonstrated in comparison to control towns, although such quasi-experimental designs require substantial numbers of individuals to show significant differences. In another city in the Netherlands, Nijmegen, single-view mammography is being used alone in a similar population study. In this study, younger women are being recruited. In both studies, recent case-control analyses have indicated a beneficial effect of screening in reducing mortality from breast cancer (Colette *et al.*, 1984; Verbeek *et al.*, 1984).

C. The United Kingdom Study

In the United Kingdom, a decision was made not to initiate an individually randomized trial. Instead, after work on pilot studies, a geographically based comparative study has been mounted (U.K. Trial Group, 1981). In two districts, population screening has been initiated; in two others, BSE teaching in clinics or groups is offered; and in four more, data are being gathered for comparative purposes, though no screening or BSE teaching has been offered. Women have been recruited for screening by letters written to them by their family physicians after age-sex registers had been created in the practices in the area. In both centers offering screening, mammography is done biennially, single-view examinations in one and two-view examinations in the other. However, annual physical examinations are offered. In one of the two screening districts, some of the practices have been randomized to a control group. Although the response has been on the order of 70% in the screening centers, there was a lower response to invitations for BSE teaching (Miller and van Slooten, 1983). It may be some years before the results of this study are available; screening is scheduled to continue for 7 years. This is one of the few studies that may provide evidence on the effectiveness of BSE.

D. The Swedish Trials

In Sweden, three large trials of mammography alone have been in progress for some years, and a fourth (in Stockholm) has recently been started. In two, single-view mammography is being used with control groups selected by randomization on a cluster sampling basis (Tabar and Gad, 1981). When single-view mammography is used alone, the oblique projection is the only view, an approach for which adequate sensitivity is claimed (Lundgren, 1979). Two examinations of the population were planned at 35- to 36-month intervals during a 5-year period that commenced in 1977, but it proved possible to offer three screenings to younger women at intervals of about 21-months. Unfortunately, the interval cancer rate was quite high, and now that screening of the control group is about to start (dictated by political considerations), there is concern about whether the studies are of sufficient power to demonstrate mortality reduction with precision. Nevertheless, at 5 years, the absolute number of advanced (stage II+) breast cancers is less in the screened group compared to the control group, although data on mortality are not yet available (Miller and van Slooten, 1983). The third project (in Malmo in southwest Sweden) uses two-view mammography and is based on randomization of individuals (Andersen *et al.*, 1979). Even here, though, there are no plans to screen the control group formally. It is known that the controls have access to mammography outside the screening center, and there is some concern over dilution. In the fourth study, recently started in Stockholm, randomization is also based on individuals, and single-view mammography is used.

If much of the age differential in mortality reduction in HIP was due to mammography, these projects are likely to teach us a great deal about the effectiveness of mammography in screening applied in the most economical way. However, they leave unanswered the question of the amount that mammography adds to the benefit of physical examination, and there is concern that the relatively high interval cancer rates noticed are at least partly due to the absence of physical examination.

E. Canadian National Breast Screening Study (NBSS)

The NBSS commenced in January 1980 (National Cancer Institute of Canada, 1980) with the following objectives:

1. To determine in volunteers aged 40–49 on entry to the study whether unselective annual screening by mammography and physical examination, when used as an adjunct to the highest standard of care in the Canadian health care system, reduces mortality from breast cancer.

2. To determine in volunteers aged 50–59 on entry to the study the additional contribution of routine annual mammographic screening to screening by physical examination alone.

3. To assess whether an appropriate combination of risk factors for breast cancer can be derived to permit restriction of screening to those at highest risk of the disease.

4. To provide the data necessary for an analysis of the cost effectiveness of breast cancer screening in Canada using current mammography techniques.

5. To provide data on the natural history of breast cancer for incorporation into computer simulation approaches in order to evaluate the optimum age at which screening should commence and its periodicity at different ages.

The NBSS plans to recruit 90,000 women into the project, 50,000 aged 40–49 and 40,000 aged 50–59. All of the planned total of 15 screening centers across the country have now been opened, with an individual recruitment target ranging from 1000 to 15,000 women. Five screening examinations were originally planned to be conducted annually, but in order to set a termination date to the study, women recruited toward the end of the recruitment phase are offered only four annual screens, as in the HIP study. After cessation of screening, follow-up will be performed by computerized record linkage with the Canadian Cancer Incidence and Mortality files, and can therefore be continued indefinitely (Miller *et al.*, 1981).

By December 31, 1984, the project had recruited over 85,000 women. However, there were initial difficulties, because it was necessary to use publicity in order to recruit participants. Recruitment through the medical profession has not been the major mechanism for a number of reasons. Many physicians appear not to be aware of the objectives of screening; some do not regard breast cancer as a particularly important condition; some are content with the ability of the approaches currently adopted, namely, BSE and physical examination, to cope with the disease; and some are concerned over the arguments used by the critics of the program on the hazards of mammography.

Slow recruitment was encountered particularly in the first center in Toronto, where the project commenced in January 1980, and subsequently in the nearby area of Hamilton, Ontario. Two sampling surveys were conducted in Toronto to assess public opinion. These revealed that there are four issues that tend to keep women away from the NBSS. One is simply ignorance, not knowing that the project exists; a second is a feeling that they are adequately cared for already by their family physicians; a third is concern over radiation; a fourth is a feeling of fear and a wish not to know. Many women are frightened of the idea that an examination might reveal breast cancer, even though there is some understanding that earlier diagnosis results in an increased probability of cure.

The controversy over radiation in the NBSS is largely related to the validity of the extrapolations from high-dose exposure to the estimated risk at low-dose levels. When, as a result of our own experience, it became clear that the dosages used in film–screen mammography were far less than had been the norm for the BCDDPs, we computed the overall risk-benefit for screening using mammography (Howe *et al.*, 1981). Even if the mortality reduction from the use of mammography was a low as 20%, our calculations suggested a clear excess of benefit over risk for women included in the NBSS at all ages.

Preliminary results from our large Canadian study of cancer following multiple fluoroscopies given for the management of tuberculosis in the 1930s and 1940s have become available (Howe, 1984). These have confirmed that there is a substantial variation in susceptibility to the effects of radiation at different ages, with maximum susceptibility when women were first irradiated in their teens or twenties and substantial reduction in risk for women first irradiated over the age of 30. This effect had first been suggested by the follow-up of women who were exposed to the atomic bomb (Land *et al.*, 1980).

With this information, it is now possible to reassure the women considering participation in studies of breast cancer screening. With mammography only being offered to women of age 40 or more, it would seem that the potential hazard in inducing breast cancer is negligible.

It is still too early to expect results from the NBSS. Recruitment is scheduled to continue through March 1985 and screening through March 1988. Thus, early mortality results cannot be expected until about 1990. Nevertheless, the detection rates by age on initial and repeat screening are of the order anticipated from the BCDDPs, although with slightly higher proportions of cancers detected on physical examination alone, possibly a reflection of more efficient physical examination. Our early recruitment difficulties now seem to be over. In Toronto, recruitment is now based largely on letters written to women in the relevant age group identified through population registers, with a response following a telephone call of around 25%. Although this seems low in comparison with the European studies, it must be borne in mind that women are being asked to consent to randomization, with no guarantee that a woman's preference on having mammography or not will be honored.

One of the features of the NBSS is that all women are taught BSE, and that this teaching is reinforced for those who return for rescreening. In addition, the frequency of practice is self-assessed ay annual questionnaires, and the efficiency of practice is assessed during the screening physical examination. This therefore raises the possibility that the effectiveness of BSE can be assessed by a case-control approach within the strata formed by randomization in the study. We are currently considering this issue in light of the use of case-control studies for the evaluation of screening, as discussed in Chapter 1.

VII. OTHER MODALITIES FOR SCREENING FOR BREAST CANCER

Although the low radiation dosage now involved in mammography suggests minimal hazard, the search continues for modalities that might replace mammography and that would be at least as sensitive and as specific. Thermography has so far not achieved high enough sensitivity and specificity to justify its use in screening (Beahrs *et al.*, 1979). In its place, interest has turned to ultrasound and diaphanoscopy.

Ultrasound of the breasts is considered in detail by Kobyashi in Chapter 7. Although ultrasound is being used for screening in Japan, it is still under active investigation in North America, although it is already being used as a diagnostic aid.

Diaphanoscopy, which involves transilluminating the breast in a darkened room with a low-powered electric light and with image detection sensitive to infrared rays using a video device, is also in an early stage of development. No data are yet available on the sensitivity and specificity of the device in a screened population. Developmental work is proceeding, and women participating in the NBSS in Winnipeg are now evaluated by diaphanoscopy if they are found to have an abnormality on the standard screening physical examination and mammography. This will help investigators to decide whether or not the test is likely to be of value in screening.

Currently, all new devices have to be evaluated in comparison with mammography and, preferably, the combination of mammography and physical examination. If devices are developed that appear to be usable for screening, it will probably be unnecessary to mount additional large-scale controlled trials to determine whether mortality reduction would follow from their use. That is, if it can be demonstrated that the new devices have equivalent or, preferably, superior sensitivity and specificity to mammography and physical examination in a healthy population being screened, it can be assumed that they will result in at least equivalent mortality reduction. Thus, although substantial numbers of healthy women, as distinct from women who present with possible symptoms of breast cancer, would have to be studied in order to reach a conclusion with precision, the investigation would not be as expensive as a long-term controlled trial and could be completed relatively rapidly. Nevertheless, difficulty will be encountered if a device is advocated for screening that does not identify a subset of the cases found on mammography, such as those in which the only radiologic sign is a cluster of fine calcifications. Since it is unlikely that any screening study using mammography can evaluate the contribution of early detection of such cancers to reduction in mortality, we will be driven to assess the importance of their early detection by surrogate measures. Nevertheless, with existing studies enabling us to assess benefits in terms of mortality reduction, and with them also providing inferences on natural history, there is some hope that survival data in future well-conducted screening studies can be assessed in relation to potential mortality reduction using mathematical models (Prorok, 1984).

VIII. FUTURE APPLICATION OF BREAST CANCER SCREENING

A. Evaluation Issues

There are several issues that will need to be borne in mind when decisions are made on whether breast cancer screening should be introduced in population projects as distinct from controlled trials. The first concerns whether screening for breast cancer is indeed effective in reducing mortality, and which modalities contribute to this reduction. Then there are questions on the type of population to be offered screening and, in this connection, the need to demonstrate that screening actually does result in the mortality reduction anticipated from controlled trials. Associated with this issue are questions on the age at which screening should start, the periodicity of rescreening, and the age at which screening should end. The final issues are related to cost-benefit considerations.

The controlled trials currently in progress will provide substantial information on mortality reduction from the modalities used. The question about the modalities to use is more difficult to answer. The Swedish studies use mammography alone; its benefit over and above that to be obtained from physical examination will be precisely determined in women aged 50–59 on entry to the Canadian trial. However, the benefit from physical examination alone will not be determined precisely from any study, and comparisons between studies will have to be conducted to produce an estimate of its effect. The controlled trials will also provide information that can be used to determine the age of onset of screening, whether or not screening can be restricted to certain readily identified high-risk groups, and the optimal level of mortality reduction that might be anticipated in practice. However, these trials will not provide information on optimal periodicity except to the extent that different controlled trials evaluate different periodicities and can be compared, a hazardous procedure at best; nor will they provide guidance on the age at which screening should cease. These issues are likely to be evaluable only through computer simulation using data on efficacy and natural history obtained from the controlled trials. Some computer simulation models are currently available (see the appendix to Beahrs *et al.*, 1979) and others are being developed. This approach has already provided guidance on periodicity and the ages at which screening for cancer of the cervix should begin and end (Yu *et al.*, 1982), and there seems little doubt that similar approaches will be feasible for breast cancer.

Some have questioned whether it will be possible to base decisions about the initiation of screening programs on studies conducted in different parts of the world, with extrapolations made to many different social circumstances. The answer is that we will have to make such extrapolations; we cannot afford to replicate studies to answer anew every question in every country (Miller and van Slooten, 1983). Providing we recognize now that such extrapolations will be required, and plan our data collection and reporting procedures appropriately, decisions should be possible, especially when we are prepared to use mathematical models appropriately.

B. Barriers in Applying Advances in Screening Detection Technology to Everyday Practice

1. General Barriers

Screening is not well adapted to application in a purely private medical care environment. Cost benefit and cost effectiveness calculations generally presuppose that the screening test is applied in a population in a manner that achieves optimal specificity and sensitivity, with sufficient prevalence of the disease to ensure that an appropriate proportion of positive tests will be found to represent disease, i.e., high predictive value positive. This is related to what some have called screening in the public health sense, which is the application of a screening test in an asymptomatic population, with a benefit that will not be immediately realizable or immediately apparent to those screened or those who apply the screen. At some stage, all screening tests for cancer require equipment that has to be procured and housed at substantial costs and that involves fairly expensive maintenance and the provision of staff who have been adequately trained in the procedures they are applying. Screening programs involving mammography for cancer of the breast need mammography machines that will deliver images of high quality but with low radiation dosage. In my opinion, this requires film–screen technology, the xerographic process resulting in nearly 10 times as much midbreast radiation, but in order to maintain high quality at low dosage, periodic monitoring of the machines and skilled maintenance are required. Physical examinations of the breast have to be conducted by skilled practitioners. Most physicians have not had the appropriate training and do not acquire the necessary experience. Nurse examiners, however, can be trained to a high level of competence over a 2- to 3-month period, and the best continue to maintain this standard year by year. Breast cancer screening also results in high costs in applying the definitive diagnostic procedure, a biopsy, and, for impalpable lesions, requires the provision of skilled practitioners to avoid mutilating biopsies.

In addition, physicians sometimes compound these difficulties by demanding fees for screening examinations equal to those for diagnostic examinations

(Dodd, 1984). This problem has generally been solved for cervical cytology, where the primary screener is the specially trained cytotechnician whose function is to recognize abnormalities but not necessarily to reach a diagnosis. Similar technicians can be trained to act as the initial screeners for physical and radiologic examination of the breast. It will almost certainly be impossible to justify screening in economic terms unless such individuals are used.

2. *Social Barriers*

In different cultures, different taboos may interfere with the application of screening tests. Although the effect of these taboos is lessening, they can lessen the willingness of women to appear for breast screening. It is important to recognize that the social barriers to acceptability of screening tests do not only apply to the person to whom the test is being offered. Spouses at times seem to have a disproportionate influence. However, they may also be an asset. For example, it seems possible that the relative failure of BSE, which can be partly attributed to the necessity for women to dissociate themselves from their own body sensations in carrying out the examination (Baines, 1983), might be overcome if their spouse or other partner was trained to carry out the examination and understood the abnormalities that were being sought. With the increasing availability of teaching models, it should be possible to ensure that training sessions incorporate both husband and wife.

3. *Behavioral Barriers*

The public at large has no real understanding of their risk of disease. This is partly because descriptions of risk are often couched in terms that the public can not understand. However, in addition, there is a widespread feeling of personal immunity—the "it can't happen to me" complex. This attitude coupled with some fatalism over the potential results of treating cancer, can substantially interfere with participation in screening programs. The public also finds it extremely difficult to weigh different types of risk. Thus, in general, there is much misconception of the risk of radiation-induced breast cancer following mammography. Some of this is caused by inappropriate advice from physicians and is inseparable from the general concern over radiation exposure from any source. In North America, it has been extremely difficult to overcome the impact of the emphasis on the risk of mammography that surfaced in the public and professional mind as a result of the BCDDPs. This is clearly a warning to avoid similar overselling of a screening procedure in the future.

4. *Influence of the Medical Profession*

I have already referred to the difficulty of applying screening when physicians are not skilled in physical examination of the breast. However, in addition, the concept of the yearly physical examination is counterproductive to the appropriate application of screening examinations. The yearly physical examination idea is under attack by a number of groups. In Canada, the Task Force on the Periodic Health Examination (1979) has emphasized the desirability of applying different examinations at different frequencies to different age and sex groups. In the NBSS in Canada, one of the barriers to participant acceptance was the women's belief that an annual physical examination provides adequate protection. This misunderstanding of screening is sometimes fostered by physicians. However, with unskilled physicians performing inadequate physical examinations of the breast, it is not surprising that there has been no indication of an effect of such procedures on mortality from breast cancer. This does not mean that adequate physical examination may not make an important contribution, as it appears to have done in women over the age of 50 in the HIP study.

Thus, whether the optimal results obtained in clinical trials can be obtained in routine practice remains an open question. There seems little doubt that it will be necessary to introduce breast cancer screening under circumstances in which its efficacy can be monitored in defined populations. Such populations include prepaid health insurance schemes, but in general will probably comprise populations with cancer registries, well-developed vital statistics systems, and epidemiologic assessment programs to measure the effectiveness of different cancer control approaches. We can anticipate some population resistance to attendance at screening centers, although it may be easier to convince women to participate once we know that the programs are effective, as distinct from the current situation, in which women are being recruited into studies with no guarantee of benefit.

5. *Economic Barriers*

Possibly as the bottom line, detailed consideration of economic issues will become very relevant. I have computed the costs and benefits of screening 100,000 women aged 40–59 annually for 5 years (Miller, 1983b). The net costs of screening were related to the years of life saved as a result of screening. The total years of life saved were 1855. Relating this figure to the net costs of screening results in a cost per year of life saved of $5697 (Table I). Using sensitivity analysis, I tested the extent to which the assumptions underlying these calculations influence the conclusions drawn. It is clear from Table 1 that the extent of mortality reduction has most influence on them.

Thus, it seems likely that effective breast screening will result in a relatively low expenditure per year of life saved. It is here that the computations cease and that one has to determine whether such an expenditure per year of life saved is justifiable. This, of course, is a moral judgment to which the public should contribute.

TABLE I

Sensitivity of Assumptions Made about Costs and Benefits from Screening 100,000 Women Aged 40–59[a]

Assumption	Alternatives assessed	Cost ($) per PYLS[b]
Cost per examination	$20	3,682
	$30[c]	5,650
	$50	9,587
Number of extra biopsies	2	5,042
	5[c]	5,650
	10	6,663
Savings per averted death	$0	6,919
	$10,000	6,458
	$27,500[c]	5,650
	$50,000	4,612
Mortality reduction	10%	26,407
	20%	12,569
	40%[c]	5,650
	60%	3,344
Screening at different ages of entry to the program	40–44	6,431
	45–49	4,810
	50–54	5,250
	55–59	7,230

[a] Reproduced, with permission, from Miller (1983b).
[b] Potential years of life saved.
[c] Used in calculations in text and for screening at different ages of entry to the program.

IX. CONCLUSION

Breast cancer screening clearly requires continued evaluation and cannot currently be adopted as a population measure. This conclusion, which I reached 6 years ago (Miller, 1977), was endorsed at the fourth meeting of the UICC project on breast cancer (Miller and Bulbrook, 1982). It also runs counter to the current American Cancer Society (1980, 1983) guidelines (Miller, 1984). Our present difficulties have partly arisen from the fact that assumptions were made regarding benefits from improving technology that could not be established in the projects initiated on the basis of these assumptions. Perhaps the most important lesson to be derived from the experience of the last decade is that we are beyond the stage when large-scale population screening programs for cancer, or indeed any disease, can be introduced on the basis of assumed benefits. Benefits will have to be established in large-scale studies. The studies that are necessary to evaluate breast cancer screening fully are now in place, and the answers we need should be available by the end of the current decade. However, one final note of caution is necessary. If, as I have inferred, the major benefit in women aged 50 or more in the HIP study derived from the physical examination, the benefit to be derived from the addition of mammography to annual physical examinations of the breasts, or even from the use of mammography alone, may be delayed. Thus, it could be many years before a significant difference in women over the age of 50 is detected in the NBSS or in the Swedish trials. If that is so, there would be no substitute for regular, efficient physical examinations of the breast by primary care physicians and the practice of BSE by women themselves.

REFERENCES

American Cancer Society (1980). Guidelines for the cancer-related check-up: Recommendations and rationale. *Ca—Cancer J. Clin.* **30,** 194–240.

American Cancer Society (1983). Mammography guidelines 1983: Background statement and update of cancer - related check-up guidelines for breast cancer detection in asymptomatic women age 40 to 49. *Ca—Cancer J. Clin.* **33,** 255.

American College of Radiology (1976). Board approves mammography policy, summary of current opinion. *Bull. Am. Coll. Radiol.* **32,** 1.

Andersen, I., Andren, L., Hildell, J., Linell, F., Ljungqvist, U., and Pettersson, H. (1979). Breast cancer screening with mammography. A population- based, randomized trial with mammography as the only screening mode. *Radiology* **132,** 273–276.

Bailar, J. C. (1976). Mammography: A contrary view. *Ann. Intern. Med.* **84,** 77–84.

Baines, C. J. (1983). Some thoughts on why women don't do breast self-examination. *Can. Med. Assoc. J.* **128,** 255–256.

Baker, L. H. (1982). Breast cancer detection demonstration project: Five-year summary report. *Ca—Cancer J. Clin.* **32,** 194–225.

Beahrs, O. H., and Smart, C. R. (1979). Diagnosis of minimal breast cancers in the BCDDP. The 66 questionable cases. *Cancer* **43,** 848–850.

Beahrs, O. H., Shapiro, S., and Smart, C. R. (1979). Report of the working Group to review the National Cancer Institute American Cancer Society breast cancer detection demonstration projects. *JNCI, J. Natl. Cancer Inst.* **62,** 640–709.

Breslow, L., Thomas, L. B., and Upton, A. C., Chairmen (1977). Final reports of the National Cancer Institute Ad Hoc working groups on mammography in screening for breast cancer and summary report of their joint findings and recommendations. *JNCI, J. Natl. Cancer Inst.* **59,** 467–541.

Canadian Task Force on the Periodic Health Examination (1979). The periodic health examination. *Can. Med. Assoc. J.* **121,** 1193–1250.

Canellos, G. P., Hellman, S., and Veronesi, U. (1982). The mangement of early breast cancer. *N. Engl. J. Med.* **306,** 1430–1432.

Cole, P., and Austin, H. (1981). Breast self-examination: An adjuvant to early cancer detection. *Am. J. Public Health* **71,** 572–574.

Collette, H. J. A., Day, N. E., Rombach, J. J., and de Waard, F. (1984). Evaluation of screening for breast cancer in a non-randomized study (the Dom Project) by means of a case-control study. *Lancet* **1,** 1224–1226.

Dales, L. G., Freidman, G. D., and Collen, M. F. (1979). Evaluating periodic multi-phasic health check-ups: A controlled trial. *J. Chronic Dis.* **32,** 385–404.

de Waard, F., Collette, H. J. A., Rombach, J. J., Baanders-van Halewijn, E. A., and Honing, C. (1984). The Dom project for the early detection of breast cancer, Utrecht, The Netherlands. *J. Chronic Dis.* **37,** 1–44.

Dodd, G. D. (1984). The continuing challenge of mammography. *Ca—Cancer J. Clin.* **34,** 57–59.

Eagan, R. L. (1964). "Mammography." Thomas, Springfield, Illinois.

Fabia, J., Bernard, P. M., and Hill, G. (1977). Recent time trends of age-specific death rates from breast cancer. Quebec and other provinces (1965 through 1974). *Can. Med. Assoc. J.* **116,** 1135–1138.

Howe, G. R. (1984). Epidemiology of radiogenic breast cancer. *In* "Radiation Carcinogenesis: Epidemiology and Biological Significance" (J. D. Boice, Jr. and J. F. Fraumeni, Jr., eds.), pp. 119–129. Raven Press, New York.

Howe, G. R., Sherman, G. J., Seminciew, R. M., and Miller, A. B. (1981). Estimated benefits and risks of screening for breast cancer. *Can. Med. Assoc. J.* **124,** 399–403.

Land, C. E., Boice, J. D., Shore, R. E., Norman, J. E., and Tokunaga, M. (1980). Breast Cancer risk from low-dose exposures to ionizing radiation: Results of parallel analysis of three exposed populations of women. *JNCI, J. Natl. Cancer Inst.* **65,** 353–376.

Leger, J. L., Naimark, A. P., Beique, R. A., McFarlane, D. V., Miller, S., and Miller, A. B. (1974). Report of the "Ad Hoc" committee on mammography. *J. Can. Assoc. Radiol.* **25,** 3–21.

Lundgren, B. (1979). Efficiency of single-view mammography: Rate of interval cancer cases. *JNCI, J. Natl. Cancer Inst.* **62,** 799–803.

Miller, A. B. (1977). Present status of breast cancer screening. *Can. Med. Assoc. J.* **117,** 845–846.

Miller, A. B. (1978a). Risk benefit in mass screening programs for breast cancer. *Semin. Oncol.* **5,** 351–359.

Miller, A. B., ed. (1978b). "Screening in Cancer," UICC Tech. Rep. Ser., Vol. 40. International Union Against Cancer, Geneva.

Miller, A. B. (1983a). Approaches to the control of breast cancer. *In* "Understanding Breast Cancer: Clinical and Laboratory Concepts" (M. Rich, J. C. Hager, and P. Furmanski, eds.), pp. 3–25. Dekker, New York.

Miller, A. B. (1983b). Screening for breast cancer. *Breast Cancer Res. Treat.* **3,** 143–156.

Miller, A. B. (1984). Routine mammography and the National Breast Screening Study. *Can. Med. Assoc. J.* **130,** 259–260.

Miller, A. B., and Bulbrook, R. D. (1982). Screening, detection and diagnosis of breast cancer. *Lancet* **1,** 1109–1111.

Miller, A. B., and van Slooten, E. A. (1983). Screening and Diagnosis in Breast Cancer; Workshop Report. *Eur. J. Cancer Clin. Oncol.* **19,** 1711–1716.

Miller, A. B., Howe, G. R., and Wall, C. (1981). The National Study of Breast Cancer Screening. *Clin. Invest. Med.* **4,** 227–258.

Moskovitz, M., and Gartside, P. S. (1982). Evidence of breast cancer mortality reduction - Aggressive screening in women under age 50. *AJR, Am. J. Roentgenol.* **138,** 911–916.

National Cancer Institute of Canada (1980). National breast-cancer screening study gets underway. *Can. Med. Assoc. J.* **122,** 243–244.

Pasternack, B. S., and Strax, P. (1979). Usefulness of statistical models to assess the benefit of breast cancer screening (letter). *JNCI, J. Natl. Cancer Inst.* **63,** 1109–1110.

Prorok, P. C. (1984). Methodological issues in randomized controlled trials of screening. *In* "Screening for Cancer" (P. C. Prorok and A. B. Miller, eds.), UICC Tech. Rep. Ser., Vol. 78, pp. 23–34. Int. Union Against Cancer, Geneva.

Prorok, P. C., Hankey, B. F., and Bundy, B. N. (1981). Concepts and problems in the evaluation of screening programs. *J. Chronic Dis.* **34,** 159–171.

Prorok, P. C., Chamberlain, J., Day, N. E., Hakama, M., and Miller, A. B. (1984). UICC Workshop on the evaluation of screening programmes for cancer. *Int. J. Cancer* **34,** 1–4.

Shapiro, S. (1977). Evidence on screening for breast cancer from a randomized trial. *Cancer* **39,** 2772–2782.

Shapiro, S. (1979). Reply to Pasternack and Strax (letter). *JNCI, J. Natl. Cancer Inst.* **63,** 1110.
Shapiro, S. (1982). Ten to fourteen-year effects of breast cancer screening on mortality. *JNCI, J. Natl. Cancer Inst.* **69,** 349–355.
Shapiro, S., Strax, P., Venet, L., and Venet, W. (1973). Changes in 5-year breast cancer mortality in a breast cancer screening program. *Proc., National Cancer Conf., 7th, 1972,* pp. 663–678.
Tabar, L., and Gad, A. (1981). Screening for breast cancer: The Swedish trial. *Radiology* **138,** 219–222.
Task Force (1979). The periodic health examination. *Can. Med. Assoc. J.* **121,** 1193–1254.
U.K. Trial of Early Detection of Breast Cancer Group (1981). Trial of early detection of breast cancer: Description of method. *Br. J. Cancer* **44,** 618–627.
Verbeek, A. L. M., Hendriks, J. H. C. L., Holland, R., Meavunae, M., Sturmans, F., and Day, N. E. (1984). Reduction of breast cancer mortality through mass screening with modern mammography. *Lancet* **1,** 1222–1224.
Walter, S. D., and Day, N. E. (1983). Estimation of the duration of a pre-clinical disease state using screening data. *Am. J. Epidemiol.* **118,** 865–886.
Yu, S. Z., Miller, A. B., and Sherman, G. J. (1982). Optimizing the age, number of tests and test interval for cervical screening in Canada. *J. Epidemiol. Commun. Health* **36,** 1–10.

18

Screening for Colorectal Cancer

SIDNEY J. WINAWER, ROBERT B. FATH, JR., DAVID SCHOTTENFELD, AND ELIZABETH HERBERT

I. Introduction 347
II. High-Risk Groups 348
A. Age and Sex 348
B. Inflammatory Bowel Disease 349
C. Familial and Hereditary Factors 350
D. History of Radiation Exposure 353
III. Screening Tests and Trials 353
A. Proctosigmoidoscopy 354
B. Clinical Trials with Fecal Occult Blood Tests 355
C. Standardization of Reporting and Trials 359
D. Other Screening Tests 359
E. Diagnostic Tests 360
IV. Guidelines for Screening and Case Finding 360
A. Average-Risk Patients 360
B. High-Risk Groups 362
C. Patient Compliance and Physician Education 363
V. Summary and Future Studies 363
References 364

I. INTRODUCTION

Incidence and mortality rates of colorectal cancer vary widely throughout the world. High rates are characteristic of highly developed countries in North America, northern and western Europe, and New Zealand. Intermediate rates are described in eastern and southern Europe, in the higher socioeconomic urban areas of Argentina, Brazil, Uruguay, and Paraguay, and among Israeli Jews born in Europe and North America. The lowest rates are found in Asia, Africa, and most countries of Latin America. In most high-risk countries, the lifetime proba-

ISBN 0-12-496720-5

bility of developing colorectal cancer varies between 4 and 5%, and one-half of the deaths due to cancers of the gastrointestinal system originate in the large bowel. Countries subject to a high incidence of colon cancer demonstrate a relatively higher frequency of sigmoid cancers, whereas in low-risk countries, cancers of the cecum and ascending colon predominate (Schottenfeld and Winawer, 1982).

An important objective in a screening intervention for a specific cancer is to ensure sufficient lead time and diminished mortality. The application of optimal treatment after diagnostic confirmation should result in improved survival and decreased morbidity when compared with treatment offered to symptomatic patients. There is considerable evidence that many, if not most, colorectal cancers arise from preexisting adenomas. Furthermore, there is evidence that the evolution of an adenoma from flat mucosa, subsequent transition to carcinoma *in situ*, and progression to invasive cancer generally requires more than 5 years. Although more colorectal cancers probably arise from adenomas, the majority of adenomas undoubtedly do not develop into cancer. The malignant potential of an adenoma may be anticipated by its size, proportion of villous elements, and degree of dysplasia (Morson, 1974). Once a frank invasive cancer has developed, there is evidence that the cancer passes through a presymptomatic early stage before progressing to a symptomatic, more advanced stage. The outcome is usually favorable (i.e., >80% survival at 5 years) when treatment is administered to patients without symptoms, because preclinical disease is generally predictive of preinvasive or early invasive disease.

II. HIGH-RISK GROUPS

The characteristics of personal and family history that are associated with increased risk should be recognized when planning screening interventions for colorectal cancer (Table I).

A. Age and Sex

In high-risk countries, the incidence of colorectal cancer increases almost exponentially between 50 and 80 years of age. The apparent decline reported after age 80 probably represents incomplete ascertainment. In the report of the United States Surveillance, Epidemiology, and End Results Program (SEER) (1978), the median age of diagnosis of *in situ* and invasive cancers of the colon (excluding the rectum) was 69.6 years, and that of the rectum 67.6 years.

In low-risk countries, where the cancers are concentrated in the cecum and ascending colon, the maximum incidence has occurred before age 60. The SEER cancer incidence data indicated that the distribution by subsites within the large

TABLE I

High-Risk Groups for Cancer of the Large Intestine

Age	
	50 years and older; asymptomatic general population
Inflammatory bowel disease	
	Chronic ulcerative colitis
	Crohn's granulomatous colitis
Familial polyposis syndromes	
	Inherited adenomatosis
	Gardner's syndrome
	Turcot's syndrome
	Oldfield's syndrome
	Juvenile polyposis
Familial cancer syndrome	
	Hereditary adenocarcinomatosis
Family history	
	Colorectal cancer or sporadic colorectal adenomas
Past history	
	Sporadic colorectal adenomas
	Colorectal cancer
	Breast or endometrial cancer
	Radiation therapy

intestine was as follows: rectum (22%), rectosigmoid (10%), sigmoid colon (25%), descending colon (6%), transverse colon including flexures (13%), ascending colon (8%), cecum (15%), and appendix (1%).

The sex ratios of colon cancer and rectal cancer differ. Rectal cancer is distinctly more common among males in most countries, whereas colon cancer affects both sexes at rather similar rates (Wynder and Shigematsu, 1967).

B. Inflammatory Bowel Disease

About 2% of the patients with chronic ulcerative colitis develop colorectal cancer. The risk of invasive carcinoma of the large intestine in patients with ulcerative colitis increases in relation to the duration of disease and the extent of mucosal involvement. Among persons with extensive ulcerative colitis of more than 10 years' duration, the risk of invasive carcinoma of the large intestine increases to approximately 20 times that expected in the general population (Devroede, 1980). The annual incidence of ulcerative colitis in countries at high risk of colorectal cancer has been estimated to vary between 2 and 7 per 100,000 (Janowitz and Sachar, 1983).

When invasive cancer occurs in patients with ulcerative colitis, it is frequently preceded by or associated with mucosal dysplasia and carcinoma *in situ* elsewhere in the large intestine. Morson (1980) has delineated the macroscopic and microscopic features of gradation of epithelial dysplasia that may appear in adenomas or in areas of flat mucosa separated from inflammatory ulcerations. The epithelial dysplasia that develops in ulcerative colitis is biologically analogous to the dysplasia that is manifested in a gastrointestinal adenoma and may serve as a marker for increased cancer risk. For this reason, Nugent (1980) recommends prospective surveillance for evidence of moderate to severe dysplasia in patients with ulcerative colitis.

Like ulcerative colitis, Crohn's granulomatous enterocolitis is more common in northern Europe, the United Kingdom, Canada, and the United States, where the annual incidence is between 2 and 4 per 100,000. In general, inflammatory bowel disease occurs more commonly in whites than in blacks and affects Jews from high-risk countries three to five times more commonly than non-Jews. However, the incidence of Crohn's disease is reported to be increasing, whereas that of ulcerative colitis is remaining stable. Of the incident cases, 70% involve the large intestine, generally in combination with involvement of the distal small intestine. In case-control studies, 10–15% of patients with Crohn's disease have at least one first-degree relative with inflammatory bowel disease or at least two to three times more frequently than the controls (Kirsner, 1980).

There is increasing evidence that Crohn's disease is associated with the development of adenocarcinomas in both the small and large intestines, although the risk does not approach the level incurred with severe forms of ulcerative colitis (Greenstein *et al.*, 1980). The risk of colorectal cancer varies in relation to the duration and severity of granulomatous colitis and is generally diagnosed under 40 years of age (Lightdale and Sherlock, 1980).

C. Familial and Hereditary Factors

Syndromes of familial polyposis include inherited adenomatosis of the colon and rectum, Gardner's syndrome, Turcot's syndrome, and Oldfield's syndrome. In the autosomal dominant familial adenomatosis syndrome, which occurs with a frequency of about 1 per 10,000 births, the probability of developing colorectal cancer is at least 50% by age 40 in untreated patients. New mutations are estimated to account for 20–30% of the cases diagnosed in the general population (Erbe, 1976). Mulvihill (1983) estimated that 425–2220 cases of heritable colorectal cancer occur each year in the United States.

Gardner's syndrome is estimated to occur about half as frequently as familial adenomatosis and also carries a high risk of intestinal cancer (McKusick, 1974). The components of the syndrome, large and small intestinal adenomatosis, bone tumors (osteomas), and soft tissue tumors (lipomas, sebaceous cysts, fibromas, fibrosarcomas) are often not expressed in a single patient, and study of the family may be necessary to separate Gardner's syndrome from familial adenomatosis. Carcinoma may occur in the stomach and small intestine (i.e., in the duodenum), as well as in the large bowel. There is evidence that tetraploidy in skin cultures containing epithelioid and fibroblastic cells occurs in most affected family members and in about half of asymptomatic family members who are at risk (Danes and Krush, 1977).

Turcot's and Oldfield's syndromes may represent variants of Gardner's syndrome or the familial adenomatosis syndrome. Turcot's syndrome represents the rare presentation of adenomas and carcinoma of the colon in association with tumors of the central nervous system. Oldfield's syndrome is another rare variant of the inherited polyposis syndromes that consists of multiple sebaceous cysts, adenomas, and adenocarcinoma of the large intestine.

Generalized juvenile polyposis (hamartomatosis) refers to an autosomal dominant syndrome characterized by hamartomatous polyps of the colon and rectum and, to a lesser extent, of the small intestine and stomach. The prevalance of juvenile polyps appears to be highest during the first decade of life and occurs more frequently in boys than in girls. No direct relationship has been demonstrated between the polyps of juvenile polyposis and adenocarcinoma of the colon or rectum. The increased risk of colorectal cancer in the family members of patients with the syndrome, in particular right-sided colonic lesions, has been attributed to an increased frequency of true adenomas and adenomatous foci within juvenile polyps in family members (Haggitt and Pitcock, 1970; Stemper *et al.*, 1975).

Members of "cancer families," in whom adenocarcinomas occur with high frequency at an early age (Fig. 1), develop colorectal carcinomas most commonly in association with adenocarcinomas of the endometrium, ovary, breast, and stomach. The cancer family syndrome with cancer of the large intestine as a major manifestation develops independently of polyposis and frequently involves the right side of the colon—cancers of the cecum and of the ascending or transverse colon (Anderson, 1982; Lynch *et al.*, 1977).

Familial aggregation of large bowel cancer occurs even among sporadic cases that are not part of defined genetic syndromes with intestinal polyposis. Studies by Woolf (1958), Macklin (1960), and Lovett (1976) concurred in estimating that the risk was approximately threefold greater in first-degree relatives of patients compared with the general population (Table II).

Whereas the inherited forms of polyposis in the aggregate probably account for less than 1% of all large bowel cancers (Lovett, 1976), the inherited types not associated with polyposis account for 12–26% (Anderson and Strong, 1974). There are at least three subgroups of inherited large bowel cancer not associated with polyposis—hereditary colonic cancer, hereditary gastrocolonic cancer, and hereditary adenocarcinomatosis. Each of these syndromes is characterized by

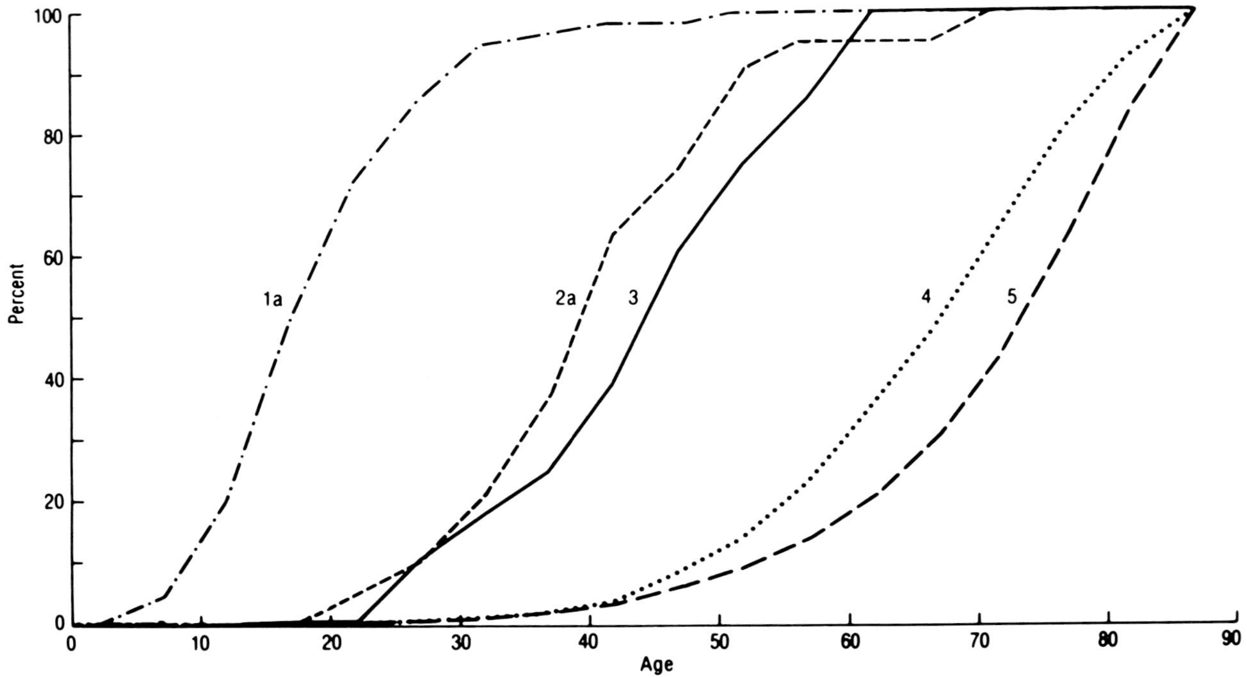

Fig. 1. Cumulative percent of incident cases at various ages having familial polyposis, compared to cumulative age incidence of colon cancer in other population groups. Curve 1a shows the onset of nonmalignant polyposis and Curve 2a the onset of cancer in familial polyposis, derived from data of 38 cases seen at Memorial Hospital. Curve 3 shows early age of onset of cancer in 28 affected individuals from Memorial Hospital series who have familial colon cancer-prone disease without polyposis. Curve 4 illustrates the age of onset of colon and rectal cancer in the general population of the United States, from the Third National Cancer Survey (NCI) and includes white and black males and females combined. Curve 5 illustrates the onset of colon and rectal cancer in males and females in Japan from data supplied by Dr. T. Hirayama. From Lipkin *et al.*, 1981.

TABLE II

Familial Aggregation in "Sporadic" Colorectal Cancer[a]

Study reference	Number of index cases	Number of first-degree relatives screened	Seen	Colon cancer expected	Ratio
St. Mark's	209	352	42	11.65	3.6:1
Macklin	145	1369	78	27.2	2.9:1
Woolf	242	763	26	8	3.2:1
Total	596	2484	146	46.8	3.1:1

[a] From Kussin *et al.*, 1979.

right-sided predominance, earlier average age at diagnosis, and multiple primary cancers, either in the large intestine or elsewhere, such as in the stomach, endometrium, or breast.

Women with colorectal cancer are at increased risk of developing independent primary carcinomas of the breast, uterine corpus, and ovary (Schottenfeld *et al.*, 1969; Schoenberg and Christine, 1974). Even in the absence of apparent familial aggregation, the proportion of colorectal cancer patients with either a previous or a simultaneous primary cancer of the large intestine is at least 5–6%. The annual incidence of subsequent multiple primary cancers of the large intestine is at least 3.5 per 1000. The presence of multiple adenomatous polyps in the resected specimen is associated with an even higher frequency of metachronous primary cancers than that just described (Schottenfeld, 1972).

D. History of Radiation Exposure

Prior radiation therapy in patients with gynecologic cancer, bladder cancer, and ankylosing spondylitis has been reported to increase the relative risk of colorectal cancer (Sandler and Sandler, 1983). Radiation as a risk factor in the natural history of colorectal cancer accounts for less than 1% of incident cases (Schottenfeld, 1983).

III. SCREENING TESTS AND TRIALS

Tests that have been evaluated or are under evaluation in the screening for colorectal cancer include proctosigmoidoscopy, fecal occult blood tests (see Chapter 13), and carcinoembryonic antigen (CEA) (Winawer and Sherlock, 1981). Additional tests under evaluation are at present considered primarily as research tools for high-risk patients and include cell proliferation studies of colonic mucosa, skin fibroblast alterations, cutaneous chromosomal abnormalities, and circulating leukocyte abnormalities. Although colonoscopy and barium enema are considered to be diagnostic tests, they have been advocated for periodic use in certain high-risk groups for the detection of adenomas and early cancers (Winawer, 1980).

A. Proctosigmoidoscopy

Proctosigmoidoscopy has not had good patient acceptance or widespread physician usage. Three studies support its possible usefulness in screening. In one study at the Strang Clinic, 58 cancers were detected in 26,000 sigmoidoscopies. In 50 determinant cases, the Dukes' staging at surgery was 80% A and B, and the 15-year survival was 90%. In a 25-year study at the University of Minnesota, periodic sigmoidoscopy in 18,000 people resulted in an 85% reduction of observed/expected cases of rectosigmoid cancers. Neither study was a controlled trial, and the completeness of the follow-up in the University of Minnesota study was not described (Winawer *et al.*, 1976). Incomplete follow-up could result in fewer than expected cancers. In a Kaiser-Permanente Hospital randomized trial, periodic screening resulted in a lower mortality for colorectal cancer over a 7-year period (Dales *et al.*, 1973). Thus, proctosigmoidoscopy has a potential value. Follow-up examination with fiberoptic instruments has shown the sensitivity of rigid proctosigmoidscopy to be approximately 80% (Bohlman *et al.*, 1977), with a specificity of 95% derived from screening programs. Greater effectiveness of the procedures could be achieved by performing them less frequently, perhaps every 3–5 years, and the cost would be lower with performance by paraprofessionals. Flexible sigmoidoscopy (with a 60-cm sigmoidoscope) has a greater yield in the hands of experts than has rigid proctosigmoidoscopy but is more costly and takes longer. A short (30- to 35-cm) flexible sigmoidoscope is under evaluation as a lower-cost substitute for the rigid scope for use by nonendoscopists. This could enhance patient compliance and improve physician utilization (Winawer *et al.*, 1982a) (Fig. 2).

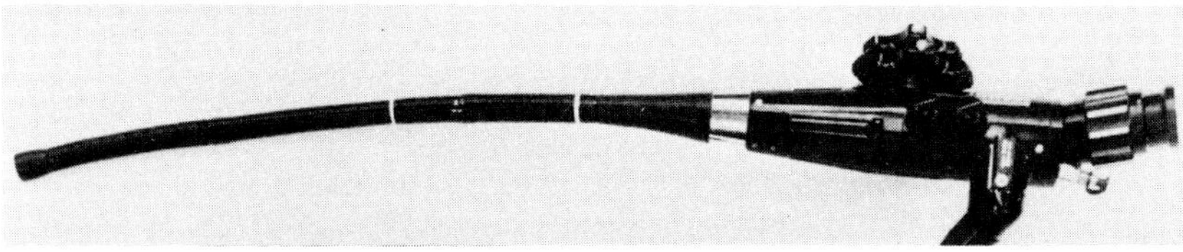

Fig. 2. This is an example of a 35 cm flexible sigmoidoscope. Instruction in the use of this instrument is usually brief. It has the potential for providing a consistent examination of the rectosigmoid with safety and patient comfort.

B. Clinical Trials with Fecal Occult Blood Tests

1. Uncontrolled Trials

Since the initial studies of Greegor, numerous community programs and trials have been implemented to determine the efficacy of the Hemoccult test (Smith-Kline Diagnostics, Sunnyvale, California) in detecting colorectal cancers. In 1972, a mass screening program offering free rectal examinations and guaiac kits was organized by Hastings (1974). Of the 2272 individuals over the age of 40 who registered for this program, 1835 returned the slide test; 114 (6.2%) of these were positive. Follow-up reports were obtained in 89 cases, but only 49 patients underwent complete examinations, 5 of whom were found to have a carcinoma. In Miller and Knight's study (1977) of 2323 patients, 39 had positive guaiac slides. Further workup revealed three patients with carcinoma and seven with polyps. Frühmorgen's screening program included 6007 individuals, with 83.5% returning the impregnated guaiac slides (Frühmorgen and Demling, 1980). A total of 136 patients had positive slides, and 117 permitted inpatient examination, including colonoscopy and air-contrast barium enema. Thirteen carcinomas and 51 adenomas were diagnosed. Colonoscopy proved to be the superior diagnostic modality. In the program organized by Gnauck in 1975, screening of 5016 patients produced 117 positive guaiac tests and the subsequent diagnosis of 13 carcinomas and multiple adenomas (Gnauck, 1977). Glober and Peskoe (1974) enlisted 1539 Japanese-American males in Hawaii for guaiac testing. A total of 344 of the 400 individuals with positive tests returned slides obtained on meat-free diets; 53 of these were positive for occult blood. Further diagnostic evaluation revealed one gastric carcinoma, three colonic carcinomas, and one colonic polyp. The frequency and predictive value for neoplasia of Hemoccult-positive slides in the before-mentioned studies ranged from 1 to 5% and 18 to 50%, respectively (Table III).

TABLE III

Recommended Methodology for Fecal Occult Blood Testing

Dietary restriction	Meat free High fiber Low peroxidase
Number of smears	6
Types of slides	Impregnated guaiac at present More specific slides under study
Rehydration	No
Storage interval	4 days preferred
Quality control	Slide window or laboratory assay

Large-scale programs utilizing the impregnated guaiac card as a screening tool were initiated by Kobayashi in Japan, Rozen in Israel, and Samec in Austria (Winawer *et al.*, 1980a). Of interest is the ongoing study in the Federal Republic of Germany, which is funded by social health insurance (Schwartz *et al.*, 1980). In 1977, Hemoccult was incorporated into the screening program and 1 year thereafter had been distributed to 2.5 million women and 1 million men; 1% of the women and 1.5% of the men had positive slides. Of the 2084 women and 2178 men who were confirmed to have undergone subsequent evaluation, 4.7% of the women and 10.7% of the men had carcinomas.

It is obvious that patient compliance in these large-scale screening programs is a major limiting factor. However, public education can offset this problem, as shown in the study of Bralow and Kopel (1979), which had a 79% compliance rate. Yet even here, follow-up could be obtained in only 30% of the individuals with positive guaiac slides.

Absent in many of the uncontrolled trials is standardization of testing methods and reporting. Frequently, little if any information is given on population characteristics, slide preparation, dietary or drug restrictions, quality control measures, or manner of further diagnostic evaluation. As a result, these studies are often difficult to compare and may not accurately depict the impact of fecal occult blood testing in the early diagnosis of colorectal carcinoma. Thus, the need for controlled studies is essential.

2. *Controlled Trials*

At present, there are two major ongoing controlled trials of fecal occult blood testing in the United States. One study is conducted at the Preventive Medicine Institute-Strang Clinic in association with the Memorial Sloan-Kettering Cancer Center (Winawer *et al.*, 1980b). Its purpose is to determine the impact of fecal occult blood testing on the mortality from colorectal cancer. The project was started in 1974 and included asymptomatic men and women over the age of 40 coming to the Strang Clinic. Patients were assigned to either the screened group or the control group by calendar periods. They all had a complete history and physical examination, along with rigid sigmoidoscopy; in addition, the screened group received guaiac-impregnated cards that were to be prepared at home within four days of their initial examination (Table IV). Patients were specifically instructed to smear two different portions of each of three different stools while adhering to a meat-free, high-fiber diet and refraining from the use of certain vitamins and medications. Those with positive slides underwent an air-contrast barium enema and colonoscopy. If a source of lower gastrointestinal bleeding was not apparent, an upper gastrointestinal series was obtained. Over 22,000 patients have participated in this study. Compliance was for 70–80% of the Hemoccult slides and 95% for sigmoidoscopy.

The overall slide positivity was 2.5%. However, this figure varied with the

TABLE IV

Fecal Occult Blood Test: Clinical Data[a]

Patient compliance	
Motivated groups	80%
Unmotivated groups	15%
Rate of positive slides (unhydrated)	1–5%
Rate of positive slides (hydrated)	Up to 20%
Predictive value for neoplasia	18–50%
Staging of detected cancers (Dukes' A and B)	60–80%
False positivity	
Unhydrated slides	2%
Hydrated slides	Up to 20%
False negativity for cancer	
Hydrated slides	9%
Unhydrated slides	31%
False negativity for adenomas	60–75%
Other	Complements sigmoidoscopy Minimal risk Colonoscopy important in workup of positive patients

[a] Summary of published result from many programs. From Winawer *et al.*, 1982b.

age group and the type of guaiac-impregnated slide. Slide positivity was 1.7% for patients in their fifties and rose to 4.4% for patients over 70 years of age (Fig. 3). One percent of the single Hemoccult slides were positive, with a predictive value of 50% for neoplasia (12% for carcinoma and 38% for adenoma). With the Hemoccult II slides, the rate of positivity increased to 3.7%, with an overall predictive value of 47%. With respect to age, the predictive value was 27% for ages 40–49, and 52% for age 70 and older.

Pertinent to the concept of smearing two slides from each bowel movement is the finding that 59% of the neoplastic lesions would have been missed if one rather than two smears per day had been examined. However, there was poor correlation between predictive value and number of positive slides.

In the last report from the Strang Clinic–Memorial Sloan-Kettering Cancer Center study, 71 cases of colon carcinoma had been diagnosed. Of the 59 cancers in the study group, 61% were detected by Hemoccult alone, 12% by both Hemoccult and sigmoidoscopy, and 10.5% by sigmoidoscopy alone. The remaining 12.5% were suggested by symptoms that led to diagnostic evaluation. The 59 cases of carcinoma in the study group can be categorized into 32 cases of prevalence and 27 cases of incidence. Fifty-nine percent of the prevalence cases

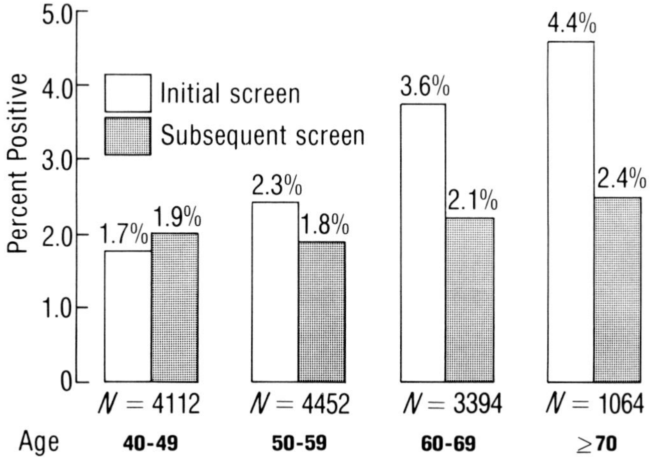

Fig. 3. This graph shows the rate of positive occult blood tests in the initial screening as compared to subsequent screening periods. It further demonstrates the correlation of the rate of positivity with age by decade. The results are based on 6 smears tested over 3 days on a meat-free, high-fiber diet without rehydrating the slide. From Winawer, S. J., Baldwin, M., Herbert, E., and Sherlock, P., "Perspectives on Prevention and Treatment of Cancer in the Elderly" (R. Yancik, P. P. Carbone, B. W. Patterson, K. Steel, and W. D. Terry, eds.). Copyright 1983 by Raven Press, New York.

and 74% of the incidence cases detected by Hemoccult slides were staged *in situ*, Dukes' A or Dukes' B lesions. However, only 33% of either the prevalence or incidence cases detected by sigmoidoscopy or evaluated because of symptoms were staged *in situ*, Dukes' A or Dukes' B lesions. Both the air-contrast barium enema and colonoscopy had a high sensitivity for carcinoma, but colonoscopy was clearly more sensitive for adenomas.

A second control trial for fecal occult blood testing was organized at the University of Minnesota (Gilbertsen *et al.*, 1980). A total of 45,000 patients over the age of 50 were randomized into three groups: those undergoing yearly Hemoccult testing, those undergoing Hemoccult testing every other year, and a control group. The positive Hemoccult was followed up with a single-column barium enema (later abandoned) and colonoscopy. Slide positivity was 2.4%, with an 8.2% predictive value for colorectal carcinoma; 78% of these cancers were either Dukes' A or Dukes' B lesions. The incidence of carcinoma was greatest in patients 63 years of age or older. Colonoscopy was significantly more sensitive than the single-column barium enema.

Clinical investigation of symptomatic patients with cancer has suggested that the sensitivity of the fecal occult blood test is 80–93%. The higher sensitivity is obtained with hydration, but this does not have the high specificity of nonhydrated slides (Macrae *et al.*, 1982). This finding remains to be verified.

The relationship of fecal occult blood testing to proctosigmoidoscopy is just beginning to be clarified. Approximately 15% of cancers detected by the fecal occult blood test are in the rectosigmoid and are detected by proctosigmoidoscopy, not by the occult blood test. Approximately 75–85% of the cancers detected in programs utilizing the occult blood test are detected above the rectosigmoid (Winawer *et al.*, 1980b; Gilbertsen *et al.*, 1980). The proctosigmoidoscope and the fecal occult blood test appear to complement each other (Winawer *et al.*, 1980b). The fecal occult blood tests appear to have better sensitivity for cancer than for polyps. The sensitivity for polyps is approximately 50% in the colon and less than 25% in the rectum. The test appears to be more sensitive for larger polyps over 2 cm in size. These larger adenomas are more likely to be malignant than smaller ones.

Early outcome variables have thus been reported with the fecal occult blood test, but issues such as cost, patient survival, and population mortality benefit have not yet been established.

C. Standardization of Reporting and Trials

It is difficult to compare the results of the various screening programs because of inadequate reporting of patient characteristics, types of slides used, interval between slide preparation and testing, type of diet used, and the presence or absence of laboratory quality control of the slide test (Winawer *et al.*, 1980b). In addition, the diagnostic workup varies greatly: some studies use sigmoidoscopy, some single-column barium enemas, some the double contrast technique, and still others colonoscopy. There is a need for standardization. Uncontrolled trials and community programs are important in determining the feasibility of these studies in terms of patient compliance, physician orientation and education, yield or diagnostic workup, staging of the cancers detected, and survival of the patients. Controlled trials are needed to determine whether screening results in a mortality reduction for colorectal cancer.

D. Other Screening Tests

Modifications of the fecal occult blood test under study include a peroxidase inhibitor, a different collection system, and various chemical and immunologic assays for blood (Winawer *et al.*, 1982b). CEA has been evaluated as an indicator of early malignancy but has been shown to have very low sensitivity and specificity and has, therefore, been given up for this purpose. It is still being evaluated as a prognosticator and in the follow-up of patients after surgery for colorectal cancer. Cell proliferation abnormalities on biopsy have shown striking changes in the presence of any neoplastic lesion in the colon but are currently a research tool. Abnormalities of circulating leukocytes have been demonstrated in families with inherited colon cancer, but this observation needs to be extended and validated. Skin fibroblast studies and skin chromosomal studies are also being used as research tools (Winawer, 1980).

E. Diagnostic Tests

It has been shown that adequate diagnostic workup of patients with a positive screening test is essential for the screening program. There is still some debate as to whether a double contrast barium enema could be used as a substitute for colonoscopy in the investigation of positive patients. Single-column barium enemas have been shown to have a low sensitivity for cancers. The double contrast barium enema is far superior to the single-column type. The sensitivity of the single-column barium enema for adenomas is even lower, especially for smaller adenomas. Colonoscopy has been demonstrated to have a high sensitivity for neoplastic lesions of the colon (97%) (Williams *et al.*, 1974; Leinicke *et al.*, 1977).

Colonoscopy has been used in the periodic surveillance of high-risk patients, including patients with nonpolyposis family cancer syndromes and ulcerative colitis (Chapter 14). When it is used in ulcerative colitis, multiple biopsies are taken to look for dysplasia of the colonic mucosa. If high-grade dysplasia is present, there is about a 50% chance that the patient already has a cancer. About 80% of the patients with ulcerative colitis and cancer have dysplasia (Lennard-Jones *et al.*, 1977).

There are screening programs in progress utilizing barium enema and/or colonoscopy for the periodic surveillance of patients at high risk. Several programs are prospectively evaluating the usefulness of biopsies for dysplasia in patients with ulcerative colitis. The results are not yet conclusive. There are many problems in the interpretation of dysplasia by pathologists.

IV. GUIDELINES FOR SCREENING AND CASE FINDING

A. Average-Risk Patients

The American Cancer Society and the International Workgroup on Colorectal Cancer have developed guidelines that address many questions regarding screening and case finding (Winawer *et al.*, 1982b). The International Workgroup felt that analysis of available data allowed the following recommendations to be made (analysis of new data will continue, which will provide a basis for modification of these recommendations):

Screening of individuals and small groups should be promoted. Persons at risk should be encouraged to enter the health care system. Relative risk should be assessed by family and personal history questionnaires.

Once patients are in the system, screening should be added to other aspects of medical evaluation.

Screening should include proctosigmoidoscopy once every three to five years, beginning between the ages of 40 and 50. Rigid proctosigmoidoscopy should be used if this is the only available instrument, but flexible proctosigmoidoscopy, using a 60 cm scope by a trained endoscopist or a 30 cm scope by a primary practicing physician or paraprofessional, is preferred.

Screening should include a fecal occult blood test annually, beginning between the ages of 40 and 50.

Diagnostic workup of patients with a positive screening test should include colonoscopy.

Screening may be encouraged for individuals and small groups but general or mass screening cannot be encouraged until firm mortality, risk, and cost data are available from ongoing programs.

Screening should be accompanied by programs to educate patients and make physicians more aware of the concepts and technology involved in screening, diagnosis, treatment, and followup.

Proper record-keeping and data collection should be part of any screening program.

Patients with a diagnosis of colorectal neoplasia should be entered into a long-range followup surveillance program with periodic direct re-examination of the colon every three to five years.

Quality control should be part of any program using fecal occult blood tests.

A program questionnaire such as that proposed by the International Workgroup on Colorectal Cancer should be used as a guide to standardize reporting of data. [From Winawer *et al.*, 1982b.]

The American Cancer Society recommends that patients over the age of 40 have a digital examination annually. The stool guaiac test should be added at age 50 on an annual basis, with sigmoidoscopy every 3–5 years after two initial negative proctosigmoidoscopies 1 year apart. The rationale is that although no single study proves the value of any particular test, there is strong suggestive evidence from several sources that detection of colon cancer prior to the onset of signs and symptoms will prolong survival. The earlier Dukes' staging detection in asymptomatic patients being screened with fecal occult blood testing appears to be similar to that seen in screening programs utilizing proctosigmoidoscopy.

It is felt that the long-term survival following detection by fecal occult blood slides will be similar to that seen after screening with proctosigmoidoscopy. This remains to be seen, of course. The screening programs with the stool guaiac slide tests have not gone on long enough to provide conclusive evidence, and until such evidence is present, as well as evidence of mortality benefit and cost effectiveness, neither the American Cancer Society, nor the International Workgroup on Colorectal Cancer, nor the National Cancer Institute is prepared to recommend mass screening with the guaiac slide test. Both the American Cancer Society and the International Workgroup on Colorectal Cancer recommend that this test be added only when a patient is already in the health care system. These recommendations are related to average-risk patients.

B. High-Risk Groups

Patients who have already undergone surgery and have been cured of colorectal cancer, as well as those with prior colonoscopic polypectomy, should have their colons cleared of additional synchronous lesions (these occur in 40–50% of patients with an index adenoma) directly, radiologically and endoscopically, initially and at periodic intervals following treatment (Winawer *et al.*, 1976).

It is possible that fecal occult blood testing may have a role as an interval examination in such high-risk groups (Table I). This is currently being studied within the framework of the National Polyp Study, with patients randomized after colonoscopic polypectomy into more aggressive and less aggressive arms. Within each group, barium enema, colonoscopy, and fecal occult blood tests are being evaluated for sensitivity and specificity. In that study, predictive factors are being examined in relation to the natural history of subsequent adenomas of various histologic types in the patients entered.

Fecal occult blood testing may have some role in the nonpolyposis, inherited colon cancer syndromes. Patients with autosomal dominant modes of inheritance in striking family histories should be directly examined by X ray or colonoscopy at periodic intervals. Fecal occult blood testing could serve as an interval examination. Patients with a suggestive family history, but not one of an autosomal dominant form, could have fecal occult blood testing and perhaps proctosigmoidoscopy performed beginning in their twenties, when their risk begins. Fecal occult blood testing has no role in patients with familial polyposis or ulcerative colitis, since they have lesions that may produce positivity without the presence

TABLE V

Application of the Fecal Occult Blood Test

Not applicable	Patients with symptoms suggesting colorectal neoplasia
	Patients with familial polyposis or Gardner's syndrome
	Patients with ulcerative colitis
As primary screen or for case finding	Asymptomatic average-risk men and women over ages 40–50
	Persons with a suggestive family history over age 20
As an adjunctive interval test	Patients with past history of adenoma
	Patients with past history of colorectal cancer
	Strong history of family cancer syndrome

[a] From Winawer *et al.*, 1982b.

of cancer. In affected families, nonaffected individuals should be screened with proctosigmoidoscopy every 6 months beginning in their teens, since this is when the polyposis becomes manifest (Table V).

C. Patient Compliance and Physician Education

Patient compliance during screening programs has been excellent when the patients have been well motivated. Those lacking the appropriate orientation and education, however, have had extremely poor compliance (Snyder-Halper *et al.*, 1980).

It has also been observed that primary care physicians who would be heavily involved in case finding, screening, diagnosis, and follow-up of such patients are not thoroughly acquainted with these techniques or with the natural history of adenomas and colorectal cancer (Dent, 1980). For case finding and screening programs to be successful, educational programs must be developed and presented to both the medical community and the lay public.

V. SUMMARY AND FUTURE STUDIES

Evidence suggests that colorectal cancer evolves from preexisting premalignant adenomas and that there is a long lead time allowing for screening. The vast majority of patients at risk can be identified only by age and have no other risk factors. There are, however, high-risk subgroups that can be identified from a risk factor questionnaire directed to the past and family history. Tests are currently available that could be useful in screening, including the fecal occult blood test and proctosigmoidoscopy. Refinement of more specific tests for occult blood and development of low cost 35-cm flexible sigmoidoscopes for the primary care physician are expected in the near future. Diagnostic tests are available with a high degree of sensitivity and specificity for use in patients with a positive screening test. Adequate treatment is better understood today and, if properly applied to early cases, could result in better survival. Diagnostic modalities could be used in follow-up programs to identify metachronous adenomas and remove them in order to maintain the benefit in the positive screenees. Demonstration of cost effectiveness, enhanced physician awareness, and public acceptance will be critical to the effective application of screening approaches.

Many issues need to be resolved before this sequence can be considered to be a valid approach, including the age at which to begin screening; the screening interval; the proper combination and interval of proctosigmoidoscopy and fecal occult blood testing; the proper workup of positive screenees; types of follow-up programs after treatment; the approach to high-risk groups as compared to average-risk patients; enhancement of patient compliance; education of physicians regarding concepts and techniques; use of radical cancer surgery in patients with cancer; and appropriate use of colonoscopic polypectomy. Some of these data may be obtained from analysis of information in the literature and from ongoing programs. Other data elements will have to be obtained from new studies. In addition to these factors, cost effectiveness and mortality data will be critical.

REFERENCES

Anderson, D. E. (1982). Familial predisposition. *In* "Cancer Epidemiology and Prevention" (D. Schottenfeld and J. F. Fraumeni, Jr., eds.), pp. 483–493. Saunders, Philadelphia, Pennsylvania.

Anderson, D. E., and Strong, L. C. (1974). Genetics of gastrointestinal tumors. *In* "Cancer Epidemiology, Environmental Factors," Excerpta Med. Congr. Ser. No. 351, Vol. 3, pp. 267–271. Excerpta Medica, Amsterdam.

Bohlman, T., Katon, R., Lipshutz, G., McCool, M., Smith, F., and Melnyk, C. (1977). Fiberoptic pansigmoidoscopy. An evaluation and comparison with rigid sigmoidoscopy. *Gastroenterology* **72,** 644–649.

Bralow, S. P., and Kopel, J. (1979). Hemoccult screening for colorectal cancer—impact study on Sarasota, Florida. *J. Fla. Med. Assoc.* **66,** 915–919.

Dales, L. G., Friedman, G. D., Ramcharan, S., Siegelaub, A. B., Campbell, B. A., Feldman, R., and Collen, M. F. (1973). Multiphasic checkup evaluation study: 3. Outpatient clinic utilization hospitalization, and mortality experience after 7 years. *Prev. Med.* **2,** 221–235.

Danes, B. S., and Krush, A. J. (1977). The Gardner syndrome: A family study in cell culture. *JNCI, J. Natl. Cancer Inst.* **58,** 771–775.

Dent, O. (1980). Physician awareness of concepts of colorectal cancer. *In* "Progress in Cancer Research and Therapy" (S. J. Winawer, D. Schottenfeld, and P. Sherlock, eds.), Vol. 13, pp. 243–244. Raven Press, New York.

Devroede, G. (1980). Risk of cancer in inflammatory bowel disease. *In* "Progress in Cancer Research and Therapy" (S. J. Winawer, D. Schottenfeld, and P. Sherlock, eds.), Vol. 13, pp. 325–334. Raven Press, New York.

Erbe, R. W. (1976). Inherited gastrointestinal polyposis syndrome. *N. Engl. J. Med.* **294,** 1101–1104.

Frühmorgen, P., and Demling, L. (1980). Early detection of colorectal cancer—a modified guaiac test—a screening examination in 6,000 humans. *In* "Progress in Cancer Research and Therapy" (S. J. Winawer, D. Schottenfeld, and P. Sherlock, eds.), Vol. 13, pp. 311–315. Raven Press, New York.

Gilbertsen, V. A., McHugh, R., Schuman, L., and Williams, S. E. (1980). The earlier detection of colorectal cancers. A preliminary report of the results of the occult blood study. *Cancer* **45,** 2899–2901.

Glober, G. A., and Peskoe, S. M. (1974). Outpatient screening for gastrointestinal lesions using guaiac-impregnated slides. *Dig. Dis.* **19,** 399–403.

Gnauck, R. (1977). Screening for colorectal cancer with the Hemoccult test. *Leber, Magen, Darm* **7,** 32–35.

Greenstein, A. J., Sachar, D. B., Smith, H., Janowitz, H. D., and Aufses, A. H., Jr. (1980). Patterns of neoplasia in Crohn's disease and ulcerative colitis. *Cancer* **46,** 403–407.

Haggitt, R. C., and Pitcock, J. A. (1970). Familial polyposis of the colon. *Cancer* **26,** 1232–1238.

Hastings, J. B. (1974). Mass screening for colorectal cancer. *Am. J. Surg.* **127,** 228–233.

Janowitz, H. D., and Sachar, D. B. (1983). Inflammatory bowel disease. *Adv. Intern. Med.* **27,** 205–246.

Kirsner, J. B. (1980). Inflammatory bowel disease—considerations of etiology and pathogenesis. *In* "Progress in Cancer Research and Therapy" (S. J. Winawer, D. Schottenfeld, and P. Sherlock, eds.), Vol. 13, pp. 319–323. Raven Press, New York.

Kussin, S., Lipkin, M., and Winawer, S. J. (1979). Inherited colon cancer: Clinical implications. *Am. J. Gastroenterol.* **72,** 448–457.

Leinicke, J. L., Dodds, W. J., Hogan, W. J., and Stewart, E. J. (1977). A comparison of colonoscopy and roentgenography for detecting polypoid lesions of the colon. *Gastrointest. Radiol.* **2,** 125–128.

Lennard-Jones, J. W., Morson, B. C., Ritchie, J. K., Shove, D. C., and Williams, C. B. (1977). Cancer in colitis: Assessment of the individual risk by clinical and histological criteria. *Gastroenterology* **73,** 1280–1289.

Lightdale, C. J., and Sherlock, P. (1980). Cancer in Crohn's disease: Memorial Hospital experience and review of the literature. *In* "Progress in Cancer Research and Therapy" (S. J. Winawer, D. Schottenfeld, and P. Sherlock, eds.), Vol. 13, pp. 341–346. Raven Press, New York.

Lipkin, M., Winawer, S. J., Sherlock, P. (1981). Early identification of individuals at increased risk for cancer of the large intestine. Part I: Definition of high-risk populations. *Clin. Bull.* **11,** 13–21.

Lovett, E. (1976). Family studies in cancer of the colon and rectum. *Br. J. Surg.* **63,** 13–18.

Lynch, P. M., Lynch, H. T., and Harris, R. E. (1977). Hereditary proximal colonic cancer. *Dis. Colon Rectum* **20,** 661–668.

Macklin, M. T. (1960). Inheritance of cancer of the stomach and large intestine in man. *JNCI, J. Natl. Cancer Inst.* **24,** 551–571.

McKusick, V. A. (1974). Genetics and large bowel cancer. *Dig. Dis.* **19,** 954–958.

Macrae, F. A., James, D., and St. John, B. (1982). Relationship between patterns of bleeding and Hemoccult sensitivity in patients with colorectal cancers or adenomas. *Gastroenterology* **82,** 891–898.

Miller, S. F., and Knight, R. A. (1977). The early detection of colorectal cancer. *Cancer* **40,** 945–949.

Morson, B. C. (1974). The polyp-cancer sequence in the large bowel. *Proc. R. Soc. Med.* **67,** 451–457.

Morson, B. C. (1980). Use of dysplasia as an indicator of risk for malignancy in patients with ulcerative colitis. *In* "Progress in Cancer Research and Therapy" (S. J. Winawer, D. Schottenfeld, and P. Sherlock, eds.), Vol. 13, pp. 347–354. Raven Press, New York.

Mulvihill, J. J. (1983). The frequency of hereditary large bowel cancer. *In* "Prevention of Hereditary Large Bowel Cancer" (J. R. F. Ingall and A. J. Mastromarino, eds.), pp. 61–75. Alan R. Liss, Inc., New York.

Nugent, F. W. (1980). Surveillance of patients with ulcerative colitis: Lahey Clinic results. *In* "Progress in Cancer Research and Therapy" (S. J. Winawer, D. Schottenfeld, and P. Sherlock, eds.), Vol. 13, pp. 375–380. Raven Press, New York.

Sandler, R. S., and Sandler, D. P. (1983). Radiation-induced cancers of the colon and rectum: Assessing the risk. *Gastroenterology* **84,** 51–57.

Schoenberg, B. S., and Christine, B. W. (1974). The association of neoplasms of the colon and rectum with primary malignancies of other sites. *Am. J. Proctol.* **17,** 41–60.

Schottenfeld, D. (1972). Patient risk factors and the detection of early cancer. *Prev. Med.* **1,** 335–351.

Schottenfeld, D. (1983). Radiation as a risk factor in the natural history of colorectal cancer. (Editorial.) *Gastroenterology* **84,** 186–187.

Schottenfeld, D., and Winawer, S. J. (1982). Large intestine. *In* "Cancer Epidemiology and Prevention" (D. Schottenfeld and J. F. Fraumeni, Jr., eds.), pp. 703–727. Saunders, Philadelphia, Pennsylvania.

Schottenfeld, D., Berg, J. W., and Vitsky, B. (1969). Incidence of multiple primary cancers: II. Index cancers arising in the stomach and lower digestive system. *J. Natl. Cancer Inst.* (*U.S.*) **43,** 77–86.

Schwartz, F. W., Holstein, H., and Brecht, J. G. (1980). Preliminary report of fecal occult blood testing in Germany. *In* "Progress in Cancer Research and Therapy" (S. J. Winawer, D. Schottenfeld, and P. Sherlock, eds.), Vol. 13, pp. 267–270. Raven Press, New York.

Snyder-Halper, M., Winawer, S. J., Brody, R. S., Andrews, M., Roth, D., and Burton, G. (1980). Issues of patient compliance. *In* "Progress in Cancer Research and Therapy" (S. J. Winawer, D. Schottenfeld, and P. Sherlock, eds.), Vol. 13, pp. 299–310. Raven Press, New York.

Stemper, T. J., Kent, T. H., and Summers, R. W. (1975). Juvenile polyposis and gastrointestinal carcinoma—a study of a kindred. *Ann. Intern. Med.* **83,** 639–646.

Williams, C. B., Hunt, R. H., Loose, H., Sakai, Y., and Swarbrick, E. T. (1974). Colonoscopy in the management of colon polyps. *Br. J. Surg.* **61,** 673–682.

Winawer, S. J. (1980). Screening for colorectal cancer: An overview. *Cancer* **45,** 1093–1098.

Winawer, S. J., and Sherlock, P. (1981). Colonic cancer: Screening for premalignant and malignant disease. *In* "Harrison's Principles of Internal Medicine" (K. J. Isselbacher, R. D. Adams, E. Braunwald, J. B. Martin, R. G. Petersdorf, and J. D. Wilson, eds.), 9th ed., pp. 115–133. McGraw-Hill, New York.

Winawer, S. J., Sherlock, P., and Schottenfeld, D. (1976). Screening for colon cancer. *Gastroenterology* **70,** 783–789.

Winawer, S. J., Andrews, M., Miller, C. H., and Fleisher, M. (1980a). Review of screening for colorectal cancer using fecal occult blood testing. *In* "Progress in Cancer Research and Therapy" (S. J. Winawer, D. Schottenfeld, and D. P. Sherlock, eds.), Vol. 13, pp. 249–259. Raven Press, New York.

Winawer, S. J., Andrews, M., Flehinger, B., Sherlock, P., Schottenfeld, D., and Miller, D. G. (1980b). Progress report on controlled trial of fecal occult blood testing for the detection of colorectal neoplasia. *Cancer* **45,** 2959–2964.

Winawer, S. J., Cummins, R., Baldwin, M. P., and Ptak, A. (1982a). A new flexible sigmoidoscope for the generalist. *Gastrointestinal Endoscopy* **28,** 233–236.

Winawer, S. J., Fleisher, M., Baldwin, M. P., and Sherlock, P. (1982b). Current status of fecal occult blood testing in screening for colorectal cancer. *Ca—Cancer J. Clin.* **32,** 100–112.

Woolf, C. M. (1958). A genetic study of carcinoma of the large intestine. *Am. J. Hum. Genet.* **10,** 42–47.

Wynder, E. L., and Shigematsu, T. (1967). Environmental factors of cancer of the rectum and colon. *Cancer* **20,** 1520–1561.

Young, J. L., Jr., Asire, A. J., and Pollack, E. S., eds. (1978). "SEER Program: Cancer Incidence and Mortality in the United States, 1973–1976," DHEW Publ. No. (NIH) 78-1837. U.S. Dept. of Health, Education and Welfare, PHS, NIH, NCI, Washington, D.C.

19

Screening for Gastric Cancer

TAKESHI HIRAYAMA, SHIGERU HISAMICHI, ISABURO FUJIMOTO, AKIRA OSHIMA, AND SUKETAMI TOMINAGA

I.	Introduction	367
II.	Rate of Screening by Age Groups	368
III.	Method of Mass Screening	369
IV.	Results of Mass Screening	370
V.	Evaluation of Mass Screening	371
VI.	Side Benefits of Mass Screening	373
VII.	Declining Detection Rate	373
VIII.	Improving the Cost Effectiveness of Mass Screening	374
IX.	Approaches Used to Minimize the Side Effects of Mass Screening	374
X.	Summary and Conclusion	375
	References	376

I. INTRODUCTION

In 1982, 30,036 men and 18,977 women died of gastric cancer in Japan. This is still the leading form of cancer in Japan. The number of deaths from gastric cancer has been increasing during the past 21 years, rising from 26,283 men and 16,467 women in 1960. The problem will remain equally serious at least up to the end of this century.

Nevertheless, much of the increase in mortality has come from an increase in population size. Thus, the age-adjusted death rate for gastric cancer has steadily come down in recent years (Hirayama, 1975, 1977a), the rate in men being 48.3 per 100,000 population in 1960, 42.1 in 1970, and 30.5 in 1981; and in women 30.1 in 1960, 26.7 in 1970 and 17.3 in 1982. This decrease is most striking at 40–69 years of age in both men and women, being nearly 50% during the past 21 years. A downward trend was also observed in incidence rates for gastric cancer

ISBN 0-12-496720-5

in the cancer registries in Osaka and Miyagi, although it was slightly less than the decline in mortality. It is important to note that gastric cancer screening has been actively developed during these periods. The purpose of this chapter is to outline the methods and to evaluate the results of such mass screening activities.

II. RATE OF SCREENING BY AGE GROUPS

Early detection programs for gastric cancer started around 1960. A governmental subsidy provided in 1966 facilitated the rapid spread of the program, as shown in Table I. About 3 to 4 million people have been screened annually by mass gastrography in Japan in recent years. This is about a fourfold growth compared to 1966. The number examined by mass radiography for gastric cancer and the number of cancers detected in 1981 were 4,350,479 and 4365, respectively, yielding an estimate of screened persons of about 9% at ages 40–69 and a detection rate of gastric cancer of 1 per 1000 screenees, respectively.

The age-specific rates of persons screened annually per 1000 population are highest at 40–59 years of age in both men and women (Fig. 1). The decline in gastric cancer death rates tends to be higher in the age groups where the coverage of mass screening is greater. For persons of age 25 and above, $r = 0.828$ in men, significant at the 1% level, and $r = 0.715$ in women, significant at the 5% level.

TABLE I

Gastric Cancer Mass Screening in Japan: Number Screened and Gastric Cancers Detected

Year	Number screened	Gastric cancer cases detected	Rate per 1000
1966	989,762	1444	1.45
1967	1,334,933	1839	1.38
1968	1,565,845	2139	1.37
1969	1,825,861	2319	1.27
1970	2,165,287	2360	1.09
1971	2,400,550	2521	1.05
1972	2,627,156	2519	0.96
1973	2,707,926	2721	1.00
1974	2,833,656	2847	1.00
1975	2,779,399	2804	1.01
1976	2,965,582	2821	0.95
1977	3,165,805	2910	0.92
1978	3,197,594	3035	0.95
1979	3,572,811	3340	0.93
1980	3,830,260	3578	0.93
1981	4,350,479	4365	1.00

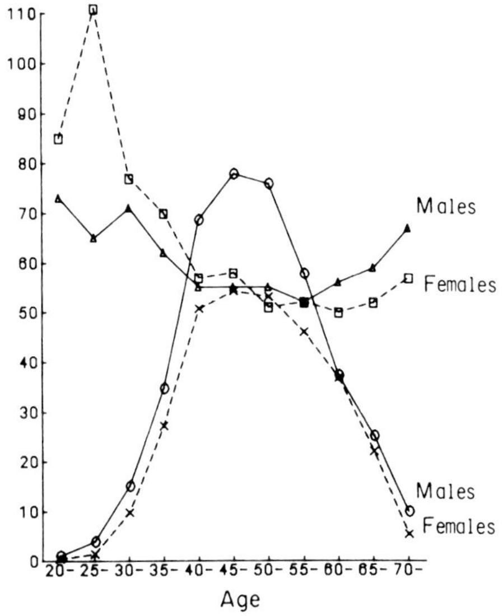

Fig. 1. Percent change in death rates from stomach cancer from 1960 to 1981 by sex and age (□--□, ▲—▲), according to the rate of mass screening for stomach cancer in 1975 (1960 = 100) (×--×, ○—○).

However, the decline in death rates is similar in men and in women, although the rate of mass screening is much higher in men.

Although the recent decline in gastric cancer death rates in Japan may be attributed to a decrease in the incidence of gastric cancer, which can be interpreted as a reflection of dietary changes made by the Japanese people, some of the decrease in mortality may also be attributed to the effect of the nationwide early detection program in recent years, since the age groups in which gastric cancer mortality has markedly decreased correspond to the age groups mainly covered by the mass screening program.

Caution is necessary in interpreting this phenomenon, since the decline in mortality started several years before the nationwide spread of mass screening took place, and also since this decline was equal in both sexes, in spite of the different rates of screening by sex (Fig. 1). In addition, the rate of screening is too low to be considered the major factor responsible for the sizable decline in mortality from gastric cancer.

III. METHOD OF MASS SCREENING

The number of persons screened and the number of gastric cancers detected were 3,889,575 and 3467 by mobile X ray units and 460,904 and 898 in cancer detection clinics in hospitals, respectively, in 1981. In nearly 90% of the mass

TABLE II

Depth of Cancerous Invasion in Operated Patients and Presence or Absence of Metastasis, 1973–1975

		Metastasis		Number	
		No	Yes	Total	Percentage
Limited to mucosa	(m)	673	37	710	21.2
Infiltrated to submucosa	(sm)	685	119	804	27.0
Up to proper muscle	(pm)	271	275	546	16.3
Pentrated to proper muscle	(ss)	117	302	419	12.5
Pentrated to serosa	(s)	174	691	865	25.9
Total		1920	1424	3344	100.0
Percentage		57.4	42.6	100.0	

screenings conducted in each prefecture by mobile X ray units, photofluorographic methods are well standardized. The examinee is asked to take effervescent granules before the examination, and six pictures are taken in various positions. This was the standard method chosen by the Japanese Society of Gastric Mass Survey to cover all aspects of the stomach.

Roll film 70–100 mm in width is used. It takes only 3–4 minutes to examine one person by this method, one unit covering 50–60 persons a day. This method is used to ensure economical expenditures and minimize X ray hazards without sacrificing diagnostic efficiency. The X ray films thus taken are examined by two specialists independently, and the cases that require further detailed examinations, such as gastrofiberscopic examination and biopsy, are selected. Early-stage cancers are found by such methods in much higher percentages than by conventional X ray diagnostic methods in outpatient departments in hospitals (Table II).

IV. RESULTS OF MASS SCREENING

Of the cases of gastric cancer detected by screening in 1973–1975, 57.4% were without lymph node metastasis (Table 2).

In terms of the extent of invasion of the gastric wall, 21.2% of lesions were limited to the mucosa (m), 24.0% infiltrated to the submucosa (sm), 16% up to proper muscle (pm), 12.5% penetrated to proper muscle (ss), and 25.9% penetrated to serosa (s). The percentages without metastases were 94.8% in m, 85.2% in sm, 49.6% in pm, 27.6% in ss, and 20.1% in ss, and 20.1% in s.

The 10-year survival rates for m and sm, pm, ss, and s were 89.6%, 68.6%,

45.3%, and 25.2%, respectively, in a follow-up study of 470 cases of gastric cancer (Hisamichi, 1978).

V. EVALUATION OF MASS SCREENING

The 5- and 10-year survival rates for gastric cancer cases detected by mass screening are significantly higher than in patients detected in outpatient clinics. The curve becomes almost flat after 5 years. Therefore, it is not likely that the better survival rate is mainly the product of so-called lead time bias.

The results of follow-up of screened persons clearly show a significantly lower gastric cancer adjusted death rate compared to that of unscreened persons: 61.9 out of 38,377.5 screened person-years versus 137.2 out of 20,653.0 unscreened person-years in males and 28.1 out of 48,888.5 screened person-years versus 53.8 unscreened person-years in females in four model areas in Miyagi Prefecture (1960–1977) (Table III). Similar results have been reported from Kanagawa Prefecture (144.32 out of 33,865 screened person-years and 176.82 out of 388,175 unscreened person-years, 1962–1971), from Tottori Prefecture (99.3 in the screened population versus 139.8 in the general population), and from Osaka Prefecture (162.4 in the screened population versus 255.2 in the general population).

Attention should, however, be paid to the fact that none of these programs was a randomized trial. A randomized trial is extremely difficult, if not impossible, to carry out when screening has spread rapidly even to remote areas of the country. The Fourth National Cancer Survey conducted in 1979 revealed that gastric cancer mass screening had been provided in 98.3% of 3278 municipalities throughout Japan. Thus, it is regarded as unrealistic to conduct a randomized trial to study the effect of gastric cancer mass screening at present or in the near future. Under such circumstances, alternative methods of evaluating the effect of screening were conducted.

In a study in Kanagawa Prefecture, the social and educational backgrounds of screened and unscreened persons were compared retrospectively; no essential difference was found. Such a postscreening comparability study could only partially remedy the drawbacks inherent in unrandomized studies.

Another alternative to a randomized trial is to compare the mortality from gastric cancer between populations with different levels of screening. Such a study was done by Kuroishi *et al.* (1983). They compared the change in gastric cancer death rates from 1969–1972 to 1973–1977 in 14 municipalities that had gastric cancer screening, with an average screening rate of 17.7% in 1969–1978, with that in 28 randomly selected comparable control municipalities, with an average screening rate of 7.7%. The death rate from gastric cancer decreased by 25.5% in the former group, being 97.5 and 73.0 per 100,000 in 1969–1972 and

TABLE III

Standardized Incidence and Mortality Rate from Gastric Cancer between the Screened and Nonscreened Groups in Four Model Areas, 40–69 Years Old, 1960–1977, Miyagi Prefecture

	Males		Females	
Age: 40–69 years	Screened group	Nonscreened group	Screened group	Nonscreened group
Number of persons at the start of the survey	2,098 (61.9%)	1,287 (38.1%)	2,227 (61.5%)	1,396 (38.5%)
Incidence cases	74	44	29	18
Person-years observed	38,125.5	20,625.0	48,819.5	21,577.0
Incidence rate (per 10^5 person-years)	187.7 (ns)[a]	201.8	58.1 (ns)	79.1
Number of deaths	25	30	14	12
Person-years	38,337.5	20,653.0	48,888.5	21,579.5
Mortality rate (per 10^5 person-years)	61.9[b]	137.2	28.1[c]	53.8

Note: standard population = world population.
[a] ns, no significance.
[b] $p < 0.005$
[c] $p < 0.01$

1973–1977, respectively, compared to a 0.7% decrease in the latter group, 84.9 and 84.3 per 100,000, respectively. The difference was statistically significant ($p<0.05$).

The following results of a natural history study of early gastric cancer also suggest the effectiveness of mass screening to prevent deaths from gastric cancer. Forty-three cases of early gastric cancer out of 56 cases detected in the Center for Adult Diseases, Osaka, were followed up without surgery for several reasons. Of these 43 cases, 27 progressed to clinical invasive cancer within 6–88 months (with a median of 27 months). It was also observed that 12 of 34 early gastric cancer patients who did not receive surgery died from gastric cancer during the observation period, having a median survival of 77 months. These results suggested that detection and surgical resection of early gastric cancer would prevent death from gastric cancer (Tsukuma *et al.*, 1983).

In summary, although attention should still be given to the possible effect of so-called lead time bias, 5- and 10-year survival rates in patients detected by mass screening are too high to be explained by this factor alone. A more serious concern is the possible influence of so-called length bias, or bias in detecting predominantly slow-growing tumors. The fact that the screened group has a significantly lower gastric cancer mortality rate compared to the unscreened group suggests that the effect of such a bias is also limited. The results of follow-up of early gastric cancers described above is also valuable in considering the effectiveness of screening on the suppression of gastric cancer deaths.

VI. SIDE BENEFITS OF MASS SCREENING

There is no doubt that the screening program has served as a strong means of public education on the need for early detection of cancer. It has also helped to increase the interest and the diagnostic capacity of practitioners on a nationwide scale. Besides, many other diseases of the stomach are detected by mass gastrography in addition to gastric cancer. In 1975, 8326 gastric polyps, 41,725 gastric ulcers, 24,430 duodenal ulcers, and 5226 gastric-duodenal ulcers were detected, in addition to 3002 gastric cancers.

Study of the detection rates by sex and age revealed interesting epidemiological patterns, such as a female preponderance of gastric polyps and a younger age peak in duodenal ulcers (Hirayama, 1978). Thus, mass screening is also useful for the early detection of these abnormalities and is valuable for thc epidemiological study of such diseases.

VII. DECLINING DETECTION RATE

As shown in Table I, the rate of detection of gastric cancer cases by mass screening has been declining in recent years. This is considered to be due to:

1. An increasing proportion of younger persons in the screened population.
2. An increasing proportion of repeatedly examined persons in the screened population.
3. A decrease in gastric cancer incidence, as recorded in the cancer registries in recent years.

Whatever the reason, one has to admit that the detection efficiency of mass screening for gastric cancer is gradually decreasing in Japan.

VIII. IMPROVING THE COST EFFECTIVENESS OF MASS SCREENING

The cost effectiveness of mass screening programs in gastric cancer control (Kitabatake *et al.*, 1973; Hirayama, 1981) should be improved by carefully studying these evaluation results and also by using local resources, funds, and facilities.

A focal attack is also necessary. One focus would be population groups never examined before. For instance, the screening program should be focused on sales workers, since the slowness of the decline in gastric cancer mortality in this group was interpreted, at least partly, as a reflection of their far lower rate of screening, especially at 40–54 years of age (Hirayama, 1977b). Thus, out of 31,205 male sales workers aged 40–54 in Kanagawa Prefecture, 21 cases of stomach cancer were registered in 1972. None of them were detected by mass screening. On the other hand, out of 421,378 persons of the same age group in other occupations, 269 cases of stomach cancer were registered. On these 269, 57 (21.2%) were detected by mass screening ($\chi^2 = 4.38$, $p<0.05$).

Another focus should be the so-called high risk groups. In order to make the current screening program more effective, it is of the utmost importance to delineate gastric cancer high-risk groups as precisely as possible and ensure that such groups are included in screening programs. Intensive epidemiological studies currently in progress to identify high-risk groups are therefore of urgent necessity, especially in Japan.

IX. APPROACHES USED TO MINIMIZE THE SIDE EFFECTS OF MASS SCREENING

To solve existing problems of possible radiation effects due to repeated mass radiography, successful efforts were made to improve X ray apparatus in order to reduce the exposure dose drastically and to enhance film sensitivity. In addition, consideration has been given to lengthening examination intervals and, as mentioned above, to concentrate mass screening on groups with the highest risk of gastric cancer and the lowest risk of leukemia and other possible radiation effects. A careful monitoring of leukemia incidence and other radiation-related conditions in the screened group is currently in progress. At this time no excess incidence of leukemia has been observed in the screened group compared to the general population in the Osaka Cancer Registry. Out of 75,981 persons screened by mass gastrography in Osaka, 30 cases of leukemia occurred during 7.2 years of follow-up, while 27.9 cases were expccted (A. Oshima, unpublished). Similar results have been reported from Miyagi Prefecture. A restrospective cohort study revealed 7 cases of leukemia out of 21,178 persons screened by mass radiography during 18 years of follow-up, while 8.4 cases were expected using the excess mortality rate of the United Nations Scientific Committee 1977 Report on the Effect of Atomic Radiation. However, in view of the somewhat rapid increase in leukemia death rates after age 40 in Japan since 1965, further careful follow-up of the effect of nation-wide mass radiography appears to be necessary.

X. SUMMARY AND CONCLUSION

The methods and results of mass screening for gastric cancer in Japan have been outlined.

The age-adjusted death rate for gastric cancer has been decreasing for the past 21 years in Japan. During the same period, mass screening for gastric cancer has been actively conducted using mass radiography (photofluorographic examination), and in recent years 3–4 million people have been screened annually. The decline in gastric cancer death rates is higher in the age groups in which the coverage rate of mass screening is greater.

Lower mortality from gastric cancer was observed in the screened group compared to the unscreened group in each of the long-term follow-up studies. The decrease in 14 municipalities with a higher rate of screening for gastric cancer was also significantly greater than in comparable control municipalities.

The observed beneficial effect of mass screening for gastric cancer does not appear to be derived mainly from either lead time bias or length bias, although the apparent effect must be influenced to some extent by both biases. Since none of the evaluations made so far are based on a randomized trial, the influence of selection bias can also not be neglected in interpreting current results.

A decline in the cost effectiveness of mass screening in recent years is shown. To enchance the efficiency and minimize any untoward effect of mass screening, it is desirable to focus screening on high-risk groups.

REFERENCES

Hirayama, T. (1975). Epidemiology of cancer of the stomach with special reference to its recent decrease in Japan. *Cancer Res.* **35,** 3460–3463.

Hirayama, T. (1977a). Changing patterns of cancer in Japan with special reference to the decrease in stomach cancer mortality. *In* ''Origins of Human Cancer, Book A'' (H. H. Hiatt *et al.,* eds.), pp. 55–75. Cold Spring Harbor Lab., Cold Spring Harbor, New York.

Hirayama, T. (1977b). Opportunities for stomach cancer control project-engineering and evaluation. *In* ''Epidemiology of Stomach Cancer: Key Questions and Answers'' (T. Hirayama, ed.), pp. 117–130. WHO-CC for Evaluation of Methods of Diagnosis and Treatment of Stomach Cancer, Tokyo.

Hirayama, T. (1978). Outline of stomach cancer screening in Japan. *In* ''Screening in Cancer'' (A. B. Miller, ed.), UICC Tech. Rep. Ser., Vol. 40, pp. 264–278. Int. Union Against Cancer, Geneva.

Hirayama, T. (1981). Methods and results (cost-effectiveness) of gastric cancer screening. *In* ''Gastric Cancer'' (J. W. Fielding *et al.,* eds.), Adv. Biosci., Vol. 32, pp. 77–84. Pergamon, Oxford

Hisamichi, S. (1978). Prognosis of the patients with gastric cancer detected by mass survey. *In* ''Principles and Practice in Gastric Mass Survey Examination'' (S. Hisamichi, ed.), pp. 91–96. Kanehara Shuppan, Tokyo (in Japanese).

Kitabatake, T., Yoneyama, M., Sakka, M., and Koga, S. (1973). Benefits and risk of stomach cancer mass screening in Japan. *Igaku no Ayumi* **84,** 445–448. (in Japanese).

Kuroishi, T., Hirose, K., Nakagawa, N., and Tominaga, S. (1983). Comparisons of trend in stomach cancer mortality between the model areas for stomach cancer screening and the control areas. *J. Gastroenterol. Mass Surv.* **58,** 45–52 (in Japanese).

Tsukuma, H., Mishima, T., and Oshima, A. (1983). Prospective study of ''early'' gastric cancer. *Int. J. Cancer* **31,** 421–426.

20

Screening for Lung Cancer

ROBERT S. FONTANA

I.	Introduction	378
	A. Magnitude and Nature of the Lung Cancer Problem	378
	B. Major Cell Types of Lung Cancer	378
	C. Detection and Localization of Asymptomatic Lung Cancer	379
	D. Aims of Current Randomized Controlled Trials in the United States	380
II.	Design of the Mayo Lung Project (MLP)	381
III.	Results of the MLP Screening Program	382
	A. Acceptance	382
	B. Suitability of Screening Procedures	382
	C. The Problem of "Contamination"	383
	D. Resources for Management of Subjects with Abnormal Test Results	384
	E. The Concept of Backdating	384
	F. Incidence Rates of Lung Cancer	385
	G. Distribution by Cell Type	385
	H. Resectability and Survival by Method of Detection	385
	I. American Joint Committee for Cancer (AJCC) Staging and Survival	387
	J. Mortality	389
IV.	Discussion	390
	A. Difficulties and Reservations	390
	B. Review of Results	391
	C. Decisions: To Screen or to Test?	392
V.	Summary	394
	References	394

ISBN 0-12-496720-5

I. INTRODUCTION

A. Magnitude and Nature of the Lung Cancer Problem

The current lung cancer pandemic continues to increase in intensity. The incidence and mortality from the disease are rising proportionally wherever cigarette smoking has become popular. Estimates for 1984 in the United States are 139,000 new cases and 121,000 deaths—about 5% of all deaths in this country (American Cancer Society, 1983).

Lung cancer risk factors are well defined. The most important one, cigarette smoking, is self-inflicted. Smoking history, age, and (to a lesser extent today) sex constitute an excellent prescreen for this tumor. The primary high-risk group consists of middle-aged and older men who have been chronic excessive smokers of cigarettes. In the technically advanced countries, more than 80% of lung cancer in men has been attributed to cigarette smoking (American Cancer Society, 1983). Although the hazards of smoking have been acknowledged for decades, and although preventive measures may be achieving some success in certain technically advanced areas, more than 4 trillion cigarettes are sold throughout the world each year.

Yet the lung cancer problem, in its present status, has not been dealt with adequately by primary prevention alone. If all smoking were to cease *now,* there would still be nearly 2 million new cases in the United States alone by the year 2000.

Today surgical resection continues to be the treatment of choice for most lung cancers, even though its effectiveness remains uncertain (Ball, 1983). Nonsurgical treatment has limited value, although some reports suggest that some patients with the small-cell type of lung cancer may derive benefit from combination chemotherapy (Aisner *et al.,* 1983).

The symptoms of early, localized lung cancer are usually insidious and nonspecific, resembling those of the chronic bronchial irritation produced by cigarette smoking. By the time that obvious symptoms, such as pain, cause the patient to seek medical care, the disease is likely to be advanced and incurable. Even in leading medical centers, only about one-fourth of all cases are resectable for cure, and less than 15% of patients with lung cancer are alive 5 years after diagnosis (American Cancer Society, 1983).

B. Major Cell Types of Lung Cancer

The term *lung cancer* encompasses a variety of diseases having a broad range of clinical manifestations, histopathologic patterns, therapeutic regimens, and prognoses (Sobin, 1979). However, 90% of lung cancers can be classified pathologically into one of four major cell types, collectively designated *bronchogenic carcinoma* (Clagett *et al.*, 1964). These are squamous (epidermoid) carcinoma, adenocarcinoma, large-cell undifferentiated carcinoma, and small-cell undifferentiated carcinoma.

About half of all squamous cancers are intrabronchial tumors that arise within the subsegmental or larger bronchi in the central or hilar regions of the lungs; the remainder are situated in the peripheral parenchymal areas. Squamous cancers tend to respond better to surgical treatment and appear to have a better prognosis than do cancers of the other major cell types (American Joint Committee for Cancer Staging and End-Results Reporting, 1979).

Adenocarcinomas and large-cell carcinomas have similar clinical manifestations. Both tend to arise in the periphery of the lungs. As a rule, their prognosis is less favorable than that of squamous cancers (American Joint Committee for Cancer Staging and End-Results Reporting, 1979).

The great majority of small-cell cancers arise in the hilar regions; about 20% are peripheral. These tumors have the least favorable prognosis of all the major cell types, because they are prone to spread early and widely (American Joint Committee for Cancer Staging and End-Results Reporting, 1979). Surgical resection alone is seldom helpful.

C. Detection and Localization of Asymptomatic Lung Cancer

It has been presumed that asymptomatic lung cancer is more likely to be localized and amenable to treatment than is symptomatic cancer. The evidence for this is tenuous, but the concept is widely accepted (Ball, 1983).

As stated in Chapter 7, there are currently only two tests capable of detecting asymptomatic, resectable, presumably early lung cancer—that is, lung cancer classifiable postresection as stage I or stage II according to the American Joint Committee on Cancer (AJCC) (1983). These are the chest roentgenogram and the sputum cytology test. They tend to complement each other: chest roentgenography is the best detector of early-stage peripheral cancers or hilar tumors of the small-cell type, and cytology is the best detector of roentgenographically inapparent (occult) cancers, which are almost invariably early, intrabronchial squamous cancers arising in the hilar bronchi (Davies, 1966; Woolner *et al.*, 1970). Full-size (36 × 43-cm) roentgenograms—either posteroanterior stereoscopic or both posteroanterior and lateral chest views—taken at 125–140 kV are favored because of their sensitivity, as are 3-day pooled or induced specimens of sputum.

The method of processing sputum developed by Saccomanno *et al.* (1963) has enhanced the detection of squamous cancer cells, which are the salient ones in occult cancer; and the flexible fiberoptic bronchoscope, devised by Ikeda *et al.*

(1968), has provided an effective means of localizing these cancers. Both of these important technologic advances were introduced in the 1960s.

In 1970, in response to concerns expressed by patients, the Division of Thoracic Diseases of the Mayo Clinic recommended that "any man aged 45 years or older who smokes one package of cigarettes or more each day should have a sputum cytology examination as well as a chest x-ray at least once a year" (Mayo Staff Newsletter, 1970). This was, and remains, a pragmatic recommendation without statistical support.

D. Aims of Current Randomized Controlled Trials in the United States

At about this same time, the United States National Cancer Institute (NCI) initiated three large, long-term, randomized controlled trials of screening for early-stage lung cancer. These trials are being conducted at the Johns Hopkins Medical Institutions, Baltimore; the Memorial Sloan-Kettering Cancer Center, New York City; and the Mayo Clinic, Rochester, Minnesota. The statistical center has been established at the University of Cincinnati. Collectively, these institutions have been designated the "National Cancer Institute (NCI) Cooperative Early Lung Cancer Group" (1979).

The major aims of the Cooperative Group are to determine:

1. Whether detection of lung cancer can be improved by adding modern sputum cytologic screening techniques to either yearly (Hopkins, Memorial) or 4-monthly (Mayo) chest roentgenography.
2. Whether the death rate from lung cancer can be reduced significantly by this type of screening program, followed by newer localizing methods and appropriate treatment of bronchogenic carcinoma.

The period of active screening was intended to be 5 or 6 years, with at least an equal period of postscreening follow-up. This aspect of the three trials has been assessed at regular intervals by the NCI.

At the time these trials were designed, it was generally accepted that routine annual chest roentgenography had no appreciable influence on lung cancer mortality. Actually, this belief has never been tested. There has never been a randomized controlled trial in which screening exclusively for lung cancer, utilizing full-sized, high-kV chest roentgenograms or modern cytologic examination of multiple-day or induced sputum—either test or both, at any interval—was compared with no testing at all. The goal of the Mayo screening program, or Mayo Lung Project, has been to determine whether such chest roentgenography and sputum cytology testing, offered every 4 months for 6 years to a group of Mayo Clinic patients at high risk for lung cancer, can reduce the lung cancer death rate appreciably below that in a control group not offered regular testing (Fontana *et al.*, 1975).

II. DESIGN OF THE MAYO LUNG PROJECT (MLP)

The MLP used Mayo Clinic outpatients as study and control subjects. There were several reasons for this, including their availability and willingness to cooperate (Fontana *et al.*, 1975). However, the principal reason for using Mayo Clinic patients was the belief that any program aimed at early detection of lung cancer could best be implemented through existing health facilities and primary physicians. In this way, patients with proved lung cancer would have their treatment expedited and patients with equivocal test results could be evaluated with a minimum of delay and worry.

In the MLP, 10,933 Mayo Clinic outpatients who were without known lung cancer but were in the high-risk group of men 45 years of age or older who smoked at least one package of cigarettes daily were screened by use of 36 × 43-cm chest roentgenograms and 3-day pooled sputum cytology tests. If either test proved positive for lung cancer on this initial screening, the patient became a "prevalence" case. There were 91 such cases, for a prevalence rate of 8.3 per 1000 offered the screening. The rate increased rapidly with age, from 1 per 1000 among men 45–49 years old to 17 per 1000 among those 65 and older.

These prevalence cases were discussed in the proceedings of a 1978 International Union Against Cancer workshop on screening for cancer (Fontana and Taylor, 1978). This presentation will be concerned with "incidence" cases, detected after initial screenings that were regarded as satisfactory and negative for lung cancer.

There were 9211 men who completed the initial screen with results that were reported as satisfactory and negative and who met certain other criteria for continued screening, including a life expectancy of at least 5 years and the mental and physical capability of withstanding pulmonary resection (at least lobectomy) if the need should arise. Subsequently, these men were studied in two randomized groups.

In the screened group, there were 4618 patients who were asked, and reminded, to have chest roentgenograms and 3-day pooled sputum cytology tests every 4 months for a period of 6 years. Intensive efforts were made to secure compliance. Noncompliant patients and those who had completed 6 years of 4-monthly screening were contacted yearly by letter.

The control group of 4593 patients received only the standard 1970 Mayo Clinic recommendation concerning yearly chest X ray films and sputum tests. No inquiries or reminders about tests were sent, but contact was maintained by annual follow-up letters.

III. RESULTS OF THE MLP SCREENING PROGRAM

A. Acceptance

Subjects in their first year of participation completed 85% of the expected number of tests. In the fifth year, compliance was 75%, and beyond that it has been between 70 and 75%. The response of the controls to the annual follow-up letter has been a constant 98% (Taylor *et al.*, 1981). While these findings compare favorably with the compliance rates observed in other screening programs, noncompliance has tended to obscure any potential difference in lung cancer mortality between the screened and control groups.

B. Suitability of Screening Procedures

Mention has been made of the fact that the chest roentgenogram and the sputum cytology test complement each other in detecting early-stage, asymptomatic lung cancers. If a roentgenographically visible lung cancer of any of the four major cell types is sufficiently advanced, cancer cells of the same type may be present in the sputum. As previously noted, occult lung cancers are usually early, intrabronchial squamous cancers originating in the hilar bronchi (Davies, 1966; Woolner *et al.*, 1970; Fontana, 1978).

Both tests are painless and safe. The radiation exposure received in making a well-collimated 36 × 43-cm chest roentgenogram at 125–140 kV is insignificant (National Cancer Institute Cooperative Early Lung Cancer Group, 1979). Both tests are cheaper than a 4-month supply of cigarettes. They are simple to perform, although admittedly interpretations can be difficult. Control of quality is essential in both procedures. Dual reading of the roentgenograms increases the detection of abnormalities, and all MLP films were interpreted at least twice (Yerushalmy, 1969; National Cancer Institute Cooperative Early Lung Cancer Group, 1979).

The effectiveness of the two tests can be studied by analysis of the data they yield, but the incidence screening is not finished yet; only the prevalence (initial) data are complete. Of the 91 lung cancers detected by the initial screening, 85 were in cases where both tests were completed and deemed satisfactory. (Six prevalence cancers were detected roentgenographically and confirmed surgically before sputum collections were completed.)

It is difficult to assess the two tests separately, because the MLP is a screening program involving complementary procedures offered to a selected high-risk population. A valid test is essential for a successful screening program, but the program may fail for other reasons, such as refusal of procedures that would confirm the diagnosis.

Further, the accuracy of the two tests cannot be analyzed definitively, because there is no way of determining precisely how many lung cancers were *not* detected by the screening. Of the 85 prevalence tumors in cases where both tests were completed satisfactorily, chest roentgenography showed 68 (80%) and sputum cytology revealed evidence of 32 (38%). The percentages may be regarded as the upper bounds of the true sensitivity of each test.

Of the 10,026 cases in which both prevalence screening tests were completed satisfactorily and lung cancer was not discovered subsequently, the chest roentgenogram was interpreted as negative in 9664 (96.4%) and sputum cytology was considered negative in 10,002 (99.8%). These percentages may be regarded as the lower bounds of the true specificity of each test.

The major problem with specificity is the definition of a negative test. For example, if all chest roentgenograms that were not interpreted as suspicious for cancer were considered negative, the specificity of roentgenography would increase to 99.2%. Similarly, if all sputum specimens that were not considered frankly positive for cancer cells were regarded as negative, the specificity of cytology would rise to 99.9% (see Chapter 7).

Sensitivity and specificity can be enhanced—and in the MLP, they were—by repeating tests with abnormal results (especially those with equivocal results) and, when possible, comparing abnormal findings with findings from previous tests.

C. The Problem of "Contamination"

A substantial proportion of the MLP control population is being tested by chest roentgenography outside of the study. This has become a source of considerable concern. It is easier to evaluate any experimental cancer screening program if, during the period of assessment, screening is not available to control subjects through other sources (such as private physicians or clinics) (Morrison, 1982).

During the controlled study of mammography as a screening device for breast cancer, that procedure was not widely used in clinical practice (Fink *et al.*, 1968). At present, cytologic examination of the sputum is not used very often to test for lung cancer in asymptomatic patients with negative chest roentgenograms. However, nearly 100 million chest X ray examinations are performed in the United States each year, and there is good evidence that middle-aged and older men who have been heavy cigarette smokers are receiving more than the average number (U.S. Department of Health, Education and Welfare, 1973). Such men are candidates not only for lung cancer but also for various other common conditions for which chest roentgenography is indicated, including coronary heart disease, hypertension, obstructive pulmonary disease, and respiratory infections.

Current data indicate that at least 50% of MLP control patients receive chest roentgenograms each year, and during a recent 2-year period approximately 80%

did so. Nearly one-third of all lung cancers in the control group have been detected in the asymptomatic phase by nonstudy chest roentgenography. Obviously, contamination of this sort reduces the contrast between the controls and the screened group.

D. Resources for Management of Subjects with Abnormal Test Results

Vital to any lung cancer screening program is the presence of easily accessible, highly qualified medical facilities where patients with suspected cancer can receive prompt diagnostic workups, appropriate treatment, and adequate follow-up. This is what makes the concept of early detection of lung cancer within the framework of the general medical examination so attractive. It allows maximal utilization of existing medical personnel and equipment, and it ensures continuity of care.

E. The Concept of Backdating

An ideal cancer screening program would detect early-stage, symptomatic, curable cancers that, in the absence of screening, would eventually be manifested as advanced, asymptomatic, and incurable.

A successful randomized controlled trial of cancer screening would proceed as follows: (1) During the screening period, the number of known cancers in the screened group would become progressively larger than the number in the control group. The excess number in the screened group would be composed primarily of early-stage cancers detected by the screen. (2) During the postscreening period, the number of cancers in the two groups would eventually equalize, as cancers in the control group attained the advanced, symptomatic stage. (3) Ultimately, there would be significantly more cancer deaths in the control group than in the screened group. At any point during the screening period, however, data would be more complete for the screened group than for the controls, because the screened group would be under closer surveillance.

The MLP randomized controlled trial of 4-monthly screening for early lung cancer has now been in progress for more than a decade. Disregarding lead time bias, it is evident that data concerning the patients in the 4-monthly screened group, who have become conditioned to notify the MLP office promptly of any change in their status, are considerably more current than are data on the controls, who are heard from only once a year. To try to compensate for this difference, the practice has been adopted of backdating by a year all information relating to the MLP incidence lung cancers. Thus, incidence data reported January 1, 1983, refer only to cancers discovered prior to January 1, 1982, but include all information known about those cancers on January 1, 1983.

TABLE I

Cell Type: 298 Incidence[a] Lung Cancers (Known January 1, 1982; Followed to January 1, 1983)

Cell type of tumor	4-monthly group (167 tumors)	Control group (131 tumors)
Squamous	57 (34%)	40 (31%)
Adenocarcinoma	45	34
Large cell	27	21
Small cell	38 (23%)	36 (27%)

[a] Detected after negative first screen.

F. Incidence Rates of Lung Cancer

From the beginning of the MLP, the incidence cases of lung cancer in the 4-monthly screened group have outnumbered those in the control group. On January 1, 1983, when MLP statistics were backdated to January 1, 1982, 167 incidence cases had been documented in the 4-monthly screened group, a rate of 5.3 per 1000 person-years of surveillance. In the control group there were 131 cases, or 4.1 per 1000 person-years. Each group had been under surveillance approximately 32,000 person-years.

G. Distribution by Cell Type

Unfortunately, 38 (23%) of the cancers in the 4-monthly group and 36 (27%) of the cancers in the control group were of the small-cell type, which has an extremely poor prognosis that is helped very little by screening (Table I). Only 57 (34%) of the 4-monthly cancers and 40 (31%) of the control cancers were of the squamous type, which tends to respond best to surgical resection. This distribution was much less favorable than had been expected, even considering the influence of length bias on the prevalence screening.

H. Resectability and Survival by Method of Detection

In the 4-monthly group, 84 (50%) of the 167 cancers were detected by the screening tests (Table II). There were 62 cancers detected by roentgenography alone, 16 by cytology alone, and 6 by both—confirming that the two screening tests do complement each other in detecting asymptomatic lung cancer.

Of the remaining 83 cancers in the 4-monthly group, 54 were detected because of symptoms of lung cancer and 29 because of nonstudy chest roentgenograms obtained for other reasons (routine medical examinations, etc.). Approximately

TABLE II

Detection and Curative Resection: Incidence of Lung Cancers (Known January 1, 1982; Followed to January 1, 1983)

Method of detection	4-monthly group		Control group	
	Cases	Resection	Cases	Resection
4-monthly screening				
Chest roentgenography	62	39	—	
Sputum cytology	16	14	—	
Both screening tests	6	4	—	
Nonstudy roentgenography	29	19	39	30
Symptoms	54	6	92	10
Total	167	82 (49%)	131	40 (31%)

one-third of these 83 cancers were detected between screenings (interval cases), one-third occurred in men who were noncompliant with screening (dropouts), and one-third were found in men who had completed their 6 years of screening.

Of the 16 incidence cancers that were detected only cytologically in the 4-monthly group, 14 (88%) were resectable for cure (all cytologically detected cancers were squamous). Of greater significance, perhaps, was the observation that 62 (64%) of the 97 cancers in the 4-monthly group that were detected roentgenographically—by either screening or nonstudy chest films—were resectable.

Of the 131 control cancers, 39 (30%) were asymptomatic and were detected by nonstudy chest films; 30 of these cancers were resectable. This contamination of the control group does not appear to have been the result of deliberate self-screening by control patients, although that might be suspected in a highly motivated population of Mayo Clinic patients. Rather, there is evidence that the control patients tended to undergo chest roentgenography because of other circumstances, including those noncancerous illnesses that are prone to occur with increasing frequency as chronic heavy smokers grow older (Fontana *et al.*, 1975).

Of the 54 cancers in the 4-monthly group that were discovered after symptoms of lung cancer had appeared, only 6 (11%) were resectable (Table II). There were 92 symptomatic cancers in the control group, and only 10 (11%) of these were resectable.

Thus, the resectable cancers amounted to 82 (49%) in the 4-monthly screened group and 40 (31%) in the control group. In clinical practice at the Mayo Clinic, between 25 and 30% of lung cancers are resectable for cure (Williams *et al.*, 1981).

Considering deaths from lung cancer only, 5-year survival among the 16 cytologically detected cases was approximately 85%, whereas among the 136

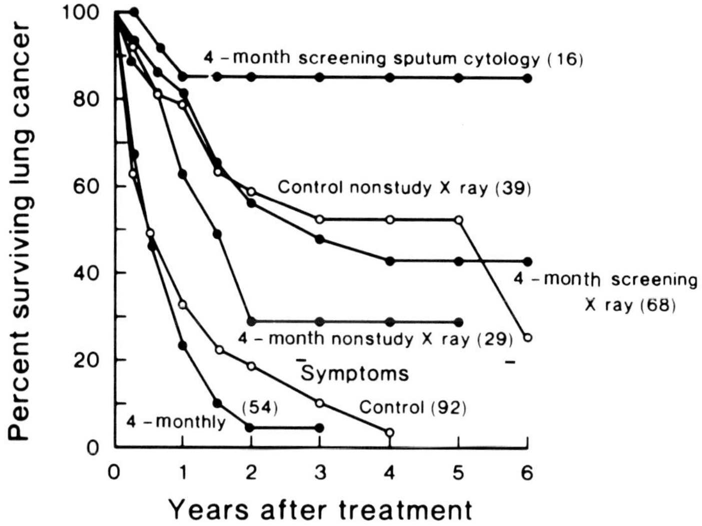

Fig. 1. Survival in 298 incidence cases of lung cancer, by method of detection. (Six cancers detected by both cytology and roentgenography in 4-monthly screening are included with the roentgenography group but not with the cytology group.) Survival is from the time of initial treatment (or refusal of treatment), and only deaths from lung cancer are considered. (Information known January 1, 1983, about cases detected before January 1, 1982.)

roentgenographically detected cases in *both* study groups it was 40–50% (Fig. 1). The survival of all of the symptomatic cases at 4 years was less than 5%. It is evident that in both study groups, the asymptomatic patients whose cancers were detected by one of the testing procedures tended to do well, but the symptomatic patients did very poorly.

I. American Joint Committee for Cancer (AJCC) Staging and Survival

Classified as postsurgical AJCC (1983) stage I or stage II were 71 (42%) of the 167 cancers in the 4-monthly screened group but only 32 (25%) of the 131 cancers in the control group (Table III). In contemporary Mayo Clinic experience, less than 20% of all lung cancers have been so classified (Williams *et al.*, 1981).

Among patients in the 4-monthly screened group who had postsurgical AJCC stage I or stage II cancers, the 5-year survival rate (lung cancer deaths only) was almost 70% (Fig. 2). It was somewhat lower in the control group, possibly because of less detailed surgical staging in this group. The 5-year survival of patients with stage III or unresected cancers was about 5% in both groups. Staging, especially postsurgical staging, seems to provide a fairly accurate basis for estimating average survival in a group of cases, but not in the individual case.

TABLE III

AJCC Stage: Incidence Lung Cancers (Known January 1, 1982; Followed to January 1, 1983)

	4-monthly group (167 tumors)		Control group (131 tumors)	
AJCC Stage	Number	Percentage	Number	Percentage
Postsurgical I	67	40	31	24
Postsurgical II	4	2	1	1
All others	96	58	99	75

It is important to remember that in a successful screening program, one should find not only more early-stage cancers in the screened group but also, eventually, *more advanced cancers in the control group.* On January 1, 1983 (backdated to January 1, 1982), there were 96 cases of AJCC stage III (and unresectable) cancers in the 4-monthly group and 99 in the control group (Table III).

The failure to observe any significant difference in the number of advanced and unresectable cancers in the two groups has been a disappointment. To the present, 36 fewer cancers have been discovered in the control group, and eventually some of those not yet discovered should be manifested as advanced,

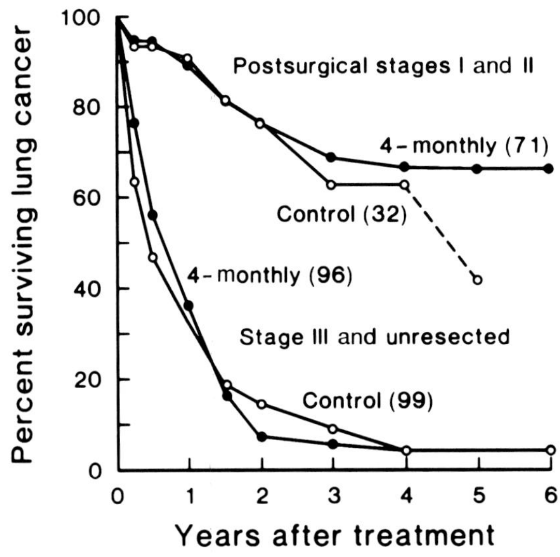

Fig. 2. Survival in 298 incidence cases of lung cancer, by stage (AJCC). Survival is from the time of initial treatment (or refusal of treatment), and only deaths from lung cancer are considered. (Information known January 1, 1983, about cases detected before January 1, 1982.)

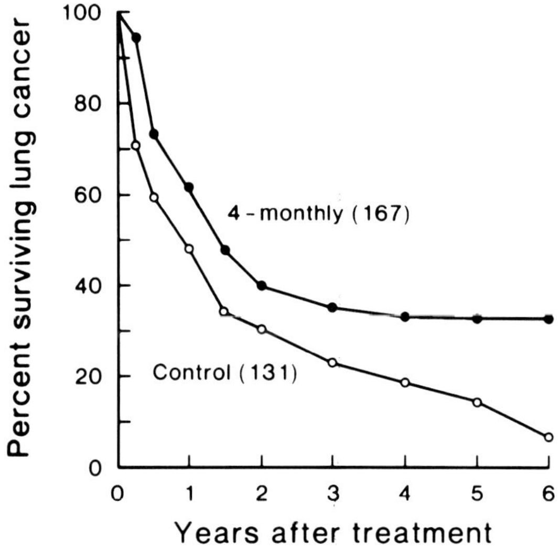

Fig. 3. Survival in 298 incidence cases of lung cancer, by study group (4-monthly surveillance versus controls). Survival is from the time of treatment (or refusal of treatment), and only deaths from lung cancer are considered. (Information known January 1, 1983, about cases detected before January 1, 1982.)

unresectable tumors. However, during the time it will take for these cancers to appear, additional advanced cases will also appear in both groups.

The variety of cell types, stages, and methods of detection of lung cancer permit conceptualization of a large group of lung cancers for which screening (or treatment) is of little value and a small group for which screening and treatment may be helpful. This hypothesis has been advanced by others (Rossing and Rossing, 1982).

Among patients with incidence cancers, 5-year survival (lung cancer deaths only) was 35% in the 4-monthly screened group and 15% in the control group (Fig. 3). These results might have been predicted from the distribution of the various cell types and AJCC stages of the cancers in the two groups.

J. Mortality

In an experimental lung cancer screening program such as the MLP, the principal benefit to the screened group should be a reduction of mortality, specifically mortality from lung cancer.

As stated above, on January 1, 1983 (backdated to January 1, 1982), both the 4-monthly screened group and the control group had been under observation for approximately 32,000 person-years. The death rate (per 1000 person-years) from all causes was 23.5 in the 4-monthly group and 23.1 in the control group—not significantly different. (Of course, the subjects of the MLP, being middle-aged or older men who have been chronic excessive smokers of cigarettes, die from a number of other smoking-related illnesses in addition to lung cancer, among which the major competing risk is ischemic heart disease.)

All deaths attributed to surgery for lung cancer have been classified as lung cancer deaths. There were 6 surgical deaths in the 4-monthly group (6% among the 98 cases with one or more thoracotomies, which were thought to be curative in 82) and 5 surgical deaths in the control group (9% among the 57 cases with one or more thoracotomies, which were thought to be curative in 40).

With these surgical deaths included, the death rate from lung cancer was 2.9 per 1000 person-years in the 4-monthly group and 2.8 in the controls. This difference is insignificant. Nor was there any appreciable difference between the cumulative lung cancer mortality rates in the two groups: after 9 years in the study, these rates were approximately 30 per 1000 patients in each group.

Thus, there is no evidence that either total mortality or lung cancer mortality can be reduced by offering 4-monthly screening to candidates who have undergone a single radiologic and cytologic test with negative results while receiving general medical examinations as outpatients at the Mayo Clinic. This is a strong statement, but it has its limitations.

The MLP subjects were men who had sought medical advice. All of those in the 4-monthly screening program had undergone initial chest roentgenography and sputum cytology tests, with results that were considered satisfactory and negative for lung cancer. All were considered to have a life expectancy of at least 5 years and were judged capable of undergoing pulmonary resection. All had been warned of the risks of smoking and had received a routine recommendation of annual chest roentgenography and sputum cytology testing. In retrospect, there are aspects of the MLP controlled trial that call to mind some of the confounding features of the Multiple Risk Factor Intervention Trial (MRFIT) on mortality from coronary heart disease (Lundberg, 1982).

IV. DISCUSSION

A. Difficulties and Reservations

It has been said that randomized controlled trials such as the MLP are time-consuming, tedious, expensive, and often outdated by the time they are completed and reported. Nevertheless, if they are well conceived and conducted, they can provide reliable information.

The MLP is now in its follow-up period; active screening ceased in late July 1982. There is still no demonstrable significant difference in total mortality or lung cancer mortality between the 4-monthly screened group and the control group. It is possible that an appreciable difference may yet develop, for there is still a substantial discrepancy between the total number of lung cancer cases in the two groups, but time appears to be running out.

It has been argued that the greater number of lung cancers in the 4-monthly group may be partly the result of overdiagnosis, or of diagnosing as a very early cancer a lesion that is not and will never become a cancer (Eddy, 1980). Data from the other two randomized controlled trials of screening for early-stage lung cancer in the United States seem to dispute this belief. These data suggest that the numerical discrepancy between the 4-monthly and control groups in the MLP might not have occurred if the control population had received annual chest roentgenography. It is generally accepted that roentgenographically visible lung cancers are truly cancers, and it is recognized that some are incurable cancers.

However, there have been other factors—not all foreseen—that have exerted a negative influence on the MLP controlled trial. There have been frustrations associated with the 25% noncompliance rate of the 4-monthly group with the screening program, the substantial contamination of the control group by examinations outside the study, the higher than expected incidence of small-cell cancer, and the lower than expected incidence of squamous cancer. There have been uncertainties due to the 12-month periods between reports on the status of the control group. There have been worries over the increasing effect of competing death risks, especially ischemic heart disease, on a steadily aging population of cigarette smokers. There have been reservations about the precision of the AJCC cancer staging system and the effectiveness of treatment, including surgical resection. In addition, there have been concerns regarding the occurrence of multiple primary lung cancers and the possibility that some lung cancers, notably roentgenographically occult cancers, may develop so slowly that they will not be discovered during the follow-up period.

B. Review of Results

Fortunately, because the MLP has been conducted conscientiously, it should be possible eventually to determine the relative importance of most of these factors. At present, the following observations seem pertinent:

1. Screening for lung cancer by chest roentgenography and sputum cytology testing has been conducted unobtrusively and effectively in a clinical setting.
2. Screening by these modalities has been accepted by Mayo Clinic patients.
3. Sputum cytology detects fewer cancers than had been expected, although sputum-detected cancers tend to have an excellent prognosis.
4. Chest roentgenography may be a more effective test for early-stage lung cancer than published reports have suggested. (Neither kind of test, however, has had its ability to reduce mortality subjected to a randomized controlled trial against *no* testing; and this would be extremely difficult to do now, especially in technically advanced areas.)

5. The resectability of cancers detected by the MLP screening program has been double that observed in clinical practice at the Mayo Clinic.

6. The proportion of postsurgical AJCC stage I or stage II cancers in the MLP 4-monthly screened group has been more than double that encountered in clinical practice.

7. The 5-year lung cancer survival has been 35% in the 4-monthly screened group and 15% in the control group.

8. There has been no significant difference in total mortality or lung cancer mortality between the 4-monthly group and the control group.

C. Decisions: To Screen or to Test?

Now is not the time to recommend large-scale radiologic or cytologic programs of screening for lung cancer. Since these programs are usually initiated by those who conduct the screening, they should benefit the persons screened by reducing lung cancer mortality. The MLP randomized trial has not demonstrated that screening can do this. Current data from this trial do not support a recommendation of screening for early-stage lung cancer as a routine public health policy.

However, it seems important to distinguish population screening from case finding in clinical practice, even though some may argue that the difference is more semantic than genuine (Eddy, 1980; Fontana and Sanderson, 1981). Case finding is initiated by the patient, who usually expects to be given a thorough examination. To withhold chest roentgenography and sputum cytology from a patient at high risk of lung cancer, when these are the only tests that can detect preclinical disease, should require proof that the procedures are unable to detect lung cancer early enough for existing therapy to cure it. This has not been demonstrated, and the design of the MLP and the substantial exposure of its control population to chest roentgenography make it impossible to address this issue.

What *has* been demonstrated is that *offering* the two screening modalities every 4 months to high-risk Mayo Clinic outpatients who already have had one negative screening appears to be no more efficacious than recommending annual chest roentgenography and sputum cytology. When the MLP began, it was assumed that annual chest roentgenography had no beneficial effect on lung cancer mortality. Yet among the 30% of lung cancers in the control group that were asymptomatic and detected by nonstudy chest roentgenograms, 75% were resectable. Moreover, among men in the control group whose tumors were discovered in this manner, the 5-year lung cancer survival rate was 50% (Fig. 1). The crucial question is, what would have happened to these men if chest roentgenography had not been available?

Like the MLP, the other two randomized controlled trials of screening for early-stage lung cancer in the United States involve large populations of high-risk subjects (men 45 years of age or older who have been chronic heavy cigarette smokers) (National Cancer Institute Cooperative Early Lung Cancer Group, 1979). Unlike the MLP, these programs offered all of their subjects annual chest roentgenography (36 × 43-cm posteroanterior and lateral views at 140 kV). In addition, half of the men in each of these trials have been allocated randomly to a group offered sputum cytology testing (induced sputum specimens every year and 3-day collections of spontaneous sputum every 4 months). Preliminary results from both trials reveal that in each of the study groups the proportion of lung cancers discovered while still in an early stage and resectable, as well as the lung cancer survivorship, was substantially better than that observed in previously reported lung cancer screening programs. However, no significant difference in lung cancer mortality has yet been observed between the two study groups in either of these trials (Tockman *et al.*, 1982).

The MLP and the other two randomized controlled trials were established to determine the value of adding sputum cytology to chest roentgenography in screening for lung cancer (National Cancer Institute Cooperative Early Lung Cancer Group, 1979). However, in all three trials, considerably more lung cancers were detected roentgenographically than cytologically. Furthermore, sizable numbers of early-stage lung cancers were detected by nonstudy roentgenography in the control population of the MLP and by annual roentgenography without sputum cytology in the other two trials.

The randomized controlled trial is ideal for evaluating new procedures, such as mammography, or new applications of procedures, such as sputum cytology testing of asymptomatic, high-risk subjects for lung cancer. However, once a procedure has become an integral part of medical practice, as the chest roentgenogram has, it may become necessary to use other, less sensitive methods to evaluate it (Morrison, 1982). One alternative that might prove useful in assessing chest roentgenography as a screening device for lung cancer is a case-control study. Although there are a number of problems associated with this type of study, at least the influence of nonstudy testing of the control population would be reduced.

In technically advanced areas of the world where adequate facilities are available, it now seems reasonable to allow chest roentgenography and sputum cytology to be applied by the individual physician caring for the individual patient. The physician may obtain the tests during the examination of a high-risk patient if he or she believes them to be indicated and the patient agrees (Tockman *et al.*, 1982). The advantages and disadvantages of testing should be discussed with the patient, as should all aspects of the medical examination. At the same time, any patients still smoking cigarettes should be informed of the risks of continuing and strongly advised to quit. Assistance in quitting should also be offered.

Finally, the decision to test in a clinical situation is an individual judgment, outside the realm of screening. Screening as a public policy requires proof of effectiveness.

V. SUMMARY

A randomized controlled trial of screening for early-stage lung cancer by periodic chest roentgenography and sputum cytology testing can be conducted expeditiously and unobtrusively in a clinical setting. Cytology testing alone detects only a small proportion of lung cancers in such a program, but cytologically detected lung cancers tend to have a favorable prognosis. Modern chest roentgenography may be a better way of detecting early-stage lung cancers than previous reports have suggested.

The resectability of lung cancers detected by the MLP screening program has been double that observed in recent clinical practice at the Mayo Clinic. The proportion of postsurgical AJCC stage I or stage II lung cancers detected by this screening program has been more than double that encountered in clinical practice.

In the MLP incidence study, 5-year lung cancer survival in the group offered rescreening every 4 months (following a satisfactory and negative prevalence screening) has been 35%. In the control group, offered standard medical care plus advice to have annual roentgenography and cytology, the 5-year lung cancer survival has been 15%. However, at this time, there is no significant difference in either total mortality or lung cancer mortality between the two groups.

ACKNOWLEDGMENTS

Supported by Research Contract NO1-CN-53886 from the National Cancer Institute.

REFERENCES

Aisner, J., Alberto, P., Bitran, J., Comis, R., Daniels, J., Hansen, H., Ikegami, H., and Smyth, J. (1983). Role of chemotherapy in small cell lung cancer: A consensus report of the International Association for the Study of Lung Cancer workshop. *Cancer Treat. Rep.* **67,** 37–43.

American Cancer Society (1983). "1984 Cancer Facts and Figures." Am. Cancer Soc., New York.

American Joint Committee for Cancer Staging and End-Results Reporting (1979). "Staging of Lung Cancer." Am. Joint Comm., Chicago, Illinois.

American Joint Committee on Cancer (1983). Lung. *In* "Manual for Staging of Cancer" (O. H. Beahrs and M. H. Myers, eds.), 2nd ed., pp. 99–105. Lippincott, Philadelphia, Pennsylvania.

Ball, W. C., Jr. (1983). The effect of surgical treatment on the natural history of lung cancer (editorial). *Am. Rev. Respir. Dis.* **127,** 1.

Clagett, O. T., Allen, T. H., Payne, W. S., and Woolner, L. B. (1964). The surgical treatment of pulmonary neoplasms: A 10-year experience. *J. Thorac. Cardiovasc. Surg.* **48,** 391–400.

Davies, D. F. (1966). A review of detection methods for the early diagnosis of lung cancer. *J. Chronic Dis.* **19,** 819–845.

Eddy, D. (1980). Guidelines for the cancer-related checkup: Recommendations and rationale. *Ca—Cancer J. Clin.* **30,** 193–240.

Fink, R., Shapiro, S., and Lewison, J. (1968). The reluctant participant in a breast cancer screening program. *Public Health Rep.* **83,** 479–490.

Fontana, R. S. (1978). The needle in the haystack (editorial). *Mayo Clin. Proc.* **53,** 616–617.

Fontana, R. S., and Sanderson D. R. (1981). Reply to letter to editor. *JAMA, J. Am. Med. Assoc.* **246,** 621–622.

Fontana, R. S., and Taylor, W. F. (1978). Screening for lung cancer: The Mayo Lung Project. *In* "Screening in Cancer" (A. B. Miller, ed.), Vol. 40, pp. 233–253. Int. Union Against Cancer, Geneva.

Fontana, R. S., Sanderson, D. R., Woolner, L. B., Miller, E., Bernatz, P. E., Payne, S., and Taylor, W. F. (1975). The Mayo Lung Project for early detection and localization of bronchogenic carcinoma: A status report. *Chest* **67,** 511–522.

Ikeda, S., Yanai, H., and Ishikawa, S. (1968). Flexible bronchofiberscope. *Keio J. Med.* **17,** 1–18.

Lundberg, G. D. (1982). MRFIT and the goals of the journal (editorial). *JAMA, J. Am. Med. Assoc.* **248,** 1501.

Mayo Staff Newsletter (1970). *Mayo Staff Newsl.* **7,** 1.

Morrison, A. S. (1982). Case definition in case-control studies of the efficacy of screening. *Am. J. Epidemiol.* **115,** 6–8.

National Cancer Institute Cooperative Early Lung Cancer Group (1979). "Manual of Procedures," 2nd ed., NIH Publ. No. 79-1972. U.S. Gov. Printing Office, Washington, D.C.

Rossing, T. H., and Rossing, R. G. (1982). Survival in lung cancer: An analysis of the effects of age, sex, resectability, and histopathologic type. *Am. Rev. Respir. Dis.* **126,** 771–777.

Saccomanno, G., Saunders, R. P., Ellis, H., Archer, V. E., Wood, B. G., and Beckler, P. A. (1963). Concentration of carcinoma or atypical cells in sputum. *Acta Cytol.* **7,** 305–310.

Sobin, L. H. (1979). The WHO histologic classification of lung tumors: Revised edition. *In* "Advances in Medical Oncology, Research and Education" (P. M. Wilkinson, ed.), Vol. II, pp. 5–8. Pergamon, Oxford.

Taylor, W. F., Fontana, R. S., Uhlenhopp, M. A., and Davis, C. S. (1981). Some results of screening for early lung cancer. *Cancer* **47,** 1114–1120.

Tockman, M. S., Becklake, M. R., Clausen, J. L., Cox, P. M., Jr., Fontana, R. S., O'Brien, R. J., Permutt, S., Petty, T. L., Reed, C., Reichman, L. B., and Stead, W. W. (1982). Screening for adult respiratory disease. *Am. Thorac. Soc. News* **8,** 15.

U.S. Department of Health, Education and Welfare (1973). "Population Exposure to X-rays, U.S. 1970." U.S. Govt. Printing Office, Washington, D. C.

Williams, D. E., Pairolero, P. C., Davis, C. S., Bernatz, P. E., Payne, W. S., Taylor, W. F., Uhlenhopp, M. A., and Fontana, R. S. (1981). Survival of patients surgically treated for stage I lung cancer. *J. Thorac. Cardiovasc. Surg.* **82,** 70–76.

Woolner, L. B., David, E., Fontana, R. S., Andersen, H. A., and Bernatz, P. E. (1970). *In situ* and early invasive bronchogenic carcinoma: Report of 28 cases with postoperative survival data. *J. Thorac. Cardiovasc. Surg.* **60,** 275–290.

Yerushalmy, J. (1969). The statistical assessment of the variability in observer perception and description of roentgenographic pulmonary shadows. *Radiol. Clin. North Am.* **7**(3), 381–392.

21

Screening for Bladder Cancer

R. A. CARTWRIGHT

I. Overview of Bladder Cancer Epidemiology as Relevant to Screening Programs . . . 398
A. Introduction . . . 398
B. Industrial Bladder Cancer, 1895–1949 . . . 398
C. Modern Bladder Cancer, 1950–1980 . . . 399
D. High-Risk Groups . . . 402
E. Are There New High-Risk Groups? . . . 403
II. Survival in Bladder Cancer . . . 403
A. Determinants of Survival . . . 403
B. What Factors of Survival Need to Be Accounted For? . . . 406
III. Screening for Bladder Cancer . . . 407
A. Early Prevention of Bladder Cancer . . . 407
B. Early Methods of Screening . . . 407
C. Overview of Papanicolaou Screening . . . 409
D. Present Position in the United Kingdom . . . 411
E. Other Screening Methods . . . 411
IV. Analyses of Bladder Cancer Screening . . . 412
A. Introduction . . . 412
B. Can Screening by MCC Alter Survival? . . . 412
C. What Effect Has Screening on the Stage of Presentation of Cases? . . . 413
V. Future of Bladder Cancer Screening . . . 415
A. Value of Screening . . . 415
B. Future of Screening . . . 416
References . . . 416

ISBN 0-12-496720-5

I. OVERVIEW OF BLADDER CANCER EPIDEMIOLOGY AS RELEVANT TO SCREENING PROGRAMS

A. Introduction

This chapter presents an overview of screening for bladder cancer by first introducing some etiologic aspects that may help define high-risk groups. Second, factors that influence survival are reviewed, because these aspects need to be considered when screening is evaluated. Third, the various screening schemes themselves, and what little evaluation is currently available, are reviewed, with a brief discussion of their deficiencies. Finally, as to the future, bladder cancer may be controllable in high-risk screened groups, but these represent only a small proportion of the totality of the disease. A future epidemiological effort will be needed to define further groups for control that can account for a greater proportion of the disease.

The bladder cancer described in this chapter is the disease experienced in the industrialized world: flat or papillary transitional cell tumors of the urothelium (Koss, 1975). The older literature distinguishes benign papilloma from carcinoma, but it is now recognized that papillomas are part of the spectrum of the carcinomas, the relatively well-differentiated, noninvasive type (UICC, 1978).

Bladder cancer accounts for some 4% of all malignant tumors in Britain, totaling 2000 female and 6000 male new cases each year [Office of Population Censuses and Surveys (OPCS), 1982]. The difference in sex ratio and the proportional incidence are similar in other parts of Europe and North America. Bladder cancer ranks among the 10 most common male cancers in Britain and the United States, but with marked regional differences, being more common in the industrial north of Britain (OPCS, 1982) and the industrial northeastern United States (Blot and Fraumeni, 1978; Staszewski, 1980).

B. Industrial Bladder Cancer, 1895–1949

Rehn (1895) was the first to report on an apparent excess of bladder cancer cases in the German aniline dye industry. He diagnosed 4 cases of bladder cancer from a workforce of about 500. This observation was followed by claims and counterclaims from Germany and Switzerland (Leichtenstern, 1898; Schedler, 1905) regarding the cause of the link between the tumors and the occupation. After World War I, production of aniline dyes spread to other parts of the world, and again apparently excessive numbers of cases were soon reported—for example, by Bridge and Henry (1928) in England, Rosenbaum and Gottlieb (1926) in Russia, Anderson (1934) in the United States, and di Maio in Italy (1937). These case reports lacked details on the total workforce or the nature of the exposure. It was debated what the carcinogenic agents might be, as well as the existence of a true excess of cases as contrasted to inflated numbers biased by specific observations. Some urologists claimed that the industrial or aniline bladder cancer was more aggressive than cancers originating from nonindustrial causes (Hueper, 1942).

Many of the uncertainties were brought to an end by the work of Case, who demonstrated a technique for calculating expected rates of disease in specific circumstances. Case studied a large number of British factories in the late 1940s (Case, 1969). His work implicated benzidine and 2-naphthylamine as major bladder carcinogens, observations substantiated by other epidemiological surveys (Monson, 1980) and laboratory research.

C. Modern Bladder Cancer, 1950–1980

Table I summarizes the results of studies on industrial bladder cancer linking the disease with occupational exposure to benzidine and 2-naphthylamine. The social and occupational experience in the United Kingdom with industrial bladder cancer is summarized by Davies *et al.* (1976) and Somerville *et al.* (1980).

Table II lists nonoccupational etiological agents. These have been uncovered by epidemiological studies or inferred from other sources. The table is confined to those etiologies for which there is at least a large element of suspicion. Cigarette smoking is a major cause and accounts from about one-quarter to one-half of all cases, the variation being due to the nature of the populations studied and the techniques employed. The relationship, however, is not a clear one. P. Vineis (unpublished observation, 1983) and Wynder and Goldsmith (1977) found a dose response between the totality of tobacco consumed and the risks of bladder cancer, while Cole *et al.* (1971) and Cartwright *et al.* (1983a) did not. Furthermore, the use of filter cigarettes reduces the risk (Cartwright *et al.*, 1983a), as may the nature of the leaf and its curing (P. Vineis, unpublished

TABLE I

Industrial Associations of Bladder Cancer

Industry	Author
Dye manufacturing	
2-Naphthylamine	Case *et al.* (1954)
Benzidine	Case and Pearson (1954)
Auramine	Mancuso and El-Attar (1967)
Coal gas	Doll *et al.* (1965)
Rubber	Case and Hosker (1954)
Cable Making	Davies (1965)
Printing	Versluys (1949); R. A. Cartwright (unpublished report, 1981)

TABLE II

Nonindustrial Associations of Bladder Cancer

Condition	Author
Bilharzia	Brand (1979)
Chronic bladder infection/ prostatic hypertrophy	Mommson *et al.* (1982)
Cigarette smoking	Wynder and Goldsmith (1977)
Acetaminophen consumption	Johansson and Wahlquist (1977)
Cyclophosphamide therapy	Beyer-Boon *et al.* (1978); Plotz *et al.* (1979)
Balkan nephropathy	Radovanovic and Krajinovic (1979)

TABLE III

Summary of New Occupational Risks Resulting from Descriptive and Case-Control Studies

Occupation	Author
Leather workers	Lockwood (1961); Wynder *et al.* (1963); Cole *et al.* (1972)
Japanese kimono painters	S. Ishizu (personal communication, 1979)
Dye users in textiles	Wynder *et al.* (1963); Anthony (1974)
Hairdressers/barbers	Wynder *et al.* (1963); Dunham *et al.* (1968)
Metal workers/machinists	Wynder *et al.* (1963); Dunham *et al.* (1968); Cartwright (1983); P. Vineis (unpublished observation, 1983)
Coal miners	Wynder *et al.* (1963)
Paint manufacturers, painters and decorators, spray shop workers	Wynder *et al.* (1963); Cole *et al.* (1972)
Textile industry (females)	Wynder *et al.* (1963); Anthony (1974)
Sailors	Dunham *et al.* (1968)
Tinsmiths and coppersmith	Dunham *et al.* (1968)
Civil engineers and other types	Dunham *et al.* (1968); Anthony (1974)
Plumbers	Dunham *et al.* (1968); Tyrrell *et al.* (1971)
Aluminum reducers	Theriault *et al.* (1981)
Carpenters	Dunham *et al.* (1968); Cartwright (1983)
Medical workers including nurses	Anthony (1974); Howe *et al.* (1980)
Tailors and tailors' pressers	Anthony (1974)
Cooks, kitchen hands, and food industry workers	Cole *et al.* (1972); Howe *et al.* (1980); Cartwright (1983)
Clerical workers	Cole *et al.* (1972); Cartwright (1983)
Photographic industry workers	Howe *et al.* (1980)
Stone masons	Tyrrell *et al.* (1971)
Truck drivers	Silverman *et al.* (1983)

observation, 1983). Bilharzia is a major cause of bladder cancer in the developing world and produces, largely but not exclusively, tumors of the squamous cell type. Screening services in areas of endemic bilharzia do exist (El-Bolkainy, 1980), but no details are given in this chapter. The links between other chronic bladder diseases, including chronic infections and prostatic disease, are hard to evaluate due to intrinsic biases in these observations. The role of acetaminophen (phenacetin) in urothelial tumors of the renal pelvis and bladder has been established.

Cyclophosphamide used as a single agent in the treatment of malignant or

TABLE IV

Human Contact with Aromatic Amines: Substances for Which There is Evidence for or against Human Carcinogenecity

Substance	Evidence	Author
Aniline	No evidence	Case and Pearson (1954); Case *et al.* (1954)
o-Toluidine	Slight evidence	
p-Chloro-*o*-Toluidine	No evidence	Ubelin and Pletscher (1954)
2,5-Diamino toluene	Slight evidence	
Anthranilic acid	No evidence	
4-Biphenylamine	Good evidence	Melick *et al.* (1955, 1971)
4-Nitrobiphenyl	Slight Evidence, but mixed with other amines	
Benzidine	Good evidence	Goldwater *et al.* (1965)
3,3′-Dichlorobenzidine	Slight evidence, but mixed with other amines	
3,3′-Dimethoxybenzidine	Slight evidence, but mixed with other amines	
4,4′-Methylene bis (2-Chloraniline)	Slight evidence	
1-Naphthylamine	Slight evidence	Case and Pearson (1954); Case *et al.* (1954)
2-Naphthylamine	Good evidence	Mancuso and El-Attar (1967)
N,N-bis (2-chloroethyl)-2-naphthylamine	Good evidence	Thiede and Christensen (1969)
N-Phenyl-2-naphthylamine	Some evidence	Fox and Collier (1976)
Auramine	Slight evidence No evidence	Case and Pearson (1954) Kirsch *et al.* (1978)
Magenta	Slight evidence, but mixed with other amines	Case and Pearson (1954)
Cyclophosphamide	Good evidence	Plotz *et al.* (1979)

autoimmune diseases, or combined with other cytotoxic agents in the treatment of many malignancies, is an aromatic amine and a proven bladder carcinogen.

A wide variety of other occupations are suggested as having excess bladder cancer cases. These are summarized in Table III and result largely from case-control studies conducted between 1965 and 1980. Many of these observations need confirmation. Some represent exposure to aromatic amines (like the paint of Kimono artists), but other associations are more obscure and some could be fortuitous. Perhaps a better approach is to examine the evidence for the bladder carcinogenicity of specific aromatic amines. This is summarized in Table IV and shows that for the majority of aromatic amines—not shown in this table—there are no data for or against their biological activity. Human studies have yet to be conducted.

In the nonoccupational area, several factors have been under study for a considerable time but have yet to be proven to be bladder carcinogens. These include viruses and rural water supplies contaminated by bracken or various halogenated compounds. In addition, coffee consumption was thought to be a factor, but this may be false, due to the link between coffee drinking and cigarette smoking. Saccharin consumption, despite animal models to the contrary, does not seem to be a major etiological factor in bladder cancer, although some small subgroups might be at risk.

D. High-Risk Groups

The history of bladder cancer control has focused on special groups of interest, largely industrial and those thought to be at high risk. There are few studies on general population screening for bladder cancer (Nemeto *et al.*, 1981), but the relative overall rarity of this disease means that it is unlikely that attempts will be made to screen an entire population without a particular exposure of some type or without other ways of identifying those who are most likely to develop the disease (Morrison, 1979).

High-risk groups are definable, but are changing with the changing etiologies of bladder cancer. To achieve success in screening, the characteristics of high-risk groups must be uncommon and readily identifiable (Morrison, 1979, also see Hakama, Chapter 4). Because the occupational groups at high risk for bladder cancer account for only a trivial proportion of the total disease, the traditional approach of screening for bladder cancer will not have a major influence on overall bladder cancer mortality.

Traditionally high-risk groups occur in the rubber and cable-making industries and in the chemical dye manufacturing industry. The aromatic amine exposure for these industries has changed since the work of Case and his colleagues, and the risks for those entering the industry after the 1950s have been reduced

(Cartwright, 1983). Cases are still occurring, however, due to the very long latent period seen in bladder carcinogenesis. These traditional groups, however, will become negligible over the next 30 years.

E. Are There New High-Risk Groups?

The classic types of industrial exposures to aromatic amines are declining in significance, while more recent exposure events may provide the high-risk groups of the future.

Cyclophosphamide, used in the treatment of malignant and nonmalignant disease, causes bladder cancers in some long-term survivors (Plotz *et al.*, 1979). The studies so far are largely case reports rather than epidemiological follow-up studies, and the exact risk has yet to be computed.

Newer *N*-substituted aryl compounds and other chemicals with affinities for the bladder mucosa exist but have not been fully evaluated for their carcinogenic potential. Some have so little contact with humans and are used in such small amounts that their evaluation is hardly worthwhile. There are exceptions, however, including methylene-*bis*-ortho-chloraniline (MBOCA), which is a proven animal bladder carcinogen that awaits full human evaluation (Committee on Amines, 1981). If MBOCA proves to be a human bladder carcinogen, screening programs may have to be introduced. MBOCA is used as an elastomer in the plastics industry. This use brings the chemical into contact with some 50,000 workers in North America alone. Furthermore, the industrial populations that have been exposed to the manufacture of this product, in Adrian, Michigan, for example, will also need to be regarded as being at high risk, along with the local nonindustrial exposed population.

Chance events in the United Kingdom have brought to light the practice by coarse fishermen of staining their maggots with powdered azo dyes, including auramine and chrysoidine. It is probably too soon to evaluate the risks of this practice (Cartwright *et al.*, 1983b), which is quite recent among most British anglers. If this habit proves hazardous, this group might require screening.

II. SURVIVAL IN BLADDER CANCER

A. Determinants of Survival

Little work has been done to determine which factors influence the overall survival of bladder cancer patients. This is of some significance with respect to evaluating a bladder screening program. Studies in the United States with the SEER program suggests that racial differences might play an important part

(Young *et al.*, 1978), with survival in blacks being significantly lower than in whites.

Work from England has indicated that the stage at presentation is the major survival factor in all types of bladder cancer. Figure 1 contrasts stages at presentation in a study of all cases occurring in specific geographic locations between 1975 and 1979. These results cannot be compared with those of other series because they represent the totality of disease: treated or untreated, of any age, and with any cause of death. This figure also shows the poor survival associated with carcinoma *in situ* lesions. Table V summarizes some of the other factors that have been investigated as possibly influencing the survival of bladder cancer patients. Tumor grade has not been investigated in this study. The analysis is by the log-rank method of Peto *et al.* (1976, 1977). No sex differences were apparent, and differences by age at diagnosis are largely explained by the probability of overall survival. The analyses found little difference between survival incorporating all causes of death with survival of those selected only as dying of

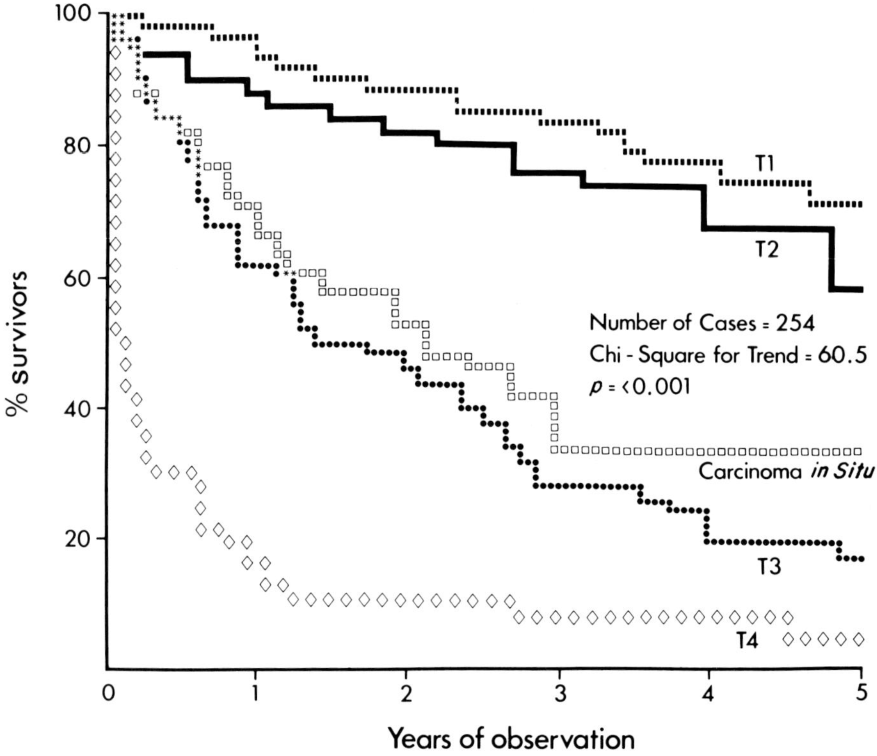

Fig. 1. Survival of bladder cancer patients from Yorkshire. Stage at diagnosis. Mixed tumors have been grouped to give preference to carcinoma *in situ* lesions.

TABLE V

Survival of Bladder Cancer in West Yorkshire (All Cases 1975–1979 Inclusive)

Factor	Number of cases	Difference within factors
Stage at presentation	611	$p = <0.01$[b]
Sex	640	$p = 0.12$[c]
Age at diagnosis	632	$p = <0.01$[b]
Cigarette smoking	398	$p = 1.00$[c]
Coffee drinking[a]	228	$p = 0.20$[c]
Saccharin consumption	398	$p = 0.48$[c]

[a] One center only.
[b] Significant.
[c] Nonsignificant.

bladder cancer. This could, in part, be due to the inappropriate addition of "bladder cancer" to all of the death certificates, irrespective of the part played in the death of the individual concerned.

A subsample of cases provided additional information that allowed a more detailed analysis of survival. The aim was to investigate what influence social or occupational contact with bladder carcinogens might have. The results for cigarette smokers, coffee drinkers, and saccharin consumption are shown in Table 5; they indicate that these habits had no detectable effect on overall survival. These results are crude, but they are identical when age, sex, and stage are accounted for.

The problem of the natural history of "chemical" bladder cancer has been anecdotally reported by many workers for over 60 years. In general, it is agreed by clinicians that industrial cases have a poorer prognosis than nonindustrial cases. Cartwright *et al.*, (1980) suggested that workers in an industrial area had a poorer prognosis, while Fox and White (1976) obliquely addressed a similar point for rubber workers but found no overall difference in survival between them and other workers with bladder cancer.

However, close analysis of the data from one dye manufacturing locality in England showed that, out of 178 patients, 35 had been involved in dye manufacturing. This subgroup had a poorer overall survival compared with the rest of the (nonindustrial) patients. This is shown in Fig. 2, but the overall difference was not significant statistically ($p = 0.07$). However, when stage and age at presentation are accounted for, the difference becomes significant at either $p = 0.04$ or $p = 0.02$, depending on how the stage was assessed in those individuals with more than one type of lesion at presentation. Most of the mixed tumors were flat carcinoma *in situ* lesions occurring along with stage T1 or T2 raised tumors.

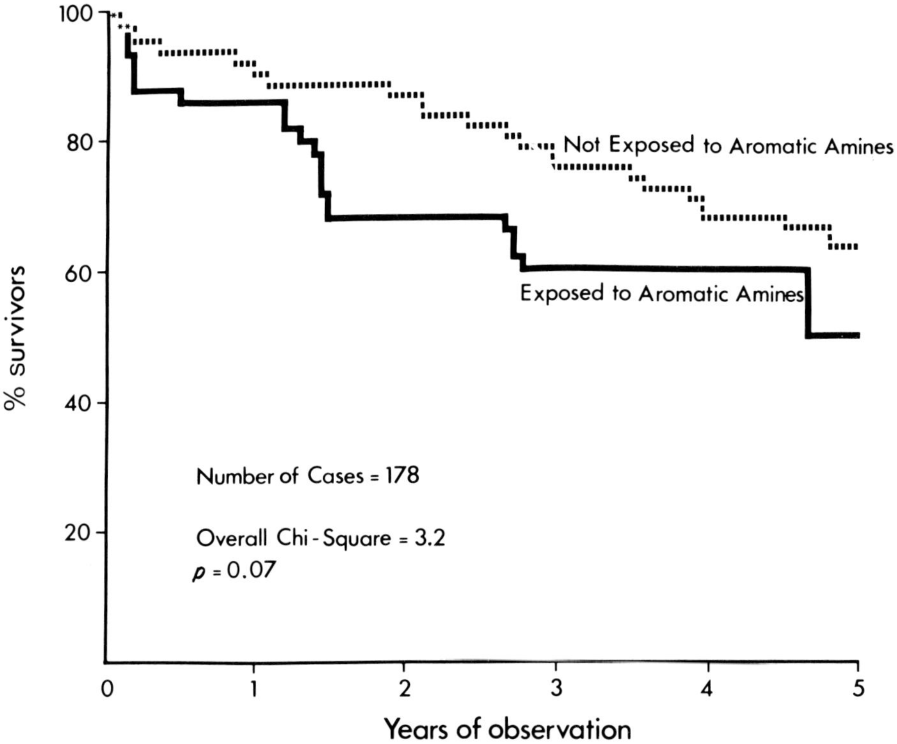

Fig. 2. Survival of bladder cancer patients from Yorkshire who were exposed or not exposed to aromatic amines.

B. What Factors of Survival Need to Be Accounted For?

Those studies described above by Cartwright and his colleagues indicate that for the factors observed, the major determinants of survival are stage at presentation and exposure to aromatic amines; those who were exposed to aromatic amines do worse, stage for stage and age for age, than those not exposed. This may be due to the nature of the bladder lesion produced by excessive aromatic amine exposure. This concept is conditional on the hypothesis that there are tumors with other behavior patterns that are the result of carcinogenic pathways not involving these aromatic amines, and that these tumors produce a less invasive proportion of cancers. There is some evidence for this with respect to the role of the enzyme *N*-acetyltransferase in bladder carcinogenesis (Cartwright *et al.*, 1982).

The invasive potential of lesions with respect to evaluation of a screening program is putatively very significant. This can be investigated by a close examination of the bladder for *in situ* lesions using intravesical staining or random bladder biopsies. In addition, the appearance of other tumors (flat or raised) and the integrity of the collagen fibers underneath the lesions (Glashan *et al.*, 1981) are helpful in making a careful overall assessment. This is discussed later in the chapter.

III. SCREENING FOR BLADDER CANCER

A. Early Prevention of Bladder Cancer

Once industrial managements acccpted the idea that a true bladder cancer excess might exist, various methods of prevention and early detection were instituted or recommended. This awareness was reflected in limited governmental regulations, which were first suggested by Leichtenstern in 1898 and introduced in Germany in 1925, Switzerland in 1920, England and Wales in 1932, and some U.S. states in the late 1930s (Hueper, 1942).

Early legislation was paralleled by industrial modernization, which started in Germany soon after the discovery of the first tumors. Such measures were designed to reduce contact between the chemicals and the workforce. These measures were singularly unsuccessful, particularly in Britain. Case and his colleagues studied the British dye manufacturing industry of 1919–1949 and found over 120 bladder tumors when they expected 4 (Case *et al.*, 1954). This lack of success with respect to preventive measures had been recognized by the industry in the 1930s and stimulated the development of methods of early detection. It also led to the control or banning of the active substances, largely identified as a result of the epidemiological work of Case, in most industrialized countries by the 1960s. Overviews of their work and screening regulations in Britain are available (Chemical Industries Association, 1976; Health and Safety Executive, 1972).

B. Early Methods of Screening

Two policies existed in the 1930s: regular examinations for microscopic hematuria and routine cystoscopies. The latter practice was advocated in continental Europe and North America, while the former was used in some British factories on the basis of a recommendation by Oppenheimer (1920). No systematic records exist on the early methods of detection. In addition, the techniques have never been critically evaluated.

1. Routine Cystoscopies

Regular cystoscopic examinations of the bladder were first instituted in U.S. factories beginning in 1931. The procedure was described by Gehrmann (1934) and Evans (1937). The cystoscopies were undertaken on an annual basis in over 500 workmen. By 1937, 83 cases of bladder cancer had been found as a result of 2868 cystoscopies. The urologists found 49 cases in the first annual round but only 1 case each on the fifth and sixth rounds. A similar procedure was started in Italy in the 1930s (di Maio, 1937) and in Switzerland in 1937 (Muller, 1945), while Billiard-Duchesne (1946–1947) describes its use in a small factory in France.

All of the research workers experienced difficulties with continued recruitment into the program and found that the detection rate became very low after the initial screen. No evaluations of the technique in terms of patient benefit or survival analysis have been published.

This form of screening was never used in the United Kingdom because it was felt that its hazards outweighed any advantages of a direct view of the bladders of unselected workmen. This approach ceased when Papanicolaou screening by malignant cell cytology (MCC) was introduced.

2. *Microscopic Hematuria*

The analysis of urine samples for microscopic hematuria was used to select individuals for cystoscopic examination. This technique, being noninvasive, was regarded as producing better compliance among the workmen. There are various

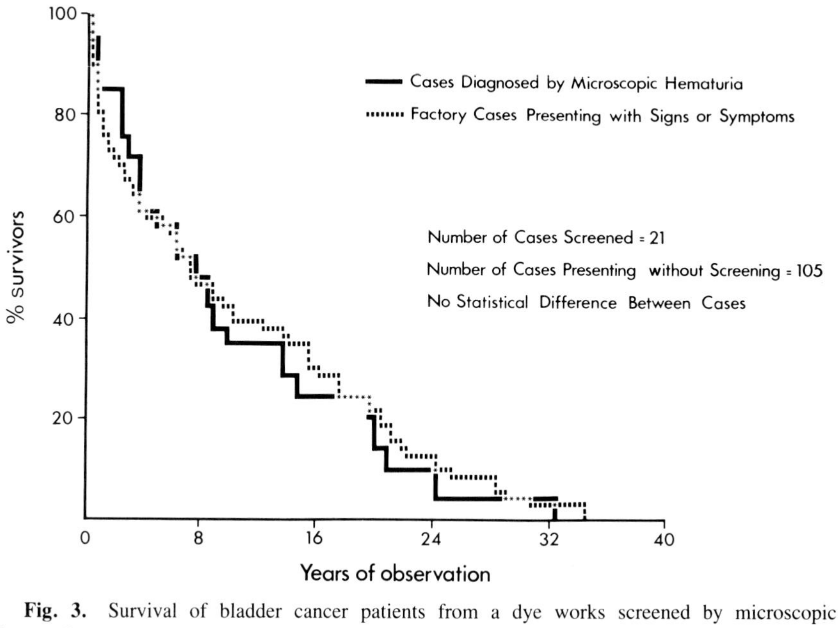

Fig. 3. Survival of bladder cancer patients from a dye works screened by microscopic hematuria.

problems associated with the interpretation of this test. Aniline toxicity itself produces hematuria. In addition, a number of normal people, perhaps 5–10% of the general population, regularly have a detectable number of red blood cells in their urine.

This method was used by Scott (1959) in a factory with a workforce of some 1800 men. He examined about 20,000 smears each year. During a 15-year period, some 40 men developed tumors, about half of which were picked up by this technique.

In a retrospective analysis of the data from 1934 to 1950, the present author has compared the crude survival of those factory cases diagnosed by microscopic hematuria (21 cases) with cases arising symptomatically in the factory over a longer period (105 cases). The results are displayed in Fig. 3 using the log-rank technique (Peto *et al.*, 1976, 1977), and although no statistics are appended, it can be seen that the survival patterns of two groups are almost identical.

The microscopic hematuria test compared unfavorably in its pick-up rate with the Papanicolaou test and has not been used to screen for bladder cancer since 1952.

C. Overview of Papanicolaou Screening

The techniques used by Papanicolaou in bladder cancer screening were described nearly 40 years ago (Papanicolaou and Marshall, 1945; Papanicolaou, 1947). This technique was introduced into Britain by Crabbe (1952), and laboratories in two dye-manufacturing plants were set up prior to 1952, using technicians trained by Crabbe or Papanicolaou.

The screening technique for chemical workers was extended to the British rubber industry by 1957 (Parkes, 1971). It was intoduced into the United States by Melicow in 1959 for the study and screening of workers exposed to xenylamine (Scott, 1962) and into Japan in 1962 (Yamaguchi *et al.*, 1982). In 1960, a screening technique became available for other workers in smaller factories in the United Kingdom not covered by the original programs. From the first, there were difficulties associated with urinary MCC. Good technical assistance was essential, together with constant cross-checking of results for consistency and for elimination of observer biases.

Until recently, little critical evaluation of this method has taken place, because most of the screening practice is based on ad hoc assessments of need, available facilities, and unpublished self-assessments. Screening intervals, for example, have varied from monthly to annually. Most of the current programs have now settled for a 6-monthly recall, but without published evidence.

The early reports on screening were aimed at comparing the Papanicolaou test with alternative methods—with which MCC compared favorably (Crabbe *et al.*, 1956). The early literature clearly shows that the techniques were gradually being improved by experience (Scott, 1962). Between 1955 and 1957, 1 false negative was found and 32 true positives (Scott, 1962) out of a total of some 1800 cases.

In another follow-up study of men of working age, some 7000 men were screened. Thirty-one tumors were picked up by the screening, together with 16 false positives and 9 false negatives. The men had not been followed once they stopped working, and there was only a short period of follow-up for some of the false positives. In addition, these data do not routinely include benign tumors. These results, therefore, are difficult to interpret, because not enough information is available about the characteristics of the cohort from which these figures are culled. Full details of the tumor stage and the appearance of the tumors in the false-negative cases are also lacking. The significance of the nine false negatives is obscure. They could involve lesions that do not shed cells or they may be interval cases, but the interval between screens is not known. Other series (Cartwright *et al.*, 1981) have found no false negatives and no interval cases when the screened workers were carefully separated from the nonparticipants or irregular participants.

Other reports record different rates of false negatives and false positives. Wiggishoff and McDonald (1972), for example, found 26% false negatives and 7% false positives in a series of 153 patients presenting to a urology unit with symptoms or signs suggestive of bladder disease. These results are fairly typical of later histopathological stage presentations (Sarnacki *et al.*, 1971; Park *et al.*, 1969), but the details on the stage of disease by mode of detection are not given. Such work indicates that a high failure rate is likely if MCC is applied to help assess the general population attending a urological clinic. This approach would not influence the overall disease pattern in any way.

The false-positive individuals are an interesting group in that they represent shedders of abnormal cells without obvious signs of disease. Traditional management consisted of observing them until tumors appeared. Of the 16 patients noted in the above study, 3 had developed observable tumors by the end of a short follow-up period. Koss *et al.* (1969) were the first to comment that these cases may well represent early lesions of bladder cancer such as carcinoma *in situ,* which could not be seen at cystoscopy.

The rubber industry (Parkes, 1975) has some 17,000 men who are periodically followed; 218 bladder tumors were found in the first 2 decades of its program. It is not clear whether the diagnosis was made by MCC in all cases, but this was certainly so for 97 workers. There were 14 false negatives reported, but further details of these is lacking.

It may be that false positives in these situations represent mixtures of lesions that include dysplasias or flat carcinomata *in situ* that at the time, were unobserved. It is also possible that the false negatives were very rapidly invasive lesions (interval cases). Alternatively, they may be the well-differentiated, fronded, carcinomatous lesions that shed malignant cells only sporadically, growing slowly and rarely causing death (Scott, 1959). These lesions most often present with hematuria and were originally termed *benign papillomata* (Umiker 1964; El-Bolkainy 1980).

It has also been suggested that recurrent bladder cancers may be diagnosed more readily than primary carcinomas (Kern *et al.*, 1968). Prior radiotherapy to the urogenital tract produces abnormal cells that are difficult for the cytologist to distinguish from truly malignant cells (Esposti *et al.*, 1970).

D. Present Position in the United Kingdom

Screening at the present time in the United Kingdom takes place in the dye manufacturing industry: the larger companies supporting their own laboratories, the smaller ones contributing to the few National Health Service laboratories that specialize in the techniques. The rubber industry operates its own national program for workers in the United Kingdom (Parkes, 1971).

All programs screen workers regularly (every 6 or 12 months) for life. Despite their backing by both unions and management, the overall uptake is rarely regular or greater than 60% of the workforce. The exact uptake of screening in the United Kingdom has been impossible to compute. In practice, although the programs are usually offered to retired workers, the incentive to be screened declines, and only a small proportion of retired workers are regularly screened.

The programs were initially offered to high-risk workers, as defined by local work practices. However, once they were underway, a general demand often occurred throughout a factory, and an almost "open door" policy would usually result.

E. Other Screening Methods

Other potential techniques of screening for bladder cancer have been suggested (Lessing, 1978, also see Chapter 8). A few have been evaluated, with largely disappointing results (Betkerur *et al.*, 1980), although the use of a tissue polypeptide antigen might be useful (Kumar *et al.*, 1978). These methods are biochemical and are not based on knowledge of the etiology of bladder cancer and the detection of epidemiologically based high-risk groups. A fuller understanding of the metabolic pathways of bladder carcinogenesis shows that there are some enzymatic variants that are found in groups more prone to aromatic amine bladder cancer (Cartwright *et al.*, 1982). This type of approach might play a helpful part in future screening programs.

IV. ANALYSES OF BLADDER CANCER SCREENING

A. Introduction

Direct evaluation of screening in the United Kingdom is not possible; the data are not available. There are a few aspects that can be addressed more fully, however, and this section contains data by the author and his colleagues on two of them. The aim of these approaches is to lead to a fuller appreciation of the problems surrounding early bladder cancer detection and control.

B. Can Screening by MCC Alter Survival?

Parkes (1969) reported that the overall 5-year survival of screened bladder cases from the rubber industry was 63%, in contrast to 50% for symptomatic cases.

This issue was tested more critically by Cartwright *et al.* (1981), who matched an industrial series of bladder cancers with those occurring in persons who were not obviously exposed to aromatic amines but who were treated by the same surgeons. The matching ratio was 1:1, those from the hospital being chosen at random from a group matched by age and year of diagnosis. The cases occurred between 1952 and 1979.

Both the hospital and factory cases fell into two groups: those diagnosed as a result of cystoscopy following signs or symptoms of bladder cancer, and those diagnosed as a result of MCC. Only one hospital case was diagnosed by screening, and was not considered further. The stage at diagnosis was not recorded in all cases. There were 88 hospital cases matched with the factory cases, and all were males. Thirty-three of the factory cases were diagnosed as a result of MCC; of these, nearly 80% were stage T1, compared to 54% for the other factory cases and 52% for the hospital cases.

Figure 4 shows the log-rank survival (Peto *et al.*, 1976, 1977) of these three groups. A nearly significant difference in survival (for all causes of death) is demonstrated ($p = 0.053$), but clear significant differences exist if the two factory groups alone are compared ($p = <0.01$). These differences in survival between the groups largely disappear when account is taken of the stage at diagnosis. Therefore, it is assumed that these are lead time differences of some 4–6 years. Stage data are available only on a subset of cases, however, and because the missing data are biased toward the unscreened factory group, the significance of these observations is not fully interpretable.

In this study, those persons diagnosed by a screen, in whom no lesions were seen at first cystoscopy, were not treated until a lesion appeared on follow-up cystoscopy. Survival times were measured from the date of the lesion rather than the date of the first abnormal cytological result.

It seems likely that when treatment of cases of bladder cancer from a screened

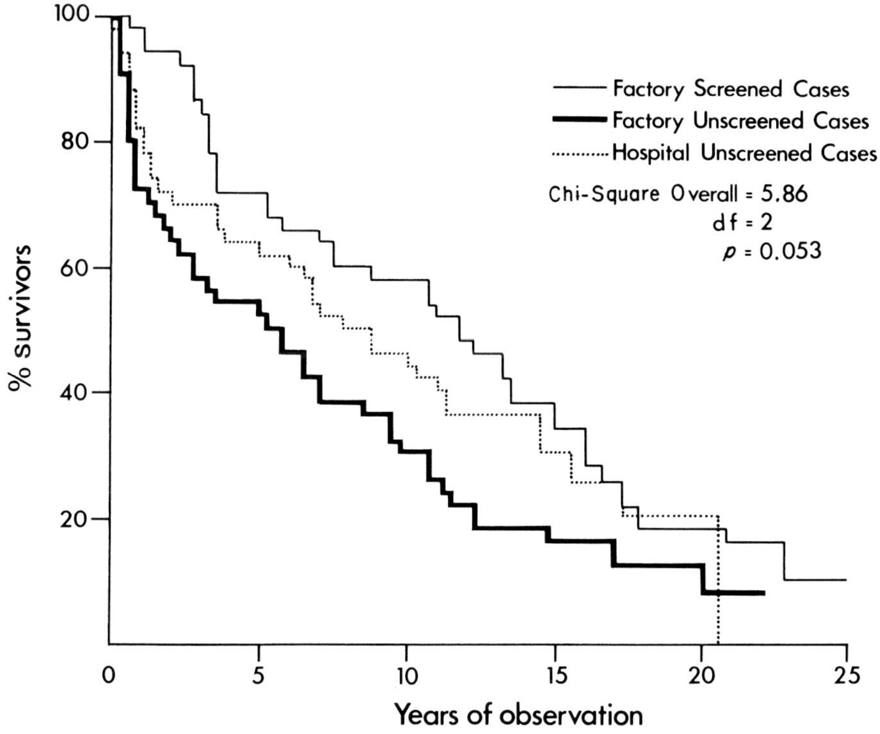

Fig. 4. Survival of bladder cancer patients from a dye works (all causes of death included). (From Cartwright *et al.*, 1981.)

group is of this conventional type, all that is achieved is lead time rather than a true modification of the natural history of the disease.

C. What Effect Has Screening on the Stage at Presentation of Cases?

In 1979 a study was set up with the long-term aim of modifying the pattern of disease in a screened population. Ths project is still underway, but it is possible to report interim results.

The population screened consisted of the employees of several local dye manufacturing companies; all have had exposure to aromatic amines. All screening was conducted at 6-month intervals, and all investigations revealing Papanicolaou grade III cells or worse were incorporated in the study. Investigations were undertaken to exclude other causes of abnormal cytology. This resulted in a group that was then cystoscoped. Random bladder biopsies were taken, irrespective of the presence of visible lesions. In addition to this group, all other persons

TABLE VI

Screening for Cases of Bladder Cancer: Results of Random Biopsies of the Bladder

Stage at diagnosis	Chemical workers with cancer (%)[a]		Nonchemical bladder cancer (%)	
	1975–1979	1980–1981	1975–1979	1980–1980
Dysplasia III	3	23	4	11
Carcinoma *in situ*	6	31	13	24
T1	24	8	44	38
T2	26	0	19	7
T3/4	32	38	21	20
Total	35	13	143	99

[a] Incorporates both screened and unscreened groups; see text.

who presented with signs or symptoms and who gave enough indication of bladder disease to be cystoscoped were entered into a parallel study. Random biopsies were also taken, with or without other observable lesions of the bladder.

The histopathology was examined for early changes in the bladder mucosa, and cases were identified with carcinoma *in situ* or its precursor lesion, dysplasia III. This process and these lesions are described by Glashan and Riley (1982). Intravesical chemotherapy was used in many of these early lesions as an attempted curative procedure. Follow-up of a few years' duration gives little evidence of the mucosal invasion of these lesions, conditional on the original abnormality being very superficial.

A comparison was made between patients identified as a result of the screen and those who presented as a direct result of their disease. No false-negative results have been found since the start of this study. In 2 years, 200 people were screened and 8 cases of early bladder cancer were found. Table VI presents these data. This table groups the industrial patients as those who participated in the screening programs and those who did not, but who were employed at the same factories. The screened patients found after 1980 all had very early disease, except for one late-stage patient (T3) who had just started to avail himself of the program. Those patients from industry who were not screened included one T1, and the rest were T3 and T4.

The results in Table VI are displayed as percentages for comparability, despite the small numbers in some columns. There is a shift in diagnostic groups at presentation in both the chemical workers and those apparently unassociated with chemicals. This is because the search for carcinoma *in situ* was not confined to the MCC-screened population; random biopsy samples were taken from all cystoscoped bladders. There are no statistically significant differences between the groups in Table VI, in part due to the small numbers. A trend may be starting, showing an overall shift to the diagnosis of very early bladder cancer in both groups, especially among the screened chemical workers. The numbers are too small at this time to allow us to examine the problem further or to extend the study to problems such as mixed tumor types.

This work would seem to reinforce the view that careful screening plus systematic biopsies and aggressive therapy may alter the outlook for those with potentially invasive, flat lesions of the bladder. The evidence to substantiate this belief is still lacking, but these small observational studies help point the way to future studies, which might be designed in a less biased way.

V. FUTURE OF BLADDER CANCER SCREENING

A. Value of Screening

A critical estimation of the value of bladder cancer screening has yet to be made. Several authors have asserted that MCC is a method of choice in high-risk groups (de Voogt, 1980). The general lack of critical evaluation may seem unusual, since screening by MCC has been underway for many years, being introduced prior to uterine cervix cancer screening.

Unfortunately, most screening has been done by private programs, with little regard for the size of the screened population. These were also "in-house" exercises and were often shrouded in confidentiality. The waters are also muddied by the lack of data about the fate of patients. Once identified, patients are often passed on either to a health service, which scatters them to numerous urologists, or to private clinics where records are unobtainable. The few exceptional situations have been utilized in this chapter.

In addition, there is some evidence, which has been presented, that screening without treatment appropriate to early, aggressive, and generalized bladder disease is of little value. In addition, studies on the natural history of bladder cancer have suggested that different etiologies are linked with different natural progressions of the disease. In particular, aromatic amine bladder carcinogenesis has been linked with more flat, invasive lesions, which have a poor prognosis, while other etiologies are linked with the papillomatous types and have an extremely good prognosis. It should be noted that flat, invasive lesions shed cells, while only some papillomata do, but the detection of the raised lesions is of lower priority (in terms of survival) than that of invasive lesions. A screening program that misses raised, well-differentiated, papillomatous-type lesions has not failed as long as all potentially highly invasive lesions, such as carcinoma *in situ*, are found. This concept has yet to be applied in the evaluation of bladder cancer screening.

The evidence presented can be criticized as containing elements of various types of bias. It is unlikely that future studies will be entirely free of bias.

Nevertheless, it seems that industrial high-risk screening selects those persons who are more likely to have aggressive bladder cancer, but screening itself has little patient benefit in terms of overall survival unless the programs incorporate the means of treatment of a generalized urothelial disease.

B. Future of Screening

The future of MCC screening will depend, first, on the identification of new groups at high risk from occupational contact with either traditional substances or new materials. Nonoccupational high-risk groups may also exist—those exposed to cyclophosphamide, for example.

Second, the future depends on the availability of automated means of screening that remove the observer biases from current methods. These could include flow cytometry (Melamed *et al.*, 1977; Collste *et al.*, 1980). The possibility of screening the general population is unlikely to be of relevance in most populations unless the population itself has had unusual exposure. Certainly, general population screening cannot possibly be done without automated techniques. Even under these circumstances, the susceptible population for the well-differentiated, fronded lesion would have to be distinguished from the group at risk from cancers with invasive potential. It is not yet clear if this can be done with sufficient accuracy, and future epidemiological studies should be directed to this issue. In addition, there are not enough data available to identify susceptible groups at high risk other than the small number of persons exposed to specific substances. Future international studies of bladder cancer epidemiology should also address this topic.

Third, a future priority should be the demonstration of effective methods to treat very early bladder disease. Techniques such as intravesical chemotherapy are still being evaluated and would be an essential part of any screening scheme.

ACKNOWLEDGMENTS

Much unpublished work in this chapter has been acquired from the cases of Mr. Robin Glashan, Huddersfield Royal Infirmary, with whom the author has collaborated for several years. I would like to thank Dr. Theo Gadian, Mr. A. Riley, and members of the Yorkshire Regional Occupational Cancer Group for their help with various parts of this chapter. Some of the work described was conducted with the help of Sylvia Bernard and Denise Barham-Hall, and was funded by the Medical Research Council of the United Kingdom.

REFERENCES

Anderson, L. W. (1934). Aniline tumors of the bladder. *J. Urol.* **31,** 148–154.

Anthony, H. M. (1974). Industrial exposure in patients with carcinoma of the bladder. *J. Soc. Occup. Med.* **24,** 110–116.

Betkerur, V., Rao, R., Hlaing, V., Rhee, H., Baumgartner, G., and Guinan, P. (1980). Screening tests for detection of bladder cancer. *Urology* **16,** 16–19.

Beyer-Boon, M. E., de Voogt, H. J., and Schaberg, A. (1978). The effect of cyclophosphamide treatment on the epithelium and stroma of the urinary bladder. *Eur. J. Cancer* **14,** 1029–1035.

Billiard-Duchesne, J. L. (1946–1947). Les amino-tumeurs de la vessie. (Tumeurs dites aniliniques). *J. Urol.* **53,** 401–422.

Blot, W. J., and Fraumeni, J. F. (1978). Geographic patterns of bladder cancer in the United States. *JNCI, J. Natl. Cancer Inst.* **61,** 1017–1023.

Brand, K. G. (1979). Schistosomiasis—Cancer: Etiological considerations—a review. *Acta Trop.* **36,** 203–214.

Bridge, J. C., and Henry, S. A. (1928). "Industrial Cancer," Report of the International Cancer Congress, p. 267. Wright, Bristol.

Cartwright, R. A. (1983). Historical and modern epidemiological studies on populations exposed to N-substituted aryl compounds. *Environ. Health Perspect.* **49,** 13–19.

Cartwright, R. A., Glashan, R. W., and Gray, B. (1980). Survival of transitional cell carcinoma in 2 Yorkshire centres. *Br. J. Urol.* **52,** 497–499.

Cartwright, R. A., Gadian, T., Garland, J. B., and Bernard, S. (1981). The influence of malignant cell cytology screening on the survival of industrial bladder cancer cases. *J. Epidemiol. Commun. Health* **35,** 35–38.

Cartwright, R. A., Glashan, R. W., Rogers, H. J., Ahmad, R. A., Barham-Hall, D., Higgins, E., and Kahn, M. A. (1982). Role of N-acetyltransferase phenotypes in bladder carcinogenesis: A pharmacogenetic epidemiological approach to bladder cancer. *Lancet* **2,** 842–846.

Cartwright, R. A., Adib, R., Appleyard, I., Glashan, R. W., Gray, B., Hamilton-Stewart, P. A., Robinson, M., and Barham-Hall, D. (1983a). Cigarette smoking and bladder cancer: An epidemiological enquiry in West Yorkshire. *J. Epidemiol. Commun. Health* **37,** 256–263.

Cartwright, R. A., Robinson, M. R. G., Glashan, R. W., Gray, B. K., Hamilton-Stewart, P., Cartwright, S. C., and Barham-Hall, D. (1983b). Does the use of stained maggots present a risk of bladder cancer to coarse fishermen? *Carcinogenesis (London)* **4,** 111–113.

Case, R. A. M. (1969). Some environmental carcinogens. *J. Soc. Med.* **62,** 1061–1066.

Case, R. A. M., and Hosker, M. E. (1954). Tumours of the urinary bladder as an occupational disease in the rubber industry in England and Wales. *Br. J. Prev. Soc. Med.* **8,** 39–50.

Case, R. A. M., and Pearson J. T. (1954). Tumours of the urinary bladder in workmen engaged in the manufacture and use of certain dyestuff intermediates in the British chemical industry. Further consideration of the role of aniline and of the manufacture of auramines and magenta (fuchsine) as possible causative agents. *Br. J. Ind. Med.* **11,** 213–216.

Case, R. A. M., Hosker, M. E., McDonald, D. B., and Pearson, J. T. (1954). Tumours of the urinary bladder in workmen engaged in the manufacture and use of certain dyestuff intermediates in the chemical industry. *Br. J. Ind. Med.* **11,** 75–104.

Chemical Industries Association (1976). "Tumours of the Bladder in the Chemical Industry," A study of their cause and prevention. Chem. Ind. Assoc., Carcinogenic Substances Committee, London.

Cole, P., Monson, R. R., and Haning, W. (1971). Smoking and cancer of the lower urinary tract. *N. Engl. J. Med.* **284,** 129–134.

Cole, P., Hoover, R., and Friedell, G. H. (1972). Occupation and cancer of the lower urinary tract. *Cancer* **29,** 1250–1260.

Collste, L. G., Darzynkiewicz, Z., Traganos, F., Sharpless, T. K., Sogani, P., Grabstald, H., Whitmore, W. F., and Melamed, M. R. (1980). Flow cytometry in bladder cancer detection and evaluation using acridine orange metachromatic nucleic acid staining of irrigation cytology specimens. *J. Urol.* **123,** 478–485.

Committee on Amines (1981). "Aromatic Amines: An Assessment of the Biological and Environmental Effects." Natl. Acad. Press, Washington D.C.

Crabbe, J. G. S. (1952). Exfoliative cytological control in occupational cancer of the bladder. *Br. Med. J.* **2,** 1072–1076.

Crabbe, J. G. S., Cresdee, W. C., Scott, T. S., and Williams, M. H. C. (1956). The cytological diagnosis of bladder tumours among dyestuff workers. *Br. J. Ind. Med.* **13,** 270–276.

Davies, J. M. (1965). Bladder tumours in the electric cable industry. *Lancet* **2,** 143–146.

Davies, J. M., Somerville, S. M., and Wallace, D. M. (1976). Occupational bladder tumour cases identified during ten years' interviewing of patients. *Br. J. Urol.* **48,** 561–566.

de Voogt, H. J. (1980). Bedeutung der urinzytologie als screening-untersuchung fur die diagnose eines harnblasenkarzinoms. *Onkologie* **5,** 233–237.

di Maio, G. (1937). Tumori e lesioni precancerose della vesica da amine o nitroderivati. *Arch. Ital. Urol.* **14,** 283.

Doll, R., Fisher, R. E. w., Gammon, E. J., Gunn, W., Hughes, G. O., Tyrer, F. H., and Wilson, W. (1965). Mortality of gas workers with special reference to cancers of the lung and bladder, chronic bronchitis and pneumoconiosis. *Br. J. Ind. Med.* **22,** 1–12.

Dunham, L. J., Rabson, A. S., Stewart, H. L., Frank, A. S., and Young, J. L. (1968). Rates, interviews and pathology study of cancer of the urinary bladder in New Orleans, Louisiana. *JNCI, J. Natl. Cancer. Inst.* **41,** 683–709.

El-Bolkainy, M. N. (1980). Cytology of bladder carcinoma. *J. Urol.* **124,** 20–22.

Esposti, P. L., Moberger, G., and Zajicek, J. (1970). The cytologic diagnosis of transitional cell tumors of the urinary bladder and its histologic basis. A study of 567 cases of urinary-tract disorder including 170 untreated and 182 irradiated bladder tumors. *Acta Cytol.* **14,** 145–155.

Evans, E. E. (1937). Causative agents and protective measures in aniline tumours of the bladder. *J. Urol.* **38,** 212–215.

Fox, A. J., and Collier, P. F. (1976). A survey of occupational cancer in the rubber and cable making industry: Analysis of deaths occurring in 1972–74. *Br. J. Ind. Med.* **33,** 249–264.

Fox, A. J., and White, G. C. (1976). Bladder cancer in rubber workers. Do screening and doctors' awareness distort the statistics? *Lancet* **1,** 1009–1011.

Gehrmann, G. H. (1934). The carcinogenetic agent—chemistry and industrial aspects. *J. Urol.* **31,** 126–137.

Glashan, R. W., and Riley, A. (1982). Intravesical therapy with Adriamycin in urothelial dysplasia and early carcinoma in situ. *Can. J. Surg.* **25,** 30–32.

Glashan, R. W., Wigesinghe, D. P., and Riley, A. (1981). The early changes in the development of bladder cancer in patients exposed to known industrial carcinogens. *Br. J. Urol.* **53,** 571–577.

Goldwater, L. J., Rosso, A. J., and Kleinfeld, M. (1965). Bladder tumours in a coal tar dye plant. *Arch. Environ. Health* **11,** 814–817.

Health and Safety Executive (UK) (1972). "Renal Tract Carcinogenesis," Employment Medical Advisory Service Notes of Guidance. H. M. Stationery Office, London.

Howe, GR., Burch, J. D., Miller, A. B., Cook, G. M., Esteve, J., Morrison, B., Gordon, P., Chambers, L. W., Fodor, G., and Winsor, G. M. (1980). Tobacco use, occupation, coffee, various nutrients and bladder cancer. *JNCI, J. Natl. Cancer Inst.* **64,** 701–713.

Hueper, W. C. (1942). "Occupational Tumours and Allied Diseases." Thomas, Springfield, Illinois.

Johansson, S., and Wahlquist, L. (1977). Tumours of the urinary bladder and ureter associated with abuse of phenacetin-containing analgesics. *Acta Pathol. Microbiol. Scand., Sect. A* **85A,** 768–774.

Kern, W. H., Bales, C. E., and Webster, W. W. (1968). Cytologic evaluation of transitional cell carcinoma of the bladder. *J. Urol.* **160,** 616–622.

Kirsch, P., Fleig, I., Frentzel-Beyme, R., Gembardt, C., Steinborn, J., Theiss, A. M., Kock, W., Seibert, W., Wellenreuther, G., and Zeller, H. (1978). Auramin Toxikulogische und arbeitsmedizinische untersuchurgen. *Arbeitsmed., Soc. Med., Praventivmed., Spec. Ed.* No. 2, p. 13.

Koss, L. G. (1975). "Tumours of the Urinary Bladder," Atlas of Tumour Pathol., Vol 11. Armed Forces Inst. Pathol., Washington, D.C.

Koss, L. G., Melamed, M. R., and Kelly, R. E. (1969). Further cytologic and histologic studies of bladder lesions in workers exposed to para-aminodiphenyl: Progress report. *J. Natl. Cancer Inst.* (*U.S.*) **43,** 233–241.

Kumar, S., Wilson, P., Brenchley, P., Taylor, G., Bjorklund, B., and Eklund, G. (1978). Frequent elevation of tissue polypeptide antigen in the sera of workers exposed to bladder carcinogens. *Int. J. Cancer* **22,** 542–545.

Leichtenstern, O. (1898). Harnblasentzundungen und Geschwulste bei Arbeitern in Farbfabriken. *Dtsch. Med. Wochenschr.* **24,** 709.

Lessing, J. A. (1978). Bladder cancer: Early diagnosis and evaluation of biologic potential. A review of newer methods. *J. Urol.* **120,** 1–5.

Lockwood, K. (1961). On the etiology of bladder tumors in Kobenhavn-Fredriksberg. An inquiry of 369 patients and 369 controls. *Acta Pathol. Microbiol. Scand.* **41** Suppl. 145, 1–166.

Mancuso, T. F., and El-Attar, A. A. (1967). Cohort study of workers exposed to beta-naphthylamine and benzidine. *J. Occup. Med.* **9,** 277–285.

Melamed, M. R., Darzynkiewicz, Z., Traganos, F., and Sharpless, T. (1977). Cytology automation by flow cytometry. *Cancer Res.* **37,** 2806–2812.

Melick, W. F., Escue, H. M., Naryka, J. J., Mezara, R. A., and Wheeler, E. P. (1955). The first reported cases of human bladder tumour due to a new carcinogen - xenylamine. *J. Urol.* **74,** 760–766.

Melick, W. F., Naryka, J. J., and Kelly, R. E. (1971). Bladder cancer due to exposure to para aminobiphenyl: 17 year follow up. *J. Urol.* **106,** 220–226.

Mommson, S., Aagaard, J., and Sell, A. (1982). An epidemiological case-control study of bladder cancer in males from a predominantly rural district. *Eur. J. Cancer Clin. Oncol.* **18,** 1205–1210.

Monson, R. R. (1980). "Occupational Epidemiology." CRC Press, Boca Raton, Florida.

Morrison, A. S. (1979). Public health value of using epidemiologic information to identify high-risk groups for bladder cancer screening. *Semin. Oncol.* **6,** 184–188.

Muller, A. (1945). Die Prophylaxe der Blasenschadigungen der in Farbstoffindustrie. *Schweiz. Med. Wochenschr.* **75,** 742–744.

Nemeto, R., Kato, T., Shibata, K., and Kano, M. (1981). Urinary cytology as a test in mass screening. *Tohoku J. Exp. Med.* **135,** 115–116.

Office of Population Censuses and Surveys (OPCS) (1982). "Cancer Statistics: Registrations 1977," MB1 No. 8 H. M. Stationary Office, London.

Oppenheimer, R. R. (1920). Zur Erkennung und behardlung der blasengeschwulste der anilinarbeiter. *Zentralbl. Gewerbe hyg. Unfallverhuet.* **8,** 105–108.

Papanicolaou, G. N. (1947). Cytology of the urinary sediment in neoplasm of the urinary tract. *J. Urol.* **57,** 375.

Papanicolaou, G. N., and Marshall, V. F. (1945). Urine sediment smears as a diagnostic procedure in cancer of the urinary tract. *Science* **101,** 519–520.

Park, C.-H., Britsch, C., Uson, A. C., and Veenema, R. J. (1969). Reliability of positive exfoliative cytologic study of the urine in urinary tract malignancy. *J. Urol.* **102,** 91–92.

Parkes, H. G. (1969). Epidemiology and etiology of human bladder cancer: Occupational bladder cancer in the British rubber industry. *J. Natl. Cancer Inst.* (*U.S.*) **43,** 249–252.

Parkes, H. G. (1971). Screening for bladder cancer. *Proc. R. Soc. Med.* **64,** 1207–1211.

Parkes, H. G. (1975). Occupational bladder cancer. *Practitioner* **214,** 80–86.

Peto, R., Pike, M. C., Armitage, P., Breslow, N. E., Cox, D. R., Howard, V., Mantel, N., McPherson, K., Peto, J., and Smith, P. G. (1976). Design and analysis of randomized clinical trials requiring prolonged observation of each patient. I. Introduction and design. *Br. J. Cancer* **34,** 585–612.

Peto, R., Pike, M. C., Armitage, P., Breslow, N. E., Cox, D. R., Howard, V., Mantel, N., McPherson, K., Peto, J., and Smith, P. G. (1977). Design and analysis of randomized clinical trials requiring prolonged observation of each patient. II. Analysis and examples. *Br. J. Cancer* **35,** 1–39.

Plotz, P. H., Klippel, J. H., Decker, J. L., Grauman, D., Wolff, B., Brown, B. C., and Rutt, G. (1979). Bladder complications in patients receiving cyclophosphamide for systemic lupus erythematosus or rheumatoid arthritis. *Ann. Intern. Med.* **91,** 221–223.

Radovanovic, Z., and Krajinovic, S. (1979). The Balkan endemic nephropathy and urnar tract tumours. *Arch. Geschwulstforsch.* **49,** 444–447.

Rehn, L. (1895). Blasengeschwulste bei fuchsin-arbeitern. *Arch. Klin. Chir.* **50,** 588–600.

Rosenbaum, N. D., and Gottlieb, J. I. (1926). Tumours of the bladder in dyers. *Gig. Tr.* **30,** 30.

Sarnacki, C. T., McCormack, L. J., Kiser, W. S., Hazard, J. B., McLaughlin, T. C., and Belovich, D. M. (1971). Urinary cytology and the clinical diagnosis of urinary tract malignancy: A clinicopathologic study of 1,400 patients. *J. Urol.* **106,** 761–764.

Schedler, D. (1905). Zur Kasuistik der blasentumoren bei Farbarbeitern. Dissertation, University of Basel.

Scott, T. S. (1959). Occupational tumours of the bladder. M.D. Thesis, Glasgow University.

Scott, T. S. (1962). "Carcinogenic and Chronic Toxic Hazards of Aromatic Amines." Elsevier, Amsterdam.

Silverman, D. T., Hoover, R. N., Albert, S., and Graff, K. M. (1983). Occupation and cancer of the lower urinary tract in Detroit. *JNCI, J. Natl. Cancer Inst.* **70,** 237–245.

Somerville, S. M., Davies, J. M., Hendry, W. F., and Williams, G. (1980). Bladder cancer as a prescribed industrial disease: A guide for clinicians. *Br. Med. J.* **1,** 540–542.

Staszewski, J. (1980). Cancer of the urinary bladder: International mortality trends. *World Health Stat. Rep.* **33,** 27–39.

Theriault, G., De Guire, L., and Cordier, S. (1981). Reducing aluminium: An occupation possibly associated with bladder cancer. *Can. Med. Assoc. J.* **124,** 419–425.

Thiede, T., and Christensen, B. C. (1969). Bladder tumours induced by chlornaphazine: A five year follow up study of chlornaphazine treated patients with polycythemia. *Acta Med. Scand.* **185,** 133–137.

Tyrrell, A. B., MacAirt, J. G., and McCaughey, W. T. E. (1971). Occupational and non-occupational factors associated with vesical neoplasms in Ireland. *J. Ir. Med. Assoc.* **64,** 213–217.

Ubelin, F., and Pletscher, A. (1954). Atiologie und prophylaxe gewerblicher tumoren in der Farbstoffindustrie. *Schweiz. Med. Wochenschr.* **84,** 917–920.

UICC (1978). "TNM Classification of Malignant Tumours," 3rd ed. Int. Union Against Cancer, Geneva.

Umiker, W. (1964). Accuracy of cytologic diagnosis of cancer of the urinary tract. *Acta Cytol.* **8,** 186–191.

Versluys, J. J. (1949). Cancer and occupation in the Netherlands. *Br. J. Cancer* **3,** 161–185.

Wiggishoff, C. G., and McDonald, J. H. (1972). Urinary exfoliative cytology in the diagnosis of bladder tumors. *Acta Cytol.* **16,** 139–141.

Wynder, E. L., Onderdonk, J., and Mantel, N. (1963). An epidemiological investigation of cancer of the bladder. *Cancer* **16,** 1388–1407.

Wynder, E. Z., and Goldsmith, R. (1977). The epidemiology of bladder cancer—a second look. *Cancer* **40,** 1246–1268.

Yamaguchi, N., Tazaki, H., and Okubo, T. (1982). Periodic urine cytology surveillance of bladder tumour incidence in dyestuff workers. *Am. J. Ind. Med.* **3,** 139–148.

Young, J. L., Asine, A. J., and Pollack, E. S. (1978). "SEER program: Cancer incidence and Mortality in the United States, 1973–1976." Natl. Inst. Health, Washington, D.C.

22

Screening for Oral Cancer

DAVID MOCK

I.	Introduction	421
II.	Epidemiology and Etiology	422
III.	Squamous Cell Carcinoma	426
	A. Lip	427
	B. Tongue	428
	C. Floor of the Mouth	428
	D. Gingiva and Alveolar Ridge	429
	E. Palate	429
	F. Buccal Mucosa	430
	G. Other Sites	430
IV.	Verrucous Carcinoma	431
V.	Characteristics of Premalignancy and Early Carcinoma	432
	A. White Lesions	432
	B. Red Lesions	433
	C. Mixed Red–White Lesions	434
VI.	Malignant Tumors of the Salivary Gland	434
VII.	Malignancies of Other Tissue	435
VIII.	Oral Examination	435
IX.	Diagnostic Procedures	436
	A. Biopsy	436
	B. Exfoliative Cytology	437
	C. Toluidine Blue Staining	439
X.	Summary and Conclusions	439
	References	440

I. INTRODUCTION

Oral cancer accounts for approximately 5% of all reported malignant tumors and 3% of cancer deaths in the average North American population. Despite the obvious accessibility of this area of the body, lesions are often not detected or

ISBN 0-12-496720-5

recognized until late in their progression. The patient is therefore subjected to mutilating surgery, often combined with debilitating radiotherapy or chemotherapy, as well as considerable risk of death. The difficulties in early recognition of oral cancer are caused by inadequate and infrequent examination of the oral tissues and confusion of malignancy with one of the many nonneoplastic lesions so common in the mouth.

Human nature dictates that each health discipline examine only those areas of interest to its specific specialty. In the oral cavity, this often means that the physician pushes the tongue down while examining the pharynx, and the dentist concentrates on the teeth and supporting structures. Thus, the two health practitioners with whom the patient may routinely come in contact avoid the other oral and perioral tissues unless the patient has a specific complaint that draws attention to these areas. Since most oral malignancies are asymptomatic until late in the disease, they often remain undetected despite regular professional health care.

A variety of tumors can and do occur in the oral cavity and its related structures. These can arise from the covering epithelium, supporting connective tissues, bone, odontogenic apparatus, and salivary glands. The mouth can also be the site of metastatic or multicentric tumors. The vast majority of oral malignancies (estimated at approximately 90%) are squamous cell carcinomas, with the bulk of the remaindcr bcing tumors of the salivary glands.

As with cancers in all other sites, the key to early detection and treatment of oral cancer is recognition of persons at greatest risk and identification of potentially premalignant and early malignant lesions. This is best accomplished by regular examination of the oral cavity and adjacent structures, with appropriate investigation of suspicious lesions.

II. EPIDEMIOLOGY AND ETIOLOGY

Epidemiological data not only suggest etiological factors but delineate those segments of the population at greatest risk of developing oral cancer. Over the years, there has been a continuous increase in the number of oral cancers (Silverberg and Holleb, 1972, 1974; Krolls and Hoffman, 1976; Silverberg, 1982, 1983, 1984). The American Cancer Society's estimate for total oral cancers was 14,200 for 1971, 23,700 for 1974, and 27,500 for 1984.

The most thorough statistical examination of oral cancer is that reported in 1976 by Krolls and Hoffman, who analyzed 14,253 cases received by the United States Armed Forces Institute of Pathology (AFIP). They found that 93% of these cases, considering all sites and 97.5% of lip carcinomas, occurred in males. The site of least male predominance was the buccal mucosa, where 78.7% of the cases occurred in men (Table I). Similar results have been reported

TABLE I

Distribution of 14,253 Cases of Oral Carcinoma by Anatomic Site, Age, Sex, and Race of Patients[a]

Anatomic site	group	Percentage of total in group	Age range (yr)	Cases in males (percentage of total)	Cases in females (percentage of total)	Cases in blacks (percentage of total)
Lower lip	5,399	38	14–99	97.5	2.5	0.6
Tongue	3,117	22	14–99	92.5	7.5	7.8
Floor of mouth	2,479	17	15–99	90.4	9.6	7.0
Gingiva	923	6	20–99	93.6	6.4	8.4
Palate	786	5.5	14–99	85.9	14.1	6.1
Tonsil	673	5	20–89	93.4	6.6	8.0
Upper lip	553	4	20–99	92.3	7.7	0
Buccal mucosa	245	2	20–99	78.7	11.3	1.7
Uvula	78	0.5	40–79	96.9	3.1	5.5
Total	14,253	100.0				

[a] From Krolls and Hoffman (1976). Reproduced with the permission of the American Dental Association and courtesy of the U.S. Armed Forces Institute of Pathology.

by other investigators, demonstrating marked male predominance (Binnie *et al.*, 1972; Silverberg and Holleb, 1972, 1974; Feldman *et al.*, 1975; Silverberg, 1982).

Although there is considerable geographic variation in the incidence of oral cancer, race itself is not an overall significant factor (Feldman *et al.*, 1975). It is notable, however, that in the study by Krolls and Hoffman (1976), the incidence of carcinoma of the lip was exceptionally low amongst blacks, supporting the concept that pigmentation offers protection from possible carcinogenic influences of actinic radiation. The annual incidence in India is quoted as 19.6 new cases per 10,000 versus 2.5 in the southern United Kingdom, demonstrating the geographic disparities (Waterhouse *et al.*, 1976). Considerable variation is also noted in countries with racially mixed populations. For example, the incidence of oral cancer in the province of Newfoundland, Canada, is approximately 3.5 times that in British Columbia (Waterhouse *et al.*, 1976). A similar geographic variation has been noted in the United States (Szpak *et al.*, 1977). It is obvious that a number of environmental, social, and dietary factors are instrumental in producing this variation, rather than racial predilection alone.

Although oral cancer is still primarily a disease of older patients, there is a trend toward its occurrence in younger individuals. Krolls and Hoffman (1976) noted that the largest number of oral carcinomas, other than those of the lower lip, accessioned from 1970 to 1973 in the AFIP, occurred in patients a decade younger than those accessioned before 1970. The case for carcinoma of the lower lip is even more convincing with approximately a 2-decade decrease. In general, however, oral carcinomas occur infrequently in persons under the age of 40 (Table II).

Tobacco has been strongly implicated as a causative factor in oral carcinoma (Wynder *et al.*, 1957; Graham *et al.*, 1977). The excessively high incidence of oral cancer in Southeast Asia is explained primarily by the predominant use of tobacco and the manner in which it is used (i.e., reverse smoking, betal nut quid). Even mild tobacco use appears to increase significantly the risk of oral carcinomas (Graham *et al.*, 1977; Wynder and Stellman, 1977). A similarly increased risk of oral cancer has been suggested in the southern United States among snuff users, particularly women (Blot and Fraumeni, 1977; Winn *et al.*, 1981). Scandinavian studies on the relationship between snuff use and oral cancer failed to demonstrate this correlation (Roed-Petersen and Pindborg, 1973; Axell *et al.*, 1976). The composition of snuff and the segment of the population using it probably varies in different parts of the world, possibly explaining these contrasting results. Histological differences in nonneoplastic snuff dippers' lesions between these geographic areas have also been noted (Axéll *et al.*, 1976; Pindborg, 1980). With the apparent increase in the use of "smokeless" tobacco, snuff may become a greater factor in the incidence of oral cancer.

The role of alcohol in oral carcinogenesis has been somewhat more controver-

TABLE II

Age Distribution of 9775 Patient with Oral Carcinomas[a]

Age range (yr)	Number of patients	Percentage
0–14	3	0.015
15–19	16	0.15
20–29	307	3.2
30–39	713	7.3
40–49	1746	17.9
50–59	2427	24.8
60–69	3113	31.8
70–79	1204	12.3
80–89	194	2.0
90–99	52	0.5
Total	9775	100.00

[a] From Krolls and Hoffman (1976). Reproduced with the permission of the American Dental Association and courtesy of the U.S. Armed Forces Institute of Pathology.

sial. Although various investigations have demonstrated a high incidence of oral cancer in heavy alcohol users, the heavy alcohol consumer usually also smokes heavily and may be malnourished, thereby confounding interpretation of statistical surveys. A synergistic effect of alcohol and tobacco has been suggested for oral carcinogenesis (Rothman and Keller, 1972; Feldman *et al.*, 1975). Feldman *et al.* (1975) combined the results of their study with those of Wynder *et al.* (1957), and the increased number of cases with varied drinking and smoking habits allowed a more detailed examination of their separate and combined effects. Their results suggest that alcohol consumption alone does not greatly increase the incidence of oral cancer, but in combination with tobacco use, it significantly increases the risk. This is supported by the lack of experimental evidence that alcohol alone is carcinogenic. There is also evidence of onset of oral cancer at an earlier age in users of alcohol and tobacco (Feldman *et al.*, 1975; Fortier, 1975; Bross and Coombs, 1976).

A number of epidemiological studies have suggested that there is a strong association between cancer of the lip and sun exposure. The incidence of lip cancer is higher in rural than in urban populations and in outdoor workers such as fishermen (Keller, 1970; Clemmesen, 1974; Spitzer *et al.*, 1975). Similarly, the risk of lip cancer is greater in countries nearer the equator (Keller, 1970; Waterhouse *et al.*, 1976). The unusually low incidence of carcinoma of the lip in countries where dark-skinned races predominate lends further support to the hypothesis that, in the absence of protective pigmentation, sun exposure influences carcinogenesis (Waterhouse *et al.*, 1976). However, a widely divergent incidence of lip cancer has been demonstrated in some areas that is unexplained by exposure to sunlight or is often inversely proportional to latitude (Spitzer *et al.*, 1975; Waterhouse *et al.*, 1976; Szpak *et al.*, 1977; Lindqvist and Teppo, 1978). Other factors such as smoking (particularly pipes), alcohol consumption, and other environmental carcinogens probably act synergistically with sunlight to produce these variable results.

Poor oral hygiene and an inadequately maintained dentition have often been implicated in the pathogenesis of oral cancer. Graham *et al.* (1977) found that patients with oral cancer had significantly more inadequate dentitions than a comparable control group and suggested that this increased the risk in such patients. They also pointed out that poor oral care might be a reflection of socioeconomic status, and oral cancer has been shown to be more common in the lower socioeconomic strata. The poorly maintained dentition would also allow trauma to the oral tissues to provide an easier portal of entry for potential carcinogens or to promote carcinogenesis initiated by other factors.

Many other factors have been suggested in the etiology of oral cancer, although the evidence is often sketchy or anecdotal. Vogler *et al.* (1962) and Binnie *et al.* (1972) found a high incidence of intraoral cancer in textile workers in the United States and Britain. This was confirmed by Moss and Lee (1974), who demonstrated an increased risk in people working in the cotton and wool industries, particularly those exposed to the dust created by the carding of raw cotton and wool. Temperature and types of foods consumed have also been implicated, but there is no statistical evidence for these beliefs (Graham *et al.*, 1977; Feldman *et al.*, 1975).

III. SQUAMOUS CELL CARCINOMA

Squamous cell carcinomas comprise the vast majority of primary oral malignancies; therefore, the statistical data on oral cancer reflect primarily the epidemiology of these lesions. Although these lesions rarely arise from salivary glands or intraosseously, they are primarily a disease of the oral mucosa. The clinical appearance of the lesion is variable, and the clinical diagnosis is often complicated by its similarity to a multitude of nonneoplastic lesions commonly seen in the mouth. The diagnosis becomes simple once the lesion becomes large or affects adjacent structures, but, of course, the prognosis then becomes more grave.

Most oral carcinomas are asymptomatic, and become painful only if infected or if there is involvement of adjacent structures, possibly producing obstruction

~~or~~ pressure. Therefore, the absence of pain in a lesion that looks ominous could be more significant than acute pain in a small, innocuous-looking lesion.

The clinical appearance of oral carcinomas is somewhat varied, with a tendency for different patterns to occur more commonly in certain sites. The lip is the most common oral site throughout most of the world, followed by the tongue and the floor of the mouth (see Table I). In parts of Southeast Asia, the palate and buccal mucosa are more commonly affected than in the Western world (Waterhouse *et al.*, 1976).

A. Lip

Carcinomas on the lower lip are most common in males and in whites. Most cases present over the age of 50. Carcinomas of the lower lip tend to occur to one side of the midline, near the vermillion border. Carcinoma of the inner labial mucosa is rare in the Western world but is more common in areas where tobacco is placed at this site.

The tumor may have a varied clinical picture, but the most common presentation is ulceration (Lynch, 1967). Carcinomas presenting as crusty, inconspicuous lesions are often disregarded in this site. It is not uncommon to note white or

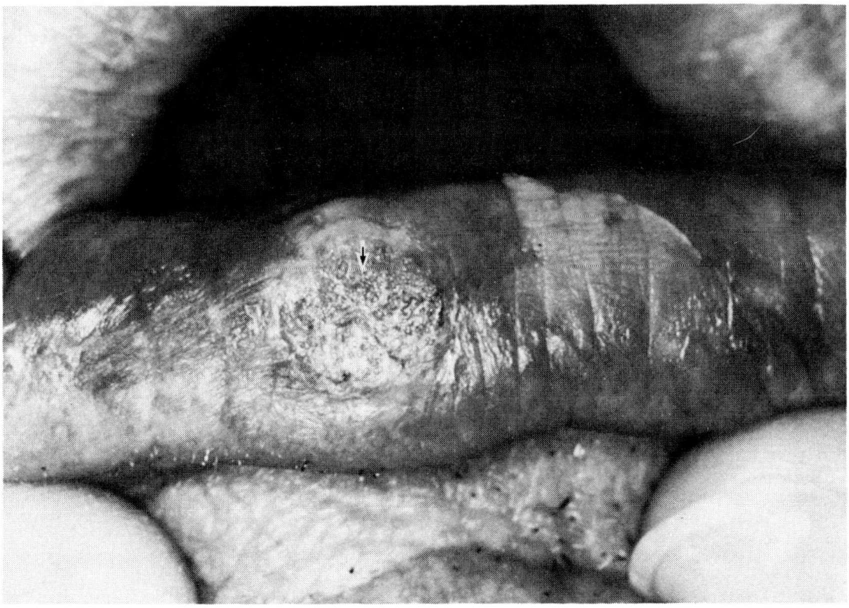

Fig. 1. Well-differentiated squamous cell carcinoma of the lower lip presenting as a crusty, flat lesion (arrow). To the right of this lesion is a triangular white area that, on biopsy, exhibited significant dysplasia.

crusty lesions on the adjacent mucosa or to elicit a history of such a preexisting lesion where the tumour has occurred (Fig. 1).

As a rule carcinomas of the lip grow slowly and metastasize late (Wurman *et al.*, 1975). Because of the apparently innocuous course of the disease, the patient often delays seeking medical attention. Out of 964 patients with lip cancers examined by Lynch (1967), 16% delayed seeking help for at least 2 years. Several investigations have found that a significant number of patients with lip cancer develop other primary malignancies of the skin, oral mucosa, or lung (Moertel *et al.*, 1961; Malmio, 1967; Newell *et al.*, 1974).

B. Tongue

Carcinomas of the tongue most often occur on the lateral borders and ventral surfaces of the anterior two-thirds (Frazell and Lucas, 1962). They rarely arise on the dorsum. When the tumor is located on the posterior aspect of the tongue, it may be painful and may decrease the mobility of the tongue if it is deeply infiltrative.

The appearance of tongue carcinomas is quite varied, ranging from large, exophytic masses to small, deeply infiltrative ulcers. Regional lymph node metastasis tends to occur much earlier than in lip carcinomas, with 35% of patients presenting with node involvement at the time of admission (Lindberg, 1972). Subdigastric nodes are most commonly affected. The diagnosis of tongue carcinomas is often confused by the common occurrence of traumatic lesions in this area.

C. Floor of the Mouth

Like cancers at other oral sites, carcinoma of the floor of the mouth shows a marked male predominance. It must be noted, however, that the ratio of men to women has markedly decreased over the last 30 years (Harrold, 1971; Easson and Palmer, 1976).

Most often these lesions initially present as white, granular lesions with areas of erythema or as innocuous-looking, painless ulcers (Fig. 2). In one study, 73 of 101 cancers of the floor of the mouth involved the orifice of the submandibular duct (Mashberg and Meyers, 1976). Deeply infiltrative lesions, particularly those near the tongue, produce a limitation of tongue movement. Lymph node metastasis tends to occur early, with one report of nodal involvement in as many as 64% of patients on admission (Correa *et al.*, 1967). Lindberg (1972) found only 30.5% of patients with nodal involvement, primarily of the submandibular nodes. Because this is rarely the site of trauma, any unexplained lesion in this site should be suspect.

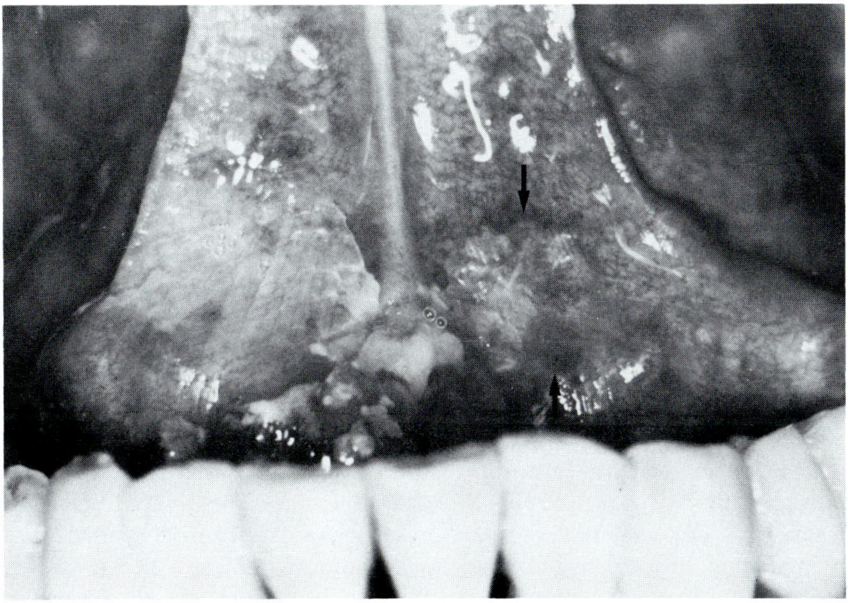

Fig. 2. An irregular, diffuse white lesion on the floor of the mouth extending onto the undersurface of the tongue. Multiple biopsies of the lesion showed a variable histological pattern ranging from mild dysplasia to carcinoma *in situ*. Small foci of erythema are noted at the periphery of the lesion (arrows).

D. Gingiva and Alveolar Ridge

The gingiva and alveolar ridge are considered together by most authors, although they represent somewhat different anatomical sites. Pindborg (1980) made a strong case for considering them separately, since their prognosis seems to vary significantly. The mandible is much more commonly affected than the maxilla, and the posterior portions of the jaws more often than the anterior areas (Cady and Catlin, 1969). This same study found that in 60% of the cases, a dentist was instrumental in detecting the lesion, although one-third of these patients underwent a dental extraction as the initial treatment. This points out a common feature of carcinomas of the gingiva: their tendency to infiltrate down the periodontium, destroying bone and causing dental mobility. These patients often present to their dentist complaining of loosening of their teeth.

E. Palate

Squamous carcinoma of the palate is rare in Western society; however, in the East and in countries where reverse smoking is practiced, it is more common.

The most common presenting symptoms are swelling and pain with ulceration. Most commonly, the lesions are exophytic, with central ulceration. The soft palate is more often affected than the hard palate, and males more frequently than females (Ratzer *et al.*, 1970; Eneroth *et al.*, 1972). The tumors tend to grow slowly and to metastasize slowly to local lymph nodes.

F. Buccal Mucosa

The buccal mucosa is not a common site for carcinoma; however, when cancer occurs in this area, its course is often insidious. Tumors of the buccal mucosa are often recognized after they have infiltrated deeply and extensively. They usually occur at or near the commissure or at the posterior of the mucosa. Generally, they occur in older patients (O'Brien and Catlin, 1965) and are often associated with habits such as tobacco chewing or snuff dipping.

The tumors near the labial commissure usually present as flat, exophytic, white lesions, often interspersed with areas of erythema. They do not ulcerate, as a rule, and have a deceptively benign appearance. The remainder of the lesions present as indurated ulcers and are usually deeply infiltrative. Verrucous carcinomas often present on the buccal mucosa but should be considered separately.

G. Other Sites

Carcinomas can occur in the more posterior portions of the mouth, including the uvula, peritonsillar tissues, and posterior oropharynx. Except for the tonsillar region, squamous carcinomas are relatively rare in these sites. Usually these tumors become symptomatic when they grow large, and the patients complain of a sore throat, a lump in the throat, or ear pain. Early tumors often escape detection because of their inflammatory appearance, commonly just foci of erythroplakia. These lesions therefore often present with extensive nodal metastasis (Lindberg, 1972).

Although it rarely involves the oral cavity directly, nasopharyngeal carcinoma (NPC) warrants mention. These cancers are somewhat unique lesions of the nasopharynx, with a high incidence among the Chinese and some native North Americans. The tumor is poorly differentiated and may be difficult to identify histologically. Its course is insidious, with extensive invasion, producing few symptoms or signs. The patient often notes symptoms only secondary to the extension of the tumor such as obstruction of the eustachian tubes. The lesion occasionally becomes obvious only after metastasis has occurred. It is one of the few tumors in which a direct link with a virus, the Epstein-Barr virus (EBV), has been demonstrated.

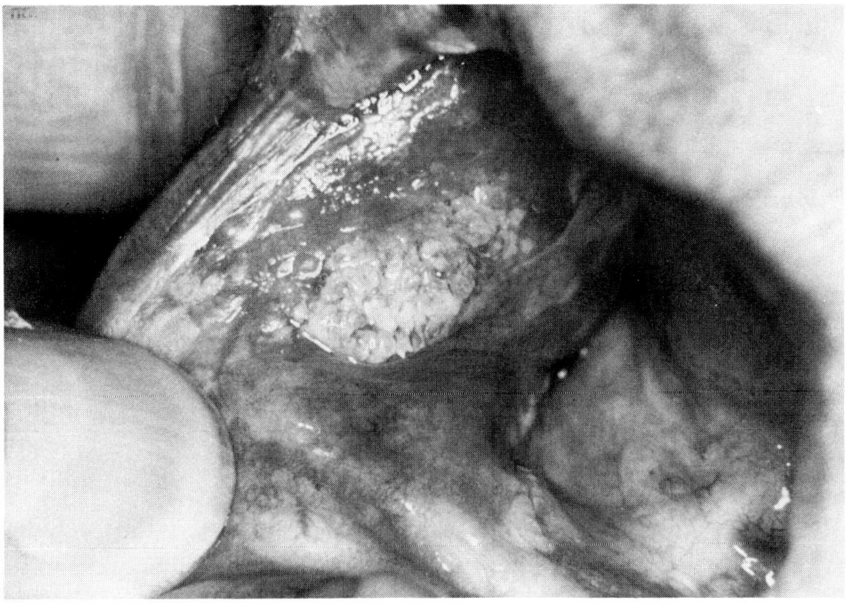

Fig. 3. Verrucous carcinoma of the buccal mucosa. Note the white, warty appearance (photograph courtesy of Dr. J. H. P. Main, University of Toronto).

IV. VERRUCOUS CARCINOMA

In 1948, Ackerman described a distinctly different carcinoma, the verrucous carcinoma, which warrants separate consideration. These lesions occur in the elderly, most often men. The most common oral sites are the buccal mucosa and the alveolar ridge or gingiva (Jacobson and Shear, 1972). Although the oral cavity is the most common site, the lesions also occur in the larynx, nose, esophagus, and external genitalia.

The lesions present as thick, white areas with either a warty or folded surface (Fig. 3). They grow very slowly, spreading superficially but widely. They are often quite large at initial presentation because of their slow, asymptomatic growth. Ultimately, invasion of local structures can occur.

The diagnosis of the oral lesions depends on their clinical as well as their histological appearance. Histologically, a verrucous carcinoma can be deceptively benign, and is often mistaken for nonneoplastic disease. Hence, the clinician must put more emphasis on the clinical presentation when considering this diagnosis in the elderly.

V. CHARACTERISTICS OF PREMALIGNANCY AND EARLY CARCINOMA

The characteristics of carcinomas specific to various oral sites have been described; however, the ideal is to detect or at least suspect neoplastic disease before the obviously recognizable tumor develops. when considering premalignant or early malignant oral mucosal lesions, three types of clinical lesions are considered:

1. The white lesion—leukoplakia
2. The red lesion—erythroplakia
3. The mixed red and white lesion—nodular or speckled leukoplakia (erythroplakia)

A. White Lesions

The term *leukoplakia* is commonly used to describe these lesions. It is best defined as an unexplained white patch or plaque on the oral mucosa that does not rub off and has historically been considered the classic premalignant oral lesion (Fig. 2).

In 1961, Shafer and Waldron examined 332 patients with clinical diagnoses suggesting this type of lesion, submitted to two oral pathology diagnostic services, probably including lesions with a speckled pattern. Of the 332 cases, 81% were histologically benign, 8.1% were invasive squamous cell carcinoma, and the remainder showed histological evidence of dysplasia or carcinoma *in situ*. A more extensive study was reported by these same authors in 1975 in which 3256 cases of oral leukoplakia were similarly examined (Waldron and Shafer, 1975). Mixed red and white lesions were definitely included in this study, but any case in which carcinoma was the primary clinical diagnosis was excluded. Of these cases, 7.6% were histologically diagnosed as squamous cell carcinoma, carcinoma *in situ,* or severe epithelial dysplasia, and 12.2% demonstrated mild to moderate dysplasia. More important, certain anatomical sites showed a greater frequency of dysplastic or carcinomatous features in clinical leukoplakia. Lesions of the floor of the mouth (42.9%), the tongue (24.2%), and the lip (24.0%) all demonstrated a higher risk than lesions at other sites.

It is generally accepted that clinical appearance is not a reliable index for predicting the significance of a leukoplakia. Certainly, the site is of assistance in determining the potential risk; however, a biopsy is necessary to determine the presence or degree of dysplasia. Although it cannot be predicted whether or not a dysplastic lesion will progress to frank malignancy, and if so at what stage, current evidence suggests a strong correlation between the severity of epithelial dysplasia and the ultimate development of a carcinoma.

B. Red Lesions

Erythoplakia generally presents as a red, velvety, well-demarcated lesion that is usually flat but may be slightly elevated. Like leukoplakia, it is asymptomatic and unexplainable by any other disease process. Although oral white lesions have been widely publicized as potential harbingers of malignancy, the red lesions have only more recently received the attention they warrant.

Mashberg *et al.*, (1973) found that 90.5% of 158 asymptomatic oral carcinomas had an erythroplastic component, and when lip lesions (which are often white or yellow) were excluded, the percentage increased to 95.8%. Shafer and Waldron (1975) examined 65 biopsy specimens from 58 cases of homogeneous oral erythroplakia. Of these, 51% were invasive carcinomas, 40% were either carcinoma *in situ* or severe epithelial dysplasia, and 9% exhibited mild to moderate dysplasia. Therefore, all samples showed some degree of dysplastic change. Thus, although an unexplained homogeneous red lesion is an uncommon oral finding, it appears that such cases are statistically likely to be either frankly malignant or premalignant.

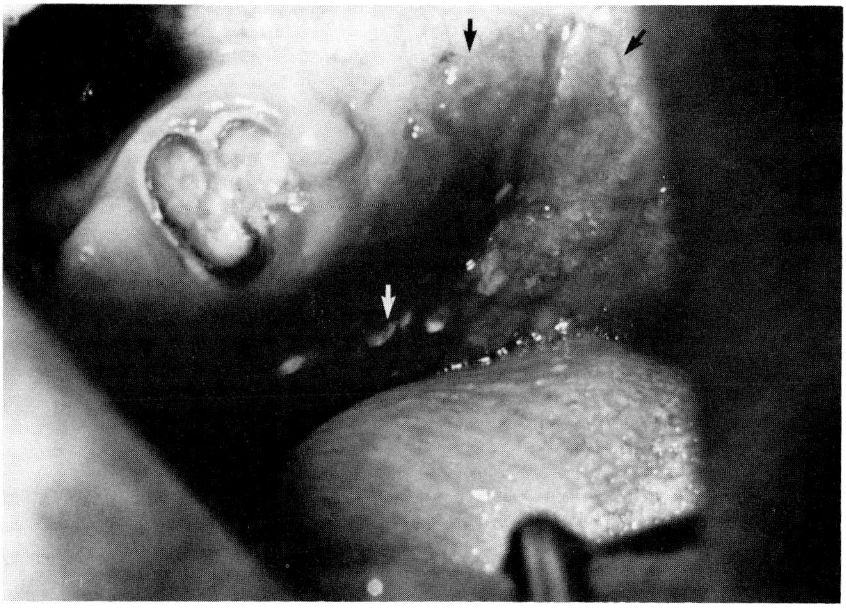

Fig. 4. An irregular red lesion on the lingual aspect of the mandible extending from the area adjacent to a carious second molar tooth into the floor of the mouth and back into the retromolar region (black arrows). Nodular white areas are speckled throughout the lesion (white arrow).

C. Mixed Red–White Lesions

Few investigators have examined these lesions separately but have included them with the erythroplakias or leukoplakias, often commenting on the probable significance of this clinical pattern (Shafer and Waldron, 1961; Waldron and Shafer, 1975; Mashberg *et al.*, 1973; Mashberg and Meyers, 1976). Pindborg *et al.* (1963) indicated that 51% of 35 lesions examined with a mixed red and white appearance showed histological evidence of dysplasia.

In reviewing the material from a previously published paper, Mashberg (1980) noted that of 207 intraoral carcinomas (excluding lip lesions), 33.3% were red, 4.9% were white, and 60% were mixed red and white. In a further examination of 169 oral lesions in high-risk sites, 64.4% of 45 red lesions, 7.5% of 53 white lesions, and 61.2% of 67 mixed red and white lesions were carcinomas. When the mixed lesions were further divided into red or white predominance, 73.3% of the red-predominant lesions were carcinomas versus 36.4% of the white-predominant ones. These results do not indicate whether the lesions that were not carcinomas showed any significant epithelial dysplasia.

In summary, any persistent, unexplained oral lesion must be investigated for possible malignancy. However, the red lesion, with or without a white component, should be considered malignant until proven otherwise (Fig. 4).

VI. MALIGNANT TUMORS OF THE SALIVARY GLAND

The oral cavity is constantly bathed by secretions of three paired major salivary glands (parotid, submandibular, and sublingual glands) and innumerable minor salivary glands. In light of the volume of glandular tissue, salivary gland tumors are relatively uncommon and most are benign. They occur primarily in adults, with a peak incidence in the sixth decade (Evans and Cruickshank, 1970). The parotid gland is most often affected.

Tumors of the major salivary glands usually present as painless lumps or swellings, making detection less of a problem than classification. A lesion in the deep portion of the parotid may not produce facial swelling, but rather oral or oropharyngeal enlargement. Pain or facial paralysis related to a parotid lesion clinically suggests the possibility of malignancy. Tumors of the sublingual glands are rare, but most are malignant. As with all salivary gland tumors, the diagnosis depends on biopsy.

Malignant tumors of the minor salivary glands usually present as exophytic lesions with or without ulceration. The palate is the most common intraoral site of salivary tumors, with the upper lip and cheek next in frequency (Fine *et al.*, 1960). Malignancy is generally more common in tumors of the minor salivary glands than in those of the major glands (Evans and Cruickshank, 1970). The experience in a multidisciplinary mouth clinic with intraoral malignant disease over 8.5 years placed oral salivary gland carcinomas in an appropriate perspective (Birt *et al.*, 1982). Out of 112 malignant tumors diagnosed in 109 patients, 6 (5.4%) were of salivary gland origin, 96 (85.8%) were squamous cell carcinomas, 4 (3.6%) were verrucous carcinomas, and the remainder were tumors originating in other tissues.

The diagnosis of malignancy in a salivary gland tumor depends on biopsy. Although certain clinical features may suggest the tumor's behavior, they can be quite misleading.

VII. MALIGNANCIES OF OTHER TISSUES

Malignant tumors of other than squamous epithelial or salivary gland origin are uncommon in the oral cavity. McCarthy and Shklar (1980) reported that for a 20-year period, their facilities had on file approximately 3000 oral carcinomas but only 27 primary mesenchymal tumors, excluding tumors of bone, and 27 metastatic tumors. Still, despite their rarity, they cannot and should not be disregarded.

Osteosarcoma, although the predominant primary malignant tumor of bone, is uncommon in the jaws. The incidence varies from approximately 4 to 6.5% of reported osteosarcomas (Dahlin, 1957; Garrington *et al.*, 1967). The jaw tumor generally affects patients slightly older than does lesion in other bones—according to the series reported by Garrington *et al.* (1967), approximately 10 years older on average. The mandible is affected more often than the maxilla. The patient most often presents with a complaint of progressive swelling, although there may also be associated pain, numbness, or loosening of teeth. The radiographic presentation is variable, depending on the amount of osteogenesis in the tumor. On dental radiographs, there is often a uniform widening of the periodontal membrane adjacent to an osteosarcoma, which, if seen, can assist in making the diagnosis.

Malignant tumors of almost all other tissues of the mouth have been reported and, as expected, are relatively rare. Those of soft tissue origin usually present as exophytic masses and those within bone as lytic lesions. Some, such as lymphomas or myelomas, when occurring in bone, can mimic dental disease.

Malignant tumors at other sites can also metastasize to the oral tissues, most often to the jaws. In a literature survey, Clausen and Poulsen (1963) found 92 cases of carcinoma metastatic to the jaws and recorded the sites of the primary tumors. They found that the breast, lung, and kidney, in order of frequency, were the major primary sites.

VIII. ORAL EXAMINATION

The examination begins when the patient enters the examining room, clinic, or dental operatory. The face, head, and neck are inspected for asymmetry, swelling, or discoloration. The shape of the mouth and the symmetry of movement during speech should be noted, since asymmetrical movement may signify a neurological deficit or a physical obstruction. The lips can then be examined, again noting symmetry and color. Specifically, any ulceration of fissure should be noted, as well as white and/or red lesions.

The intraoral examination requires very few instruments, but a good light source is mandatory. Although a hand-held light can be used, a direct light (i.e., dental light), headlight, or head mirror is preferable. Mouth mirrors or laryngeal mirrors are necessary to visualize obstructed areas. Two mouth mirrors are useful, since one can be used for retraction while the other is used for examination. Gauze facilitates grasping of the tongue.

All intraoral mucosal surfaces must be examined carefully, and a variety of examination systems have been described. It is usually easiest for each individual to develop his own system, but ensuring that the less obvious and obstructed areas are seen. The lips and cheeks must be retracted such that the vestibules are visualized. A mirror is necessary to examine the lingual and palatal gingiva and lingual surface of the mandible. The tongue should be retracted, allowing examination of the medial aspect of the posterior mandibular gingiva, posterior floor of the mouth, and medial aspect of the mandibular ramus. The tongue should be grasped and pulled forward, allowing direct examination of the posterior dorsal surface, and then drawn and twisted to either side to examine the lateral and ventral surfaces. The floor of the mouth and the ventral tongue can be directly visualized, as can the hard and soft palates. It is also useful to ask the patient to stick out the tongue and then put it into each cheek to note any limitation of movement. The lips, floor of the mouth, and cheeks can also be readily palpated. Further examination of the pharynx and larynx is possible, with practice, using a laryngeal mirror. Any abnormality should be examined and investigated.

Finally, the patient's neck should be palpated. Both the submandibular and parotid glands can also be felt extraorally, and the submandibular glands can be bimanually palpated with one finger in the mouth and the other below and medial to the posterior mandible.

IX. DIAGNOSTIC PROCEDURES

A. Biopsy

The removal and subsequent microscopic examination of an adequate sample of any suspicious oral lesion is the only way to make or eliminate the diagnosis of malignancy. A biopsy of most oral surface lesions can be adequately performed by any physician with appropriate facilities and familiarity with the technique. A dentist is certainly capable of obtaining an adequate specimen because of familiarity with the oral anatomy and the availability of appropriate instruments in the office. Lesions in inaccessible areas, vascular lesions, or those in deeper structures or tissues may require a medical or dental specialist and/or a hospital environment.

Depending on the size and site of the lesion, a biopsy may be incisional or excisional. Occasionally, mention is made of the potential hazard of spreading a tumor locally or even causing metastatic dissemination by incisional biopsy. Certainly, local spread along an incision is a possibility and has been reported in other sites with deep tumors; however, if the biopsy confirms malignancy, the treatment would involve the entire region, making this possible sequela insignificant. There has been no evidence that incisional biopsy will lead to metastatic spread of an oral cancer. The diagnosis must be made, and a biopsy is therefore necessary to avoid undue delay in treatment.

Obtaining a biopsy of the oral mucosa is a relatively simple task. Most often a scalpel is used, but a biopsy punch, if properly handled, is quite adequate. In most cases, local anesthesia via infiltration is adequate, and the wound can be closed with sutures. Scarring is rarly a concern in the oral mucosa. The sample must be adequate. Hence, in large lesions, multiple biopsy specimens may be required to get a representative sample (Fig. 2). The most common complaints made by surgical pathologists examining oral biopsy specimens concern their inadequate depth or their distortion by mishandling. Areas of obvious necrosis should be avoided, and the sample should be placed into the fixative, usually 10% neutral buffered formalin, as quickly as possible.

B. Exfoliative Cytology

The introduction and extensive use of cytology in medicine, and particularly the demonstrated value of exfoliative cytology in detecting neoplasia of the uterine cervix, stimulated an interest in applying these techniques in the oral cavity. The use of oral exfoliative cytology as a diagnostic tool for malignancy has been controversial, whereas its use for the diagnosis of viral and fungal disease is well accepted.

Exfoliative cytology samples and examines exfoliated, or scraped-off, superficial cells of the oral mucosa. Cells from a malignant lesion exhibit alterations that can be recognized and associated with a neoplastic process. It is therefore apparent that this technique will not aid in the diagnosis of subepithelial lesions unless the surface is ulcerated. The success of the technique depends upon three factors: the sample must be adequate and representative of the lesion; the pathologist must be experienced in examining this type of specimen; and the tumor cells must be morphologically altered to such an extent that the changes are apparent. All three of these requirements can potentially present problems in arriving at the correct interpretation. Many oral carcinomas are very well differentiated (e.g., lip carcinoma), and individual cell morphology may not show the severity of alteration that the tissue itself would demonstrate. This problem is amplified if the pathologist has not had enough experience with oral cytology to assign appropriate significance to minor changes. The acquisition of an adequate sample also often depends on the loss of intercellular cohesiveness in a carcinoma, which is less characteristic of a well-differentiated tumor. Therefore, a report on an exfoliative cytology specimen is not a diagnosis, and a negative cytology report does not preclude malignant disease.

Unlike cytology of the uterine cervix and other sites, oral cytology is primarily used when a lesion has been noted on examination. A mouth rinse technique applicable to mass screening has been investigated but has not been widely accepted as valid (Helsper *et al.*, 1963, 1966; Folsom *et al.*, 1972). This technique is burdened not only with the complications of the smear technique but with its own sampling errors as well. If the clinical presentation of a lesion suggests malignancy, a biopsy should be performed in most cases. Exfoliative cytology may be useful where a surgical procedure is medically contraindicated, if a patient refuses biopsy, for follow-up examinations, or as additional insurance for lesions in which there is no suspicion of malignancy.

The reliability of oral exfoliative cytology is variable and questionable. In two reports of a 5-year prospective study in which oral lesions were examined by both biopsy and cytologic techniques, the false-negative rate for oral cytology was 14.6% and 13.9% (Shklar *et al.*, 1968, 1970). In another extensive study of oral exfoliative cytology, a false-negative rate of 31% was recorded (Folsom *et al.*, 1972). False positives also occur but are considerably less significant. The reliability rate also varies according to the oral site of the lesion. In the study by Folsom *et al.* (1972), the reliability rate (i.e., the percentage of correct diagnoses) for the lip was 38%, the oral pharynx 56%, the buccal mucosa 60%, the tongue 71%, the palate 73%, and the floor of the mouth 89%. In this same study, it should also be noted that cytologic examination revealed three carcinomas that would not otherwise have been biopsied.

The advantages of the cytology technique are its simplicity and its lack of complications. The mouth rinse method is not widely used because it is so unreliable. The other technique requires only obtaining a sample of cells by scraping the surface of the lesion and spreading the product on a glass slide. After fixation, the slide is submitted to a pathologist for staining and examination. Staats and Goldsby (1963) demonstrated that the use of a dental spatula for obtaining the sample yielded a better specimen than a wooden tongue blade. Because of the possibility of false negatives, certain guidelines are necessary for the use of oral exfoliative cytology. An obviously malignant or suspicious lesion should be biopsied, because cytologic sampling will, at best, only delay treatment and, at worst, yield a false-negative result. Lip lesions or thick white lesions are best biopsied for diagnosis. In addition, a negative report on a cytology specimen should not imply the absence of malignant disease. Continued observation and repetition of the test are necessary to rule out malignancy or premalignancy. Still, when used as an adjunct to careful oral examination and when these guidelines are followed, this technique can be useful for mass screening programs where the population size may make biopsy of all oral lesions too monumental a task.

C. Toluidine Blue Staining

The aim of this technique is similar to that of exfoliative cytology: to develop a means of identifying malignant or premalignant lesions without subjecting the patient to unnecessary surgery and with a minimal armamentarium. The concept of a topical marker has obvious appeal, since the results are immediately apparent. Toluidine blue has been shown to stain oral carcinomas and not normal oral mucosa (Myers, 1970; Sabes *et al.*, 1971). Inflammatory lesions have also been shown to give a positive reaction with the dye (Iwano *et al.*, 1965). As with exfoliative cytology, false positives do not present a significant problem; however, false negatives decrease the value of the procedure significantly.

Sabes *et al.* (1971) tested this technique on carcinogen-treated hamster cheek pouch mucosa. They found a 21.4% incidence of false negatives in younger lesions, which increased to 39.6% in older lesions. It could be argued that in this experimental situation the tumors are very well differentiated and slow-growing, explaining the high incidence of false-negative results; however, many human oral carcinomas and most premalignant oral lesions would present the same problem.

This test has therefore not been shown to be of significant value in screening for oral cancer, and it has not been widely used. The procedure can certainly be valuable in helping to determine surgical resection margins or for follow-up after radiation therapy, along with careful clinical examination.

X. SUMMARY AND CONCLUSIONS

Unlike cancer of the visceral organs, oral cancer can usually be identified or suspected after careful clinical examination while it is still at a relatively treatable stage. Often, early malignant changes can be suspected by clinically detectable alterations but are missed because the patient's mucosa is not examined. The death rate from oral cancer would be significantly lower if all physicians and dentists included a systematic examination of the oral cavity and mucosa in their procedures. The majority of patients with undetected oral cancer or premalignant lesions would probably not voluntarily enter screening programs; hence, the opportunity to carry out an oral examination must be seized whenever they enter the health care system.

For mass population screening, clinical examination of the oral cavity would be the procedure of choice. This can be done efficiently and quickly by trained personnel. Once an abnormality is identified, a biopsy should be performed.

Exfoliative cytology can be used if a biopsy is medically contraindicated, or physically impossible, or if the biopsy site needs clarification. Such mass screenings have been performed effectively in the past.

A screening program for oral cancer should concentrate on those segments of the population at greatest risk. Pindborg (1984) summarized the reported results of screening programs for oral cancer and demonstrated the poor yield from unselected population groups. Such a program would therefore be most effective if it were made available to the lower socioeconomic strata, particularly encouraging participation by abusers of alcohol, users of tobacco in any form, and those who spend a great deal of time outdoors exposed to excessive sunlight. Since oral cancer is relatively uncommon below age 40, this would be an efficient lower age limit for mass screening programs.

The primary difficulty in the early diagnosis of malignancy is to identify premalignancy histologically. At present, this depends on a subjective evaluation by a pathologist, and there is considerable difference in the significance various pathologists put on specific histological characteristics. The ideal time to identify such a lesion is before a frankly invasive tumor is present. Therefore, considerable research is warranted in order to identify various immunological or biochemical markers for early malignant transformation.

Epidemiological studies have delineated a number of factors that seem to predispose people to oral cancer. Some of the data have also demonstrated regional differences that remain unexplained. Further research is necessary in these regions of high oral cancer incidence to examine the influence of specific factors that might have eluded the broader studies. The unusually high incidence of lip carcinoma in Newfoundland, Canada, is an example of a situation worthy of careful analysis. An intensive investigation of such variables as the incidence in various occupational groups, prevalence of tobacco use and alcohol consumption, length of time spent outdoors, and diet could provide valuable data further defining the groups at risk. This seems a natural advancement on the broader statistical studies.

A number of high-risk groups for the development of oral cancer have already been defined. These groups can be screened by medical, dental, or trained auxiliary personnel with little more equipment than a light, mirrors, and gauze. The oral cavity can be readily examined clinically and premalignant or early malignant lesions detected. Therefore, the techniques already exist for mass screening of this accessible site.

REFERENCES

Ackerman, L. V. (1948). Verrucous carcinoma of the oral cavity. *Surgery* (*St. Louis*) **23,** 670–678.

Axéll, T., Mörnstad, H., and Sundstrom, B. (1976). The relationship of the clinical picture to the histopathology of snuff dippers lesions in a Swedish population. *J. Oral Pathol.* **5,** 229–236.

Binnie, W. H., Cawson, R. A., Hill, G. B., and Soaper, A. E. (1972). Oral cancer in England and Wales: A national study of morbidity, mortality, curability and related factors. "Office of Population Census and Surveys: Studies on Medical and Population Subjects," No. 23. H. M. Stationery Office, London.

Birt, D., From, L., and Main, J. H. P. (1982). Profile of malignant disease in the mouth clinic. *J. Otolaryngol.* **11,** 365–370.

Blot, W. J., and Fraumeni, J. F. (1977). Geographic patterns of oral cancer in the United States: Etiologic implications. *J. Chronic Dis.* **30,** 745–757.

Bross, I. D. J., and Coombs, J. (1976). Early onset of oral cancer among women who drink and smoke. *Oncology* **33,** 136–139.

Cady, B., and Catlin, D. (1969). Epidermoid carcinoma of the gum. A 20 year survey. *Cancer* **23,** 551–569.

Clausen, F., and Poulsen, H. (1963). Metastatic carcinoma of the jaws. *Acta Pathol. Microbiol. Scand.* **57,** 361–374.

Clemmesen, J. (1974). Statistical studies in the aetiology of malignant neoplasms: IV. Denmark 1943–67. *Acta Pathol. Microbiol. Scand., Suppl.* 247.

Correa, J. W., Bosch, A., and Marcial, V. A. (1967). Carcinoma of the floor of the mouth. *Am. J. Roentgenol., Radium Ther. Nucl. Med.* **99,** 302–312.

Dahlin, D. C. (1957). "Bone Tumors: General Aspects and an Analysis of Cases." Thomas, Springfield, Illinois.

Easson, E. C., and Palmer, M. K. (1976). Prognostic factors in oral cancer. *Clin. Oncol.* **2,** 191–202.

Eneroth, C. M., Hjertman, L., and Moberger, G. (1972). Squamous cell carcinoma of the palate. *Acta Oto-Laryngol.* **73,** 418–427.

Evans, R. W., and Cruickshank, A. H. (1970). Epithelial tumors of the salivary glands. *In* "Major Problems in Pathology" (J. S. Bennington, ed.), Vol. 1, pp. 11–26. Saunders, Philadelphia, Pennsylvania.

Feldman, J. G., Hagen, M., Nagarajan, M., and Kissin, B. (1975). A case control investigation of alcohol, tobacco and diet in head and neck cancer. *Prev. Med.* **4,** 444–463.

Fine, G., Marshall, R. B., and Horn, R. C. (1960). Tumors of the minor salivary glands. *Cancer* **13,** 653–669.

Folsom, T. G., White, C. P., Bromer, L., Canby, H. F., and Garrington, G. E. (1972). Oral exfoliative study. Review of the literature and report of a three year study. *Oral Surg., Oral Med. Oral Pathol.* **33,** 61–74.

Fortier, R. A. (1975). Etude sur les facteurs étiologiques des cancers buccaux-pharyngés dans la province de Québec. *J. Can. Dent. Assoc.* **41,** 235–241.

Frazell, E. L., and Lucas, J. C. (1962). Cancer of the tongue. Report of the management of 1554 patients. *Cancer* **15,** 1085–1099.

Garrington, G. E., Scofield, H. H., Cornyn, J., and Hooker, S. P. (1967). Osteosarcoma of the jaws. Analysis of 56 cases. *Cancer* **20,** 377–391.

Graham, S., Dayal, H., Rohrer, T., Swanson, M., Sultz, H., Shedd, D., and Fischman, S. (1977). Dentition, diet, tobacco and alcohol in the epidemiology of oral cancer. *J. Natl. Cancer Inst. (U.S.)* **59,** 1611–1618.

Harrold, C. C. (1971). Management of cancer of the floor of the mouth. *Am. J. Surg.* **22,** 487–493.

Helsper, J. T., Sharp, G. S., and Bullock, W. K. (1963). The mouthwash technic. A method of screening for intra-oral carcinoma. *Am. J. Surg.* **106,** 802–806.

Helsper, J. T., Sharp, G. S., and Bullock, W. K. (1966). Experiences with the tissue culture solution mouthwash method for the early detection of oral cancer. *Acta Cytol.* **10,** 179–181.

Iwano, T., Yanagizawa, T., and Iwayanagi, T. (1965). An in vivo staining test using toluidine blue for oral cytodiagnosis. *Shika Gakuho* **65,** 66–67.

Jacobson, S., and Shear, M. (1972). Verrucous carcinoma of the mouth. *J. Oral Pathol.* **1,** 66–75.

Keller, A. Z. (1970). Cellular types, survival, race, nativity, occupation, habits and associated diseases in the pathogenesis of lip cancer. *Am. J. Epidemiol.* **91,** 486–499.

Krolls, S. O., and Hoffman, S. (1976). Squamous cell carcinoma of the oral soft tissues: A statistical analysis of 14,253 cases by age, sex and race. *J. Am. Dent. Assoc.* **92,** 571–574.

Lindberg, R. (1972). Distribution of cervical lymph node metastases from squamous cell carcinoma of the upper respiratory and digestive tracts. *Cancer* **29,** 1446–1449.

Lindqvist, C., and Teppo, L. (1978). Epidemiological evaluation of sunlight as a risk factor of lip cancer. *Br. J. Cancer* **37,** 983–989.

Lynch, G. A. (1967). Cancer of the lip. *Ulster Med. J.* **36,** 44–50.

McCarthy, P. L., and Shklar, G. (1980). "Diseases of the Oral Mucosa," 2nd ed. Lea & Febiger, Philadelphia, Pennsylvania.

Malmio, K. (1967). Occurrence of primary multiple cancer in patients with cancer of the lip. *Ann. Chir. Gynaecol. Fenn.* **56,** 332–337.

Mashberg, A. (1980). Clinical features of oral malignancy in relation to prognosis. *In* "Oral Premalignancy. Proceedings of the First Dows Symposium" (I. C. MacKenzie, E. Dabelsteen, and C. A. Squier, Eds.), pp. 292–303. Univ. of Iowa Press, Iowa City, Iowa.

Mashberg, A., and Meyers, H. (1976). Anatomic site and size of 222 early asymptomatic oral squamous cell carcinomas. A continuing prospective study of oral cancer. *Cancer* **37,** 2149–2157.

Mashberg, A., Morrissey, J. B., and Garfinkel, L. (1973). A study of the appearance of early asymptomatic oral squamous carcinoma. *Cancer* **32,** 1436–1445.

Moertel, C. G., Dockerty, M. B., and Baggenstoss, A. H. (1961). Multiple primary malignant neoplasms: III. Tumors of multicentric origin. *Cancer* **14,** 238–248.

Moss, E., and Lee, W. R. (1974). Occurrence of oral and pharyngeal cancers in textile workers. *Br. J. Int. Med.* **31,** 224–232.

Myers, E. N. (1970). The toluidine blue test in lesions of the oral cavity. *Ca—Cancer J. Clin.* **20,** 135–139.

Newell, G. R., Krementz, E. T., and Roberts, J. O. (1974). Multiple primary neoplasms in blacks compared to whites: II. Further cancers in patients with cancer of the buccal cavity and pharynx. *JNCI, J. Natl. Cancer Inst.* **52,** 639–642.

O'Brien, P. H., and Catlin, P. (1965). Cancer of the cheek (mucosa). *Cancer* **18,** 1392.

Pindborg, J. J. (1980). "Oral Cancer and Precancer." Wright, Bristol.

Pindborg, J. J. (1984). "Screening for Oral Cancer with Special Reference to Problems in Developing Countries," UICC Tech. Rep. Ser. Vol. 78, pp. 174–183. Int. Union Against Cancer, Geneva.

Pindborg, J. J., Renstrup, G., Poulsen, H. E., and Silverman, S. (1963). Studies in oral leukoplakias. V. Clinical and histological signs of malignancy. *Acta Odontol. Scand.* **21,** 407–414.

Ratzer, E. R., Schweitzer, R. J., and Frazell, E. L. (1970). Epidermoid carcinoma of the palate. *Am. J. Surg.* **119,** 294–297.

Roed-Petersen, B., and Pindborg, J. J. (1973). A study of Danish snuff-induced oral leukoplakias. *J. Oral Pathol.* **2,** 301–313.

Rothman, K., and Keller, A. (1972). The effect of joint exposure to alcohol and tobacco on cancer of the mouth and pharynx. *J. Chronic Dis.* **25,** 711–716.

Sabes, W. R., Singer, R. E., and Kuhn, T. (1971). Effectiveness of toluidine blue as an aid to biopsy in the diagnosis of D.M.B.A. induced hamster pouch dysplasia and carcinoma. *Cancer* **29,** 1584–1589.

Shafer, W. G., and Waldron, C. A. (1961). A clinical and histopathological study of oral leukoplakia. *Surg., Gynecol. Obstet.* **112,** 411–420.

Shafer, W. G., and Waldron, C. A. (1975). Erythroplakia of the oral cavity. *Cancer* **36,** 1021–1028.

Shklar, G., Meyer, I., Cataldo, E., and Taylor, R. (1968). Correlated study of oral cytology and histopathology. Report on 2,052 oral lesions. *Oral Surg., Oral Med. Oral Pathol.* **25,** 61–70.

Shklar, G., Cataldo, E., and Meyers, I. (1970). Reliability of cytologic smear in diagnosis of oral cancer. *Arch. Otolaryngol.* **91,** 158–160.

Silverberg, E. (1982). Cancer statistics, 1982. *Ca—Cancer J. Clin.* **32,** 15–31.

Silverberg, E. (1983). Cancer statistics, 1983. *Ca—Cancer J. Clin.* **33,** 9–25.

Silverberg, E. (1984). Cancer statistics, 1984. *Ca—Cancer J. Clin.* **34,** 7–23.

Silverberg, E., and Holleb, A. I. (1972). Cancer statistics, 1972. *Ca—Cancer J. Clin.* **22,** 2–20.

Silverberg, E., and Holleb, A. I. (1974). Cancer statistics 1974 - worldwide epidemiology. *Ca—Cancer J. Clin.* **24,** 2–21.

Spitzer, W. O., Hill, G. B., Chamber, L. W., Helliwell, B. E., and Murphy, H. B. (1975). The occupation of fishing as a risk factor in cancer of the lip. *N. Engl. J. Med.* **293,** 419–424.

Staats, O. J., and Goldsby, J. W. (1963). Graphic comparison of intraoral exfoliative cytology technics. *Acta Cytol.* **7,** 107–110.

Szpak, C. A., Stone, M. J., and Frenkel, E. P. (1977). Some observations concerning the demographic and geographic incidence of carcinoma of the lip and buccal cavity. *Cancer* **40,** 343–348.

Vogler, W. R., Bross, I. J., and Milmore, B. K. (1962). A retrospective study of etiological factors in cancer of the mouth, pharynx and larynx. *Cancer* **15,** 246–258.

Waldron, C. A., and Shafer, W. G. (1975). Leukoplakia revisited. A clinicopathologic study 3256 oral leukoplakias. *Cancer* **36,** 1386–1392.

Waterhouse, J., Muir, C., Correa, P., and Powell, J. (1976). "Cancer Incidence in Five Continents," Vol. 3. Int. Agency Res. Cancer, Lyon.

Winn, D. M., Blot, W. J., Shy, C. M., Pickle, L. W., Toledo, A., and Fraumeni, J. F. (1981). Snuff dipping and oral cancer among women in the southern United States. *N. Engl. J. Med.* **304,** 745–749.

Wurman, L. H., Adams, G. L., and Meyerhoff, W. L. (1975). Carcinoma of the lip. *Am. J. Surg.* **130,** 470–474.

Wynder, E. L., and Stellman, S. D. (1977). Comparative epidemiology of tobacco-related cancers. *Cancer Res.* **37,** 4608–4622.

Wynder, E. L., Bross, I. J., and Feldman, R. M. (1957). A study of the etiological factors in cancer of thc mouth. *Cancer* **10,** 1300–1323.

Index

A

Acetaminophen, carcinogenicity, 400, 401
N-Acetyltransferase, carcinogenicity, 406
Adenocarcinoma
  of bladder, 130
  colorectal, 351
  Crohn's disease and, 350
  pulmonary, 115, 184, 379
Adenoma, colorectal, 33
  barium enema detection, 261
  blood loss from, 241
  as cancer precursor, 348
  familial polyposis coli and, 252–253
  fecal occult blood test detection, 355, 359
  resected, 254
Adenomatosis, 350, 351
Adenosis, 149
Alcohol use, oral cancer and, 424–425, 426
Alkaline phosphatase test, 36, 137
Alveolar ridge cancer, 429, 431
American Cancer Society
  colorectal cancer screening guidelines, 360–361
  Pap smear guidelines, 55
  physician-based screening recommendations, 5
American Joint Committee for Cancer staging, 387–389
Aniline dyes, carcinogenicity, 398–399
Aromatic amines, as bladder carcinogens, 398–399, 401, 402, 406, 411, 413–414
Asbestos exposure, 31
Attributable benefit, 20
Atypia, squamous
  marked, 112, 113
  moderate, 112, 113, 117–118
  slight, 112
Auramine, carcinogenicity, 403
Azo dyes, carcinogenicity, 403

B

Backdating, 384
Barium enema, *see* Radiography, double contrast
Benzidine exposure, 399, 401
Bias, in survival evaluation, 16–18
Bilharzia, bladder cancer and, 400, 401
Biological error, 299
Biopsy, of oral mucosa, 437
Bladder cancer, 397–406
  classification, 129–131
  epidemiology, 398–403
  incidence, 121, 398
  industrial-related
    early screening programs, 407–409
    prognosis, 406
  mortality rate, 35, 121
  nonpapillary carcinoma *in situ,* 130, 134
  papillary, 127–128, 130, 131, 132
  population at risk, 35, 133–134, 398–403
  prognosis, 121, 406
  recurrent, 411
  risk factors, 398–403
    industrial, 399–402, 401, 402–403, 405–406, 410–411
    nonindustrial, 399–402, 403
    tobacco smoking, 399, 400, 401, 402, 405
  sex ratio, 398
  survival determinants, 403–406
  transitional cell, 128–129, 130, 131, 132
Bladder cancer screening, 121–140
  biochemical methods, 411
  cancer control phases, 28

Bladder cancer screening (*cont.*)
enzyme tests, 137
flow cytometry, 135–136
high-risk groups, 402–403, 415, 416
history, 406–409
of industrial populations, 402–403, 407–409, 410–414
mortality reduction and, 35
national policy, 27
routine cystoscopy, 407–408
tumor markers, 136–137
urinary cytology, 121–134, 409–411
classification system, 129–131
cytologic examination, 123–129
diagnostic accuracy, 131–133
evaluation, 412–415
methodology, 122–123
screening programs, 133–134
stage at presentation, 412–413
survival effects, 412–413
terminology, 131
value of, 415–416
urinary occult blood, 134–135, 408–409
Bone cancer, oral, 435
Breast(s)
aging effects, 222
benign changes, 149—152
cysts, 150, 151, 152
echography of, 224, 225, 226
cytosarcoma phylloides, 225, 226
endocrine-related changes, 149
fibroadenoma, 150, 151, 224, 226
fibrocystic, 149, 151, 273
lipoma, 150, 151, 152
palpation, 141, 143, 144, 149, *see also* Breast physical examination; Breast self-examination
papilloma, 150, 151
structure types, 149, 150
Breast cancer
calcification in, 152–153, 155–157, 160
clinical examination, 141, 142, 143, 157, *see also* Breast physical examination
conservative therapy, 331–332
colorectal cancer and, 353
incidence, 10, 325, 327–328
mortality, 327
premature, 10, 11
nonpalpable stage, 141
overdiagnosis, 331, 332
palpable, 143
postmenopausal, 330
primary signs, 152–154
radiation-related, 148, 331, *see also* Mammography, radiation hazard
secondary signs, 154–155
survival rates, 30
Breast Cancer Detection Demonstration Projects, 158, 330–332
Breast cancer screening, 30–31, 325–345, *see also* Mammography
acceptibility, 13
age factors, 329–330
Canadian National Breast Screening Study, 334–336
computed tomography in, 147
cost–benefits, 339, 341–342
costs, 14, 339–340
diaphanoscopy in, 158, 337
evaluation problems, 326–328
future applications, 338–342
Kaiser-Permanente Study, 332–333
lead time, 328, 329
length bias, 17
mortality rate effects, 328–329
in Netherlands, 333
physician's role, 339, 340–341
population at risk, 15, 41–42
quality control, 9
randomized trials, 30–31
selection bias, 17
self-selection, 326
in Sweden, 334
thermography in, 15, 37, 158, 337
UICC Workshop recommendations, 332
ultrasonography in, 158, 215–236, 337
advantages, 215
collagen fiber content effects, 230, 231, 232
diagnostic accuracy, 228, 229
diagnostic criteria, 223–225
equipment, 218–219
expanded, 228–229
history, 216–218
of malignant disease, 226–230
of medullary carcinoma, 227–228, 230, 231
of normal breast, 220–222
programs, 231–234
of scirrhous carcinoma, 226–227, 229–230, 231
screening program methods, 232–234

screening program results, 234
ultrasonic tissue characterization, 229–230
water-bag approach, 218–220
in United Kingdom, 333
Breast cancer screening centers, 157–158
Breast physical examination, 271–284
efficacy, 284
evaluation, 327
mortality reduction and, 329
nipple discharge and, 283–284
oblique position, 282–284
palpation techniques, 273–274, 276–279
physician ineptitude in, 271, 339, 341
supine position, 279–282
upright position, 272, 274–279
inspection, 274–276
palpation, 276–279
Breast self-examination, 30, 31, 284–286
evaluation, 327
frequency, 285
by sex partner, 340
technique, 286–290
British Columbia Cohort Study, 298–301
Bronchogenic carcinoma, 182, 183, 379, *see also* Lung cancer
Bronchoscope, flexible fiberoptic, 379–380
Buccal mucosa cancer
clinical features, 430
diagnosis, 439
incidence, 422, 423, 424
verrucous, 431

C

Calcification, of breast, 152–153, 155–157, 160
Canadian National Breast Screening Study, 334–336
Cancer, *see also* specific cancers
natural history, 11–12
premature mortality, 10, 11
smoking and, 27
Cancer control, 25–48
definition, 26
morbidity reduction and, 26
research, 27–29
screening programs and, 29–44
Cancer registries, 304
Carcinoembryonic antigen test (CEA), 13
for bladder cancer, 136–137
for colorectal cancer, 353, 359
Carcinoma *in situ*
cervical
diagnostic criteria, 94–95
duration, 297
dysplasia as precursor, 301–302
incidence increase, 96–98
microinvasive, 95
progression, 296–301
recurrence, 96
regression, 296, 297, 300
treatment, 98
variants, 96
transitional cell, 128–129
Cardiovascular studies, 74
Case-control studies, 19–20
Case finding
in lung cancer, 392
screening versus, 4
Cervical cancer
carcinoma *in situ*
diagnostic criteria, 94–95, 96
duration, 297
dysplasia as precursor, 301–302
incidence increase, 96–98
microinvasive, 95
progression, 296–301
recurrence, 96
regression, 296, 297, 300
treatment, 98
variants, 96
detectable preclinical phase, 7
high-risk population, 29
incidence, 10, 34, 96–98
invasive, 296–301
mortality rate, 34
oral contraceptives and, 313
precursor lesion site, 88
premature mortality, 10, 11
regression, 12, 96
Cervical cancer screening, 295–323, *see also* Papanicolaou smear screening
acceptibility, 13
behavioral barriers to, 319
cancer control phases, 28
cancer natural history and, 296–302
British Columbia Cohort Study, 298–301
dysplasia as precursor, 301–302
early studies, 296–298
colposcopy in, 34–35, 96, 97–98, 305
efficacy, 3–4
optical screening schedules, 313–319

Cervical cancer screening (*cont.*)
outcome evaluation, 303–312
case-control study, 311–312
incidence effects, 303–306
mortality reduction effects, 303, 304, 306–311
patient compliance, 318–319
population at risk, 15, 29, 42–43, 312–313
quality control, 34
selection bias, 17
selective screening, 42–43
self-collection devices in, 35
uterine cancer mortality and, 306–307, 308, 310
Cervical cytology, *see* Papanicolaou smear
Cervical intraepithelial neoplasia, 94–96
Cervical spatula, 88–89
Chest radiology, 32, 163–191
cancer cell types and, 179, 180
cancer growth rates and, 187
clinical severity and, 181
detected cancer incidence, 32, 175, 176
digital, 172–173
false negatives, 176, 177
frequency of performance, 163, 383
full-size, 379
indications for, 380
lateral view, 169, 182–183
missed cancers, 183, 184–185, 187
mortality effects of, 380
observer error, 186
posteroanterior view, 168–172, 183, 184, 186, 187
quality control, 173–174, 183
radiation dosage, 382
randomized controlled trials, 381–390
screening applications, 174–182
sensitivity, 176, 177, 183, 186, 188, 383
specificity, 176, 177, 188, 383
sputum cytology and, 114, 379, 382, 386
stage distribution, 176, 178, 179
techniques, 164–173, 182
antiscatter measures, 166–167
beam energy, 165–166
film–screen combinations, 167–168
filtration, 166
focal spot size, 166
number of views, 168–172
optimization, 163–164
prior methods, 164
Chromium radioassay, 241–242
Chrysoidine, carcinogenicity, 403
Coffee, carcinogenicity, 402, 405
Cohort effect, 298, 299
Colectomy, subtotal, 255
Colon cancer, *see* Colorectal cancer
Colonoscopy
bowel preparation, 259–260
complications, 258, 260–261
contraindications, 259
double contrast barium enema and, 263–264
efficacy, 355
equipment, 259
indications, 258
screening frequency, 252
as screening tool, 354, 360
sedation for, 260
sensitivity, 263–264, 358, 360
specificity, 263–264
Colo-Rect test, 244
Colorectal cancer
adenoma precursors, 254, 348
blood loss from, 241
breast cancer and, 353
cancer control phases, 28
cell proliferation abnormalities, 359
incidence, 10, 347
inherited nonpolyposis, 252
leukocyte abnormalities, 359–360
ovary cancer and, 353
premature mortality and, 10, 11
probability of developing, 347–348
prognosis, 348
resected, 254
resected adenoma and, 254
risk factors, 252–255, 348–353
age, 348–349
familial/hereditary, 252–254, 350–353
geographic, 347
inflammatory bowel disease, 254–255, 349–350
radiation, 353
sex, 349
sites, 348–349
skin chromosomal studies, 360
skin fibroblast studies, 360
survival rate, 33
uterine cancer and, 353
Colorectal cancer screening, 249–269, 347–366
acceptibility, 13
of average-risk populations, 250–251, 360–361

carcinoembryonic antigen test (CEA), 353, 359
case findings, 360–362
chromium radioassay, 241–242
colonoscopy
bowel preparation, 259–260
complications, 260–261
equipment, 259
sedation, 260
sensitivity, 358
specificity, 263–264
cost–benefits, 54
criteria, 33–34
diagnostic tests, 360
double contrast barium enema, 261–262
fecal occult blood tests, 33, 34, 237–247, 353, 355–359
available tests, 244–246
for average-risk populations, 361
characteristics, 238–239
controlled trials, 356–359
dietary factors, 240–241, 242
error sources, 238–239
false negatives, 33
false positives, 33, 240, 242
guidelines, 361, 362
for high-risk populations, 362
immunochemical tests, 244–245
methodology, 245, 355
positivity, 356–358
proctosigmoidoscopy and, 357, 359
quality control, 242–243
reactants, 237
rehydration, 242
sensitivity, 238, 239, 241–242, 358, 359
storage, 242
uncontrolled trials, 355–356
guidelines, 360–363
life prolongation and, 50
logistics, 264–265
mortality reduction and, 33
patient compliance, 356, 363
physician education for, 363
population at risk, 252–255, 348–353, 362
proctosigmoidoscopy, 353, 354
for average-risk populations, 361
complications, 258–259
controlled trials, 357, 359
equipment, 256–257
fecal occult blood test and, 357, 359
guidelines, 361, 362
for high-risk populations, 362
procedure, 257
proctosigmoidoscopy, flexible, 251, 257–258, 354
for average-risk populations, 361
of colorectal adenomas, 252–253
complications, 258–259
efficacy, 251
guidelines, 361
prevalence of use, 251
procedure, 257–258
sensitivity, 262
training for, 265
sensitivity, 262, 263–264
serological tests, 250
specificity, 263–264
technical aspects, 256–262
test technique choice, 250–255
for average-risk populations, 250–251
for high-risk populations, 252–255
tests, 353–360
Coloscreen test, 243, 244
Colposcope, 97
Colposcopy, 34–35, 96, 97–98
cervical cancer and, 305
Computed tomography, 36, 37
of breast cancer, 147
Computer models, of cost–benefit decisions, 54–56
Cone biopsy, 98, 99
Controlled intervention trials, 27
Cost–benefit analysis, 49–57
average versus marginal, 53–55
of breast cancer screening, 339, 341–342
externalities and equity, 52
of gastric cancer screening, 374, 375
models, 54–56
societal costs versus charges, 53
Creatine phosphokinase test, 36
Crohn's disease, 210, 350
Cyclophosphamide, carcinogencity, 401–402, 403
Cyst(s), of breast, 150, 151, 152
ultrasonography of, 224, 225, 226
Cystic mastitis, 149
Cystoscopy, routine, 407–408
Cytologic examinations, *see* specific type of cytology
Cytosarcoma phylloides, 225, 226
Cytotechnologists, slide screening load of, 92

D

Defined population studies, 27
Denominator error, 298, 299
Deoxyribonucleic acid histograms, 135, 136
Detecatest, 244
Detectable preclinical phase, 7, 9
Developing countries, screening programs in, 14–15
Diagnosis, screening and, 15–16
Diaphanography, 36, 158, 337
Dyes, as bladder carcinogens, 398–399, 401, 402, 403, 406, 407
Dysplasia
  of breast, 149
  cervical, 111
    as carinoma *in situ* precursor, 301–302
    incidence, 296, 297
    mild, 94, 95
    moderate, 94, 95
    severe, 94, 95
  colorectal, 255
  detectable preclinical phase, 7, 9
  oral, 433, 434

E

Echography, *see* Ultrasonography
Edema, of breast, 152
Educational programs
  for breast cancer screening, 327
  for colorectal cancer screening, 363
Electrosurgery, colorectal, 258, 260
Endometrial cancer, 34, 308
Enzyme tests
  for bladder cancer, 137
  for prostate cancer, 36
Epidermoid carcinoma, 130
Epstein-Barr virus, 430
Erythoplakia, 433
Ethics, 13–15

F

False negatives
  biological component, 8
  in cervical cytology, 8, 29, 44, 100–101, 299, 409, 410
  in chest radiology, 176, 177
  in fecal occult blood tests, 33
  in oral cytology, 438, 439
  retesting and, 7–8
  in toluidine blue staining, 439
False positives
  in breast physical examination, 284
  in fecal occult blood tests, 33, 240, 242
  in oral cytology, 438
  test accuracy and, 75–76
  in urinary cytology, 409, 410
Fecal occult blood tests, 33, 34, 237–247, 353, 355–359, *see also* specific test names
  available tests, 242–246
  for average-risk populations, 361
  characteristics, 238–239
  controlled trials, 356–359
  dietary factors, 240–241
  error sources, 238–239
  false negatives, 33
  false positives, 33, 240, 242
  guidelines, 361, 362
  for high-risk populations, 362
  immunochemical tests, 245
  methodology, 245, 355
  positivity, 356–358
  proctosigmoidoscopy and, 357, 359
  quality control, 242–243 '
  reactants, 237
  rehydration, 242
  sensitivity, 238, 239, 241–242, 358, 359
  storage, 242
  uncontrolled trials, 355–356
Fecatest, 244
Fecatwin test, 244
FeCult test, 244
Fibroadenoma, of breast, 150, 151, 224, 226
Fibrocystic breast disease, 149, 151, 273
Fibrocystic mastopathy, 149
Fibrosis, pleural, 185
Fine needle aspiration, of breast, 283
Flow cytometry, 135–136
Follow-up, 15–16, 74, 96–99
Framingham Heart Study, 74

G

Galactocele, 152
Galactosyl transferase isoenzymes, 137
Gardner's syndrome, 252, 350–351

Gastric cancer
  dietary factors, 369
  early detection, 198–208
  incidence, 194, 367–368, 372
  intestinal metaplasia, 197, 198
  metastatic, 370
  mortality rates, 367, 369
  resected, 201, 203
  superficial depressed, 200–201, 202
  superficial elevated, 198–199
  superficial flat, 198
  survival rate, 207–208
Gastric cancer screening, 367–376, *see also* Radiography, double contrast
  age-specific rate, 368–369
  cost effectiveness, 374, 375
  detection rate, 208, 368
    declining, 373–374
  evaluation, 371–373
  lead time bias, 373
  length bias, 373
  methodology, 369–370
  mortality rate and, 371–373
  radiation side effects, 374–375
  results, 370–371
  side benefits, 373
  survival rates and, 370–371
Genitourinary cancer screening, 28, *see also* Bladder cancer screening
Gingiva cancer, 429, 431
β-Glucuronidase, urinary, 137
Guaiac cards, *see* Fecal occult blood tests

H

Haemoscreen, 244
Hamartoma, 253
Hamartomatosis, 351
Health Insurance Plan of Greater New York Study, 27, 144, 157, 158, 328–329
Health questionnaire, 72
Hema-Check, 244
Hematest, 237
Hematuria, urinary, 134–135, 408–409
Hemoccult test, 244, 355–359, *see also* Fecal occult blood tests
  controlled trials, 356–359
  dietary factors, 240–241, 242
  quality control, 243
  rehydration, 242
  uncontrolled trials, 355–356
Hemofec, 244
Hemoquant, 245
Hemorrhage, gastrointestinal, 241
Herpes simplex virus-specific markers, 137
High-risk populations, *see* Population at risk
Hysterectomy, cervical cancer mortality and, 306, 307, 308–309

I

Infectious disease, screening for, 70
Inflammatory bowel disease, 210, 349–350
Instrument calibration, 80
International Union Against Cancer (UICC) Workshop, 8–12, 16, 21–22
Interventions, 26

J

Jaw, cancer of, 435–436
Johns Hopkins Lung Project, 174–182

K

Kaiser-Permanente Medical Care Program, 70, 76
Kaiser-Permanente mammography study, 332–333

L

Lactic dehydrogenase test, 36, 137
Large-cell undifferentiated carcinoma, 379
Large intestine cancer, 349, 351, 353
Lead time bias, 17
  in breast cancer screening, 328, 329
  in gastric cancer screening, 373
Length bias, 17, 18
  in gastric cancer screening, 373
Leukemia, mass radiography and, 375
Leukoplakia, 432
Life
  quality of, 50–51
  value of, 52, 53
Life expectancy, 10, 11
Lip(s), leukoplakia, 432
Lip cancer
  diagnosis, 439
  risk factors, 422, 423, 424, 425, 426
  squamous cell carcinoma, 427–428

Lipoma, of breast, 150, 151, 152
Lumpectomy, 51
Lung cancer
  asymptomatic, 379–380
  benign, 188
  chemotherapy, 378
  control methods, 31
  detection, 379–380
  incidence, 10
    among smokers, 188, 378
  localization, 379–380
  mortality, 378
    chest radiology effects, 380
    premature, 10, 11
  prognosis, 379
  risk factors, 378
  smoking-related, 10, 31, 32, 65–66, 188, 378
  treatment, 51, 378
  types, 378–379
Lung cancer screening, 377–395, *see also* Chest radiology; Sputum cytology
  cancer control phases, 28
  case finding and, 392
  clinical trials, 32
  Mayo Lung Project findings, 106, 380, 381–394
    American Joint Committee for Cancer staging, 387–389
    backdating, 348
    cancer cell type distribution, 385
    curative resection effects, 385–387
    follow-up resources, 384
    implications of, 390–394
    incidence rates, 384–385
    mortality, 389–390
    nonstudy chest radiographs and, 383
    screening procedure suitability, 382–383
    sputum cytology, 106–117
    subject acceptance, 381–382
    survival time, 386–387, 388, 389, 392, 394
  mortality reduction and, 32
  occult cancer incidence, 115, 116, 117
Lymphoma, oral, 436
Lysozymes, urinary, 137

M

Mammography, 141–161
  age factors, 330
  benign changes and, 149–152
  breast calcification and, 152–153, 155–157, 160
  breast structure and, 330
  Canadian National Breast Screening Study, 334–336
  cost versus risk, 53
  efficacy, 30–31, 142–143, 155, 157–158, 160, 330, 332
  history, 143–144
  indications for, 159
  Kaiser-Permanente Study, 332–333
  malignant changes and, 152–155
    primary signs, 152–154
    secondary signs, 154–155
  mammogram interpretation, 148–159
  observer variation, 8–9
  population at risk, 15
  radiation dose, 146–147, 148, 332
  radiation hazard, 13, 30, 53, 147–148, 331, 336
  rationale for, 142–143
  screening applications, 157–159
  sensitivity, 31, 37
  specificity, 31
  Swedish study, 334
  technical factors, 144–147
  thermography and, 15
  ultrasonography and, 229
Mandible cancer, 435
Mastectomy, 51
  unnecessary, 331
Maxilla cancer, 435
Mayo Lung Project, 106, 380, 381–394
  American Joint Committee for Cancer staging, 387–389
  backdating, 384
  cancer cell type distribution, 385
  curative resection effects, 385–387
  follow-up resources, 384
  implications of, 390–394
  lung cancer rates, 384–385
  mortality results, 389–390
  nonstudy chest radiographs and, 383
  screening procedure suitability, 383–383
  sputum cytology
    abnormal specimen follow-up, 112–113
    cell type distribution, 114–117
    cytologic reports, 110–112
    processing methods, 379–380
    randomized controlled trials, 381–390
    techniques, 106–110

subject acceptance, 382
survival time, 385–390, 392, 394
Mazoplasia, 149
Medical care decision-making, 50–51
Medullary carcinoma, of breast, 227–228, 230, 231
Mesenchymal cancer, oral, 435
Metaplasia
intestinal, 197
squamous, 111
Metastatic cancer, oral, 435, 436
Methylene-*bis*-ortho-chloraniline, 403
Microadenoma, 253
Microcalcification, of breast, 152–153, 160
Mortality, *see also* Mortality rate under specific cancers
premature, 10, 11
reduction, 26
Mouth floor, leukoplakia, 433
Mouth floor cancer
clinical features, 428–429
diagnosis, 439
Mouth floor posterior cancer, 430
Multiple discriminant analysis, of risk factors, 64–65
Myeloma, oral, 436

N

2-Naphthylamine, carcinogenicity, 399, 401
Nasopharyngeal cancer, 430
National Cancer Institute Division of Resources, Centers and Community Activities, 26
Nipple changes, 154, 155
Nipple discharge, 283–284
Nuclear magnetic resonance, 36, 53

O

Occult blood
fecal, *see* Fecal occult blood tests
urinary, *see* Hematuria, urinary
Occultest, 237–238
Occupational exposure
bladder cancer and, 398–400, 401, 402–403, 404–406, 410–411
lung cancer and, 31
oral cancer and, 426
Octoson, 218
Oldfield's syndrome, 350, 351
Opportunity costs, 52
Oral cancer
alcohol use and, 424–425, 426
of bone, 435
clinical appearance, 426–431
diagnosis, 436–439
biopsy, 436–437
cytology, 437–439
oral examination, 35–36, 440, 441
toluidine blue staining, 439
epidemiology, 422–426
etiology, 422–426
incidence, 421, 422
metastatic, 435, 436
mortality, 421
premalignant lesions, 432–434
primary mesenchymal, 435
risk factors, 422–426, 441
of salivary glands, 434–435
smoking and, 424, 425, 426
squamous cell carcinoma, 426–431
alveolar ridge, 429
buccal mucosa, 430
gingiva, 429
lip, 427–428
mouth floor, 428–429
mouth posterior, 430
nasopharyngeal cancer and, 430
palate, 429–430
tongue, 428
subsite incidence, 422–424
verrucous, 431
Oral cancer screening, 36, 439–440
Oral contraceptives, cervical cancer and, 313
Oral cytology, 438–439
Oral examination, 435–436, 440, 441
Osteosarcoma, oral, 435–436
Ovary cancer, colorectal cancer and, 353

P

Paget's disease, 154
Palate cancer, 429–430
Papanicolaou smear
abnormal, 93–99
cervical cancer mortality and, 34
cost, 52
cost effectiveness, 50, 53–54, 55–56
false negatives, 8, 29, 44, 100–101, 299, 409, 410
history, 87–88
reporting terminology, 93–96

Papanicolaou smear (*cont.*)
sensitivity, 100
specificity, 100
Papanicolaou smear screening
American Cancer Society guidelines, 55
case-control study, 311–312
national policy, 51
optimal screening schedule, 313–319
quality control, 92, 99–102
requirements, 88–102
follow-up system, 96–99
interpretation, 92
reporting of findings, 93–96
screening, 92, 93
smear collection, 88–90
smear processing, 90–92
Papanicolaou urinary screening, *see* Urinary cytology
Papillary carcinoma, of bladder, 127–128
classification, 130
urinary cytology of, 127–128, 130, 131, 132
Papilloma
of bladder, 129–130
of breast, 150, 151
Papillomata, of bladder, 411, 415
Patient identification, 79
Patient preferences, 51, 54
Patient satisfaction, 75
Pelvic examination, 315
Personnel training, 80
Peutz-Jegher syndrome, 253
Pharynx cancer, 439, *see also* Nasopharyngeal cancer
Photofluorography, 164, 183
Physician office visits, screening during, 4, 5, 28
Polyp(s)
colorectal, 239, 359
gastric, 373
Peutz-Jegher, 253
upper gastrointestinal, 253
Polypectomy, 251
Polypeptide antigen test, 411
Polyposis
familial, 252–255, 350–355
adenoma and, 252–253
juvenile, 253–254, 351
Population at risk, 15, *see also* Selective screening; Target populations
for bladder cancer, 35, 133–134, 398–403
for breast cancer, 15, 41–42
for cervical cancer, 15, 29, 42–43, 312–313
for colorectal cancer, 252–255, 348–353, 362
for oral cancer, 422–426, 440, 441
risk factors and, 62–65
selection, 41–43, 59–67
selective screening, 65–66
self-selection, 63
Positive discrimination performance, 101
Positive test, predictive value, 9
Precursor conditions, 7, 9
Predictive value, 6, 9, 75
Present value, 51
Prevention, 27
Proctosigmoidoscopy, 353, 354
for average-risk populations, 361
complications, 258–259
controlled trials, 357, 359
equipment, 256–257
fecal occult blood test and, 357, 359
flexible, 354
for average-risk populations, 361
of colorectal adenomas, 252–253
complications, 258–259
efficacy, 251
guidelines, 361
prevalence of use, 251
procedure, 257–258
sensitivity, 262
60-cm, 251, 256, 257
30-cm, 251
of ureterosigmoidostomy, 255
guidelines, 362
for high-risk populations, 362
procedure, 257
rigid, 251
sensitivity, 262, 263–264
serological tests and, 250
specificity, 263
training, 265
Prostate cancer screening, 35–36
cancer control phases, 28
Pseudo variables, 19

Q

Quality control, 8–9, 29, 43–44
breast cancer screening, 9
cervical cancer screening, 34
chest radiology, 173–174, 183

error correction and, 82
fecal occult blood tests, 242–243
instrument calibration, 80
linkage of test results, 79
multiphasic screening, 79–82
Pap smear screening, 92, 99–102
patient identification, 79
personnel performance, 80
personnel training, 80
problem reporting, 80–82
sputum cytology, 109–110
test results, 80
Quality-adjusted year of life saved (QAYLS), 51, 53
Quasi-experimental studies, 19
Quik-Cult, 244

R

Radiation exposure
colorectal cancer and, 353
as mammography hazard, 13, 30, 53, 147–148, 331, 336
Radiography, double contrast, 195
colorectal, 261–262, 354, 360
colonoscopy and, 263–264
complications, 262
sensitivity, 263–264, 360
specificity, 263–264
gastric, 193–214, 368–375
detected cancer incidence, 194
diagnostic results, 207–208
efficacy, 193
evaluation, 209
film findings, 196–206
inflammatory bowel disease, 210
methodology, 194–195, 210–213
radiation side effects, 374–375
of ulcers, 195, 209
Randomized trials, 18–19
Receiver operating characteristic curves, 6
Rectal cancer, *see* Colorectal cancer
Relative risk, 62
Retesting, false negative results and, 7–8
Ribonuclease test, 36
Risk factors, *see also* under specific cancers
combined, 63–65
selective screening and, 62–65
Risk versus benefit, 20–21
Risks, 53

S

Saccharin, carcinogenicity, 402, 405
Salivary gland cancer, 434–435
Sarcoma, of bladder, 130
Scirrhous carcinoma, ultrasonography of, 226–227, 229–230, 231
Screening
cancer control and, 25–48
cost–benefits, 49–57
average versus marginal, 53–55
discounting, 51
externalities and equity, 52
models, 54–56
present value, 51
societal costs versus charges, 53
costs, 52
definition, 4–5, 29
diagnosis and, 15–16
ethics, 13–15
follow-up, 15–16, 74, 96–99
history, 70–71
of infectious disease, 70
multiphasic, 70–73
criteria, 71
definition, 70
implementation principles, 76–77
patient satisfaction, 75
problems, 77–78
provider satisfaction, 75–76
quality control, 79–82
screening test selection, 74
secondary advantages, 71–73
specialized health examinations, 78–79
target population recruitment, 74
target population selection, 73–74
new methods, 28, 36–37
population at risk, *see* Population at risk
principles, 9–13
acceptibility, 13
cancer natural history, 11–12
safety, 13
treatment efficacy, 12
quality of life and, 50–51
selective, *see* Selective screening
self-selection, 63
sensitivity, 60, 61, 62, 63
specificity, 60, 61, 62, 63
treatment and, 15–16

Screening programs, 29–30, *see also* specific cancer screening programs
costs, 38, 40
data management, 44–45
design, 38–41
disease factors, 41
disease importance, 10–11
evaluation, 16–22, 37–41
case-control studies, 19–20
classification of approaches, 18
quasi-experimental studies, 19
randomized trials, 18–19
risk versus benefit, 20–21
survival evaluation bias, 16–18
financing, 44–45
health outcome and, 38–39, 40
implementation, 43–45
low attendance, 63
mathematical models, 40–41
quality control, 43–44
resources, 43
screening population recruitment, 43
screening population selection, 41–43
self-selection, 63
sensitivity, 60, 61, 62, 63
specificity, 60, 61, 62, 63
Screening test(s), *see also* specific tests
acceptibility, 13
linkage of test results, 79
predictive value, 6, 9, 75
purpose, 216
safety, 13
selection, 74
sensitivity, 59–60, 61
specificity, 59, 60, 61
validity, 5–9
Sedation, for colonoscopy, 260
Selection bias, 17
Selective screening, *see also* Population at risk; Target populations
cervical cancer, 42–43
definition, 59
of high-risk populations, 29
cost-yield, 61–63
lack of efficacy, 65–66
risk factors, 62–65
subject selection, 59–67
multiphasic screening, 73
during physician visits, 28
screening test validity and, 59–61
Self-selection, 63, 326
Sensitivity
chest radiology, 176, 177, 183, 186, 188, 383
colonoscopy, 263–264, 358, 360
definition, 59–60
double contrast radiography, 263–264, 360
fecal occult blood test, 238, 239, 241–242, 358, 359
mammography, 3, 37
Pap smear, 100
proctosigmoidoscopy, 262
screening programs, 60, 61, 62, 63
screening tests, 5–9, 59–60, 61
sputum cytology, 117–118, 382, 383
Sensitivity analysis, 54
Sigmoid colon cancer, 255
Sigmoidoscopy, *see* Proctosigmoidoscopy
Skin cancer screening, 36
Small-cell undifferentiated carcinoma, 379
Smoking, cancer and, 27
bladder cancer and, 35, 399, 400, 401, 402, 405
lung cancer and, 31, 32, 65–66, 188, 378
oral cancer and, 424, 425, 426
sputum production and, 108–109
Snuff, oral cancer and, 424
Societal costs, of screening, 52, 53
Somascope, 218
Specificity
chest radiology, 176, 177, 188, 383
colonoscopy, 263–264
colorectal cancer screening, 263–264
definition, 60
double contrast radiography, 263–264
mammography, 31
Pap smear, 100
proctosigmoidoscopy, 263
screening programs, 60, 61, 62, 63
screening tests, 5–9, 59, 60, 61
sputum cytology, 117, 118
Sputum cytology, 105–119
abnormal specimen follow-up, 112–113
cell type distribution, 114–117
chest radiology and, 114, 379, 382, 385
cytologic reports, 110–112
abnormal findings, 111–112
negative results, 110–111
efficacy, 32
importance, 118

indications, 380
microscopic screening, 109–110
occult cancer detection, 379
"pooled" sputum collection, 108
processing methodology, 107–108, 379–380
quality control, 109–110
randomized controlled trials, 381–390
sensitivity, 117–118, 382, 383
slide preparation, 109
specificity, 117, 118
specimen adequacy, 108–109
technical aspects, 106–107
Squamous cell(s)
pulmonary, 111
atypia, 112, 113, 117–118
urinary, 123
Squamous cell carcinoma
bladder, 130
cervical, 88
oral, 426–431
alveolar ridge, 429
buccal mucosa, 430
gingiva, 429
lip, 427–428
mouth floor, 428–429
mouth posterior, 430
nasopharyngeal cancer and, 430
palate, 429–430
tongue, 428
pulmonary, 379
detection, 379–380
screening incidence, 114–117
Stoma, urinary, 255
N-Substituted aryl compounds, 403
Survival, bias in evaluating, 16–18

T

Taker error, 299
Target populations, 69–83, *see also* Population at risk; Selective screening
recruitment, 74
screening follow-up compliance, 16
selection, 73–74
Testicular cancer screening, 36
Thermography, 15, 36, 37, 158, 337
Thyroid cancer screening, 28, 36
Time-varying Markov models, 54
Toluidine blue staining, 439–440
Tongue, leukoplakia, 433
Tongue cancer, 428, 439
Transitional cell carcinoma, 130
in situ, 128–129
papillary, 127–128
urinary cytology of, 127, 128–129, 131, 132
Transitional epithelial cells, 123, 124, 125–129
Treatment, screening and, 12, 15–16
Tuberculosis, intestinal, 195, 209
Tumor markers, 13, 136–137
Tumor registries, 45
Turcot's syndrome, 350, 351

U

Ulcer(s)
gastric-duodenal, 373
peptic, 193
tuberculous, 195, 209
Ulcerative colitis
colorectal cancer and, 254–255, 349–350
double contrast radiography, 210
Ultrasonography, 36, 37, 218
in breast cancer screening, 158, 215–236, 337
advantages, 215
collagen fiber content, 230, 231, 232
cyst, 224, 225, 226
cytosarcoma phylloides, 225, 226
diagnostic accuracy, 228, 229
diagnostic criteria, 223–225
equipment, 218–219
expanded, 228–229
fibroadenoma, 224, 226
history, 216–218
malignant disease, 226–230
medullary carcinoma, 227–228, 230, 231
normal breast, 220–222
scirrhous carcinoma, 226–227, 229–230, 231
screening program methods, 232–234
screening program results, 234
screening programs, 231–234
ultrasonic tissue characterization, 229–230
water-bag approach, 218–220
mammography compared with, 229
Ultrasonotomography, 218

United States Breast Cancer Detection Demonstration Projects, 5
Ureter, sigmoid colon cancer and, 255
Ureterosigmoidostomy, 255
Urinary cytology, 121–134, 408–411
  bladder cancer survival rates and, 412–413
  cancer stage at presentation, 413–415
  classification, 129–131
  cytologic examination, 123–129
  detection rate, 35
  diagnostic accuracy, 131–133
  evaluation, 414–415
  future of, 415–416
  methodology, 122–123
  screening programs, 133–134
  terminology, 131
Urothelial cells, 123
Uterine cancer, *see also* Cervical cancer
  cervical cancer screening and, 306–307, 308, 310
  colorectal cancer and, 353
Uterine cancer screening, 28, 34–35
Utility analysis, 51

V

Vaginal irrigation technique, 88
Verrucous cancer, oral, 431

X

Xenylamine, 409
Xeromammography, 144, 145